Pathophysiology & Pharmacology in Nursing

Sara Miller McCune founded SAGE Publishing in 1965 to support the dissemination of usable knowledge and educate a global community. SAGE publishes more than 1000 journals and over 800 new books each year, spanning a wide range of subject areas. Our growing selection of library products includes archives, data, case studies and video. SAGE remains majority owned by our founder and after her lifetime will become owned by a charitable trust that secures the company's continued independence.

Los Angeles | London | New Delhi | Singapore | Washington DC | Melbourne

2nd Edition

Pathophysiology & Pharmacology in Nursing

Sarah Ashelford,
Justine Raynsford
& Vanessa Taylor

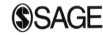

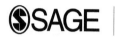

Learning Matters
An imprint of SAGE Publications Ltd
1 Oliver's Yard
55 City Road
London EC1Y 1SP

SAGE Publications Inc.
2455 Teller Road
Thousand Oaks, California 91320

SAGE Publications India Pvt Ltd
B 1/I 1 Mohan Cooperative Industrial Area
Mathura Road
New Delhi 110 044

SAGE Publications Asia-Pacific Pte Ltd
3 Church Street
#10-04 Samsung Hub
Singapore 049483

Editor: Donna Goddard
Development editor: Eleanor Rivers
Senior project editor: Chris Marke
Project management: Swales & Willis Ltd, Exeter,
Devon
Marketing manager: George Kimble
Cover design: Wendy Scott
Typeset by: C&M Digitals (P) Ltd, Chennai, India

Library of Congress Control Number: 2019935711

British Library Cataloguing in Publication Data

A catalogue record for this book is available from
the British Library

ISBN 978-1-5264-3210-0
ISBN 978-1-5264-3211-7 (pbk)

Contents

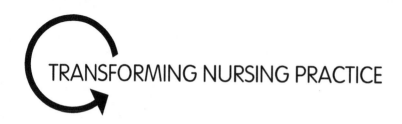

TRANSFORMING NURSING PRACTICE

Transforming Nursing Practice is a series tailor made for pre-registration students nurses. Each book in the series is:

 Affordable

 Mapped to the NMC Standards of proficiency for registered nurses

 Full of active learning features

 Focused on applying theory to practice

Each book addresses a core topic and they have been carefully developed to be simple to use, quick to read and written in clear language.

An invaluable series of books that explicitly relates to the NMC standards. Each book covers a different topic that students need to explore in order to develop into a qualified nurse... I would recommend this series to all Pre-Registered nursing students whatever their field or year of study.

LINDA ROBSON,
Senior Lecturer at Edge Hill University

Many titles in the series are on our recommended reading list and for good reason - the content is up to date and easy to read. These are the books that actually get used beyond training and into your nursing career.

EMMA LYDON,
Adult Student Nursing

ABOUT THE SERIES EDITORS

DR MOOI STANDING is an Independent Nursing Consultant (UK and International) and is responsible for the core knowledge, adult nursing and personal and professional learning skills titles. She is an experienced NMC Quality Assurance Reviewer of educational programmes and a Professional Regulator Panellist on the NMC Practice Committee. Mooi is also Board member of Special Olympics Malaysia, enabling people with intellectual disabilities to participate in sports and athletics nationally and internationally.

DR SANDRA WALKER is a Clinical Academic in Mental Health working between Southern Health Trust and the University of Southampton and responsible for the mental health nursing titles. She is a Qualified Mental Health Nurse with a wide range of clinical experience spanning more than 25 years.

BESTSELLING TEXTBOOKS

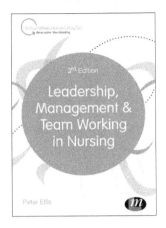

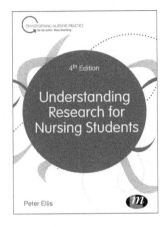

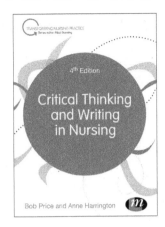

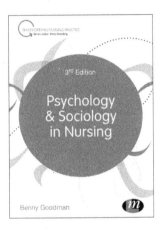

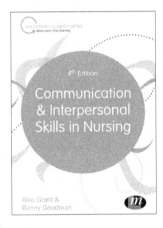

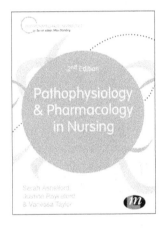

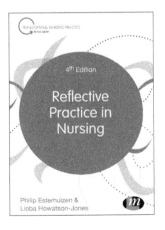

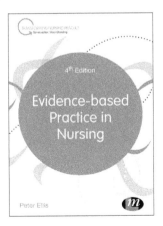

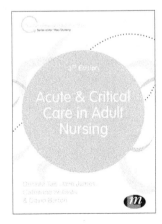

You can find a full list of textbooks in the
Transforming Nursing Practice series at

https://uk.sagepub.com

About the authors

Dr Sarah Ashelford is a lecturer in biological sciences within the Department of Health Sciences, University of York. Prior to this, Sarah worked at the University of Lincoln and University of Bradford leading the biosciences and pathophysiology themes for all nursing fields and post-registration programmes. Sarah has a BSc in Genetics and a PhD from the University of Edinburgh.

At the University of York, Sarah lectures on a range of programmes including Nursing Associate, pre-registration undergraduate and postgraduate nursing and midwifery programmes. She leads the Biological Basis of Illness module for the MSc Advanced Clinical Practice award. A member of the Biosciences in Nursing Education (BiNE) Steering Group, Sarah led the development of the pathophysiology outcomes for the BiNE Quality Assurance Framework (B-QAF). She undertakes research to enhance teaching, learning and assessment of the biosciences.

Justine Raynsford is a pharmacist and currently works as a lecturer within the School of Nursing and Healthcare Leadership at the University of Bradford. She is joint programme leader for non-medical prescribing and also leads on the Applied Pathophysiology and Pharmacology module for advanced practitioners. Both courses encourage interdisciplinary learning, welcoming students from nursing, pharmacy, paramedic science, radiography and physiotherapy. Justine has a clinical background in mental health and for many years she combined a role as a pharmacist prescriber with her academic role.

Dr Vanessa Taylor is Senior Lecturer in the Department of Nursing and Midwifery at the University of Huddersfield. Prior to this, Vanessa worked at the University of York, University of Manchester and University of Bradford. She also held a UK-wide role as Discipline Lead for Nursing and Midwifery at the Higher Education Academy. Vanessa has extensive teaching, curriculum design and development experience. Vanessa is Chair of the Bioscience in Nurse Education (BiNE) Steering Group, leading the BiNE Quality Assurance Framework (B-QAF). She is also Chair of the BiNE group and has undertaken projects evaluating bioscience teaching in pre-registration curricula. Vanessa has a clinical background in cancer and palliative care. Her research interests also focus on the evaluation of cancer, palliative and end of life education, workforce development and service evaluation. Vanessa has developed End of Life Care Outcomes for Health Education England (Yorkshire and the Humber), the Career and Education Framework for Cancer Nursing (with the RCN/UKONS) and is a member of the RCN Cancer and Breast Care Forum.

Contributor

Margaret Bannister RGN, RM, BSc (Hons), MSc Nurse Consultant and Diabetes BSc/ MSc Pathway Lead, University of Bradford. Margaret has 30 years' experience in diabetes care including 13 years as a diabetes specialist nurse and 15 as nurse consultant in Bradford. She was a member of the RCN diabetes forum 2004–2012 and Chair 2006–2010, Chair of the National Nurse Consultant Group 2008–2010 and nurse representative in the 2008 NICE type 2 diabetes guideline consensus group.

As the nurse consultant in Bradford and Airedale from 2002 to 2017 she clinically led the community diabetes team that supports the intermediate care service across the district. She was clinically based in the community but worked across all levels of the service. Her particular areas of clinical interest are patient-focused care delivery and education, particularly of other healthcare professionals. Her lecturing commitments at the university include leading the BSc and MSc diabetes pathways including delivery of diabetes specific modules and structured diabetes related input into pre-registration nurse training. Multidisciplinary working and the delivery of integrated diabetes care remains the primary focus for her work. Her clinical focus was predominately with patients with type 2 diabetes experiencing problems with treatment regimes, resistance to therapy change or adherence challenges. Since retiring from her full time NHS clinical role in 2017 she has been working with diabetes teams across Yorkshire providing clinical leadership and support for a variety of projects aimed at improving access to care for people living with diabetes plus education and development of healthcare professionals involved in diabetes care delivery.

Acknowledgements

We would like to thank students and colleagues who have used the first edition of this book and provided enthusiastic feedback. Your feedback has informed the development of this second edition. We have included additional content and chapters, and all content has been reviewed and references updated where available. Any inaccuracies we acknowledge as our own.

We would like to thank our editor Donna Goddard, and Alex Clabburn for proposing the idea of this book and for his continued drive and enthusiasm during the writing of the first and this second edition. We thank our patient and thorough editor Eleanor Rivers for her editorial work keeping us on track with the vision and style of Learning Matters. We would like to thank the detailed and rigorous feedback we received from our anonymous reviewer.

SA would like to thank in particular Emma Waters for her advice on Lola's fracture as it would be managed at A&E. Again any inaccuracies are our own.

Introduction

Who is this book for?

This book is an introductory textbook written for pre-registration nursing students in all fields of nursing (mental health, learning disability, adult and children's nursing). It is also useful for those health professionals undertaking continuing professional development and post-registration postgraduate programmes.

Why *Pathophysiology and Pharmacology in Nursing*?

Pathophysiology and pharmacology are the two subjects which form the focus of this book. We know from our students, pre- and post-registration, that it can be challenging to learn, understand and apply pathophysiology and pharmacology knowledge. This requires an understanding of diseases, but also an ability to apply these types of knowledge to inform nursing or clinical assessment, care and management of patients in your practice. Our aim, therefore, is to provide you with an understanding of pathophysiology and pharmacology as they relate to clinical practice. Throughout each chapter, we apply this underpinning knowledge using case studies and scenarios to diseases and conditions that patients in all fields of nursing can present with.

The demonstration of the application of pathophysiology and pharmacological knowledge to case studies and real-life events is the strength of this book. Through this application, you will develop your knowledge, understanding and skills to inform your clinical decision-making in practice. As part of the holistic care of your patients, this knowledge will enable you to communicate effectively with the multi-professional team and your patients to promote their health, facilitate early diagnosis, recovery, rehabilitation or to provide palliative and end of life care.

Book structure

The book is divided into three sections:

Section 1: Core concepts and key pathophysiological processes – Chapters 1–5

Section 2: Protective mechanisms – Chapters 6 and 7

Section 3: Systems diseases and conditions – Chapters 8–14

The focus of each section and the chapters are described more fully below.

Section 1 introduces key principles, concepts and processes laying the foundations necessary for the study of subsequent chapters in the book.

Chapter 1 introduces you to pathophysiology and pharmacology. Pathophysiology concerns the nature of diseases, and seeks to explain the processes or mechanisms by which a condition develops and progresses, and results in the signs and symptoms of illness that affect your patients. You will be introduced to the key concepts of **pharmacology: pharmacokinetics** and **pharmacodynamics**. Pharmacokinetics describes how the body affects drugs following administration, including the mechanisms and chemical changes of absorption and distribution, and the routes of excretion for the metabolites of the drug. Pharmacodynamics, in contrast, focuses on how drugs affect the body.

Chapter 2 explains the way in which our bodies respond to injury and infection through the process of inflammation. The inflammatory response is a core concept of pathophysiology and applies widely to understanding the disease or condition your patient may present with. We consider the ways the body may become injured through events including direct trauma, burns and infection, as well as through disease-processes such as tumour formation, **atherosclerosis** and **hypersensitivity**. The acute inflammatory response is short-lived and a protective response that helps to remove the cause of injury and start the healing process. However, by contrast, chronic inflammation is long-lasting, and one of the major causes of injury and damage to the body. In this chapter you will learn how many diseases and conditions involve injury through inflammation. You will be introduced to steroids which are important drugs used for reducing inflammation. Steroids are particularly important in reducing the effects of chronic inflammation.

Chapter 3 introduces you to the main infectious microorganisms that can cause disease. These are bacteria, viruses, fungi and protozoa. As with inflammation, infection is a core pathophysiology concept. We will examine the nature of these microorganisms, how they are transmitted and how they can cause disease. We introduce the key drugs used to help treat infections: antibacterials, antivirals and antifungals. We also look at ways in which healthcare professionals can reduce the spread of microorganisms and examine the increasingly important issue of antibiotic resistance. Finally, in this chapter, we examine the pathophysiology of sepsis and its treatment.

Chapter 4 follows on from Chapters 2 and 3 to examine in greater detail the role of the immune system in both responding to infections and as a possible cause of disease and injury. You will be introduced to the cells and molecules of the adaptive immune system and how these work together to fight infections. You will then learn about how the immune system can 'over-react' to cause hypersensitivity and **autoimmune** diseases. We look at immunodeficiency disease which occurs in people whose immune systems are not strong enough to fight infections. We examine the nature of vaccines and the use of **monoclonal antibodies** as targeted therapies for a variety of diseases. This chapter is one of the most technical and may take more time to understand than the others in this book. It is fundamental to understanding our resistance to infections, and in understanding the many diseases which involve inflammation and hypersensitivity.

Chapter 5 focuses on cancer. There are more than 200 different types of cancer. This chapter identifies the risk factors for cancer and the strategies for prevention and early detection of the four most common cancers in the UK. The chapter also demonstrates the importance of understanding cancer biology and the development of personalised treatment to enhance survival and limit the side-effects of drugs experienced by people affected by cancer. The process of carcinogenesis can help us understand how a normal cell becomes a cancer cell and acquires the capabilities known as the hallmarks of cancer. Understanding carcinogenesis also helps us to understand why people develop the signs and symptoms that they present with, and how drugs such as hormones, chemotherapy, targeted therapies and other interventions are used to treat, manage or palliate cancer and its effects.

Section 2 focuses on the protective mechanisms of pain, nausea and vomiting.

Chapter 6 introduces the physiology of pain. Pain in response to tissue injury is a protective mechanism alerting us that we have a damaged or diseased tissue. Pain is also a serious and significant symptom and one in which the nurse has a key role in assessing and managing its effects. We examine the different types of medicines to help reduce pain. These are collectively referred to as **analgesics**. We focus on the class of medicines called non-steroidal anti-inflammatory drugs (NSAIDs) and **opioid** analgesics, which include codeine and morphine.

Chapter 7 focuses on nausea and vomiting, which cause distress, anxiety and reduced quality of life as well as other complications such as dehydration, malnutrition and electrolyte imbalance. Despite their distressing and debilitating effects, nausea and vomiting are as important as biological systems for our survival. They act as protective mechanisms against ingestion of toxins from drug side-effects and as additional symptoms to other diseases which may be occurring. In this chapter, we discuss the vomiting response. This includes the organs, systems and multiple neurotransmitters responsible for processing the information and co-ordinating nausea and vomiting. We identify the neurotransmitters which are involved in stimulating the vomiting response which are important when you are deciding which anti-emetic to administer. This chapter also discusses clinical assessment and the pharmacological options.

Section 3 focuses on systems diseases and conditions. 'Systems diseases' are those affecting a particular body system such as the respiratory system or cardiovascular system. It can be useful to classify diseases by body system, although it is important to recognise that most diseases and conditions also involve other systems and body components, especially the immune system and inflammation. Our focus on diabetes and depression also demonstrates the impact of a disease on different systems and body components.

Chapters 8–14 focus on a small number of conditions and the pharmacological therapies. We have usually selected the most common or most significant examples for each body system. This approach has been taken to help you apply your knowledge of the relevant physiology and pathophysiological processes and pharmacological interventions to case studies and scenarios. **Chapter 8**, for example, examines cardiovascular disease and hypertension. **Chapter 9** examines respiratory disease, in particular asthma and chronic obstructive pulmonary disease. **Chapter 10** focuses on two common symptoms of gastrointestinal (GI) disorders – constipation and diarrhoea – and on examples of 'infection and inflammatory GI disorders' including peptic ulcer and inflammatory bowel disease (IBD). Diabetes is the focus of **Chapter 11**. Diabetes is a metabolic disease which means it alters the body's ability to use, store or process some of the important chemical components needed for effective **metabolism**. With diabetes, the primary problem is with glucose regulation and glucose use by the body cells as an energy source. You are introduced to the two main types of diabetes: type 1 and type 2. In **Chapter 12**, we focus on Parkinson's disease, epilepsy and Alzheimer's as three common neurological conditions. We cover the current drugs to treat these conditions. **Chapter 13,** considers one of the most common mental health conditions: depression. We focus on the possible underlying biology that leads to the symptoms of depression such as low mood, poor concentration and lack of enjoyment. Some of the biological theories are explored such as neurotransmitter levels, stress and dysregulation of the HPA axis and inflammation. **Chapter 14** examines renal conditions, namely acute kidney injury and chronic kidney disease. We cover the main presentations and pharmacological management.

It is important to appreciate that all the chapters of this book are interlinked. The human body functions as a whole with all its individual components working together. (This is called **integration** and is examined in Chapter 1.) It is, therefore, somewhat artificial to divide the workings of the human body in health and in disease into different parts or systems. However, as a student learning about these ideas for the first time, separating out the different systems is helpful. To assist you to integrate your learning, you will be asked to make links between chapters, and refer back to material covered in previous chapters as well as to look ahead to where a particular idea may be examined more closely in a subsequent chapter.

A note on terminology: There are a range of terms used to describe people who are recipients of healthcare across different fields of practice. Choosing the correct term can be challenging. Patient is a common expression used in the National Health Service (NHS). We recognise that not everyone supports the use of 'patient'. However, it is widely understood and can apply to people who are recipients of health and social care in hospitals, in the person's own home, in the primary care setting and in the voluntary, charitable and independent sectors. We could have used terms such as service user or client. However, throughout this book, for ease of reading and brevity of writing, we use the term 'patient' to refer to all groups and individuals who have direct or indirect contact with health and social care providers. The term 'carer' is used to describe someone of any age who provides unpaid support to a family member or friend who could not manage without this help. In selecting diseases, we have tried to be mindful of the different fields of nursing practice, balancing acute and long-term conditions, the place of care delivery and the contribution of nursing to primary and secondary prevention, health promotion, acute and long-term care, rehabilitation, palliative and end of life care. In this book, we use the term 'disease' and 'condition' to refer to any abnormal condition or illness that impairs normal functioning.

Requirements for the NMC *Standards of Proficiency for Registered Nurses* (NMC, 2018)

In 2018, the Nursing and Midwifery Council (NMC) reviewed and published the new standards of proficiency it expects for registered nurses. The proficiencies specify the core knowledge and skills that registered nurses must demonstrate when caring for people of all ages and across all settings. The *Future Nurse: Standards of Proficiency for Registered Nurses* (NMC, 2018) apply to all NMC registered nurses. These are the standards the NMC considers necessary in order to deliver safe, compassionate and effective nursing care. In addition to knowledge proficiencies, two annexes provide a description of skills which registered nurses should be able to demonstrate that they can do at the point of registration to provide safe nursing care. This book is structured so that it will help you to understand and meet the proficiencies required for entry to the NMC register.

This book includes the latest standards of proficiency taken from the *Standards of Proficiency for Registered Nurses* (NMC, 2018) and supports the following proficiencies:

Platform 1: Being an accountable professional

1.8 demonstrate the knowledge, skills and ability to think critically when applying evidence and drawing on experience to make evidence informed decisions in all situations;

1.9 understand the need to base all decisions regarding care and interventions on people's needs and preferences, recognising and addressing any personal and external factors that may unduly influence their decisions;

1.18 demonstrate the knowledge and confidence to contribute effectively and proactively in an interdisciplinary team;

1.19 safely demonstrate evidence-based practice in all skills and procedures stated in Annexes A and B.

Platform 2: Promoting health and preventing ill health

2.2 demonstrate knowledge of epidemiology, demography, genomics and the wider determinants of health, illness and wellbeing and apply this to an understanding of global patterns of health and wellbeing outcomes;

2.11 promote health and prevent ill health by understanding and explaining to people the principles of pathogenesis, immunology and the evidence-base for immunisation, vaccination and herd immunity;

2.12 protect health through understanding and applying the principles of infection prevention and control, including communicable disease surveillance and antimicrobial stewardship and resistance.

Platform 3: Assessing needs and planning care

3.1 demonstrate and apply knowledge of human development from conception to death when undertaking full and accurate person-centred nursing assessments and developing appropriate care plans;

3.2 demonstrate and apply knowledge of body systems and homeostasis, human anatomy and physiology, biology, genomics, pharmacology and social and behavioural sciences when undertaking full and accurate person-centred nursing assessments and developing appropriate care plans;

3.3 demonstrate and apply knowledge of all commonly encountered mental, physical, behavioural and cognitive health conditions, medication usage and treatments when undertaking full and accurate assessments of nursing care needs and when developing, prioritising and reviewing person-centred care plans;

3.5 demonstrate the ability to accurately process all information gathered during the assessment process to identify needs for individualised nursing care and develop person-centred evidence-based plans for nursing interventions with agreed goals;

3.11 undertake routine investigations, interpreting and sharing findings as appropriate;

3.12 interpret results from routine investigations, taking prompt action when required by implementing appropriate interventions, requesting additional investigations or escalating to others.

Platform 4: Providing and evaluating care

4.3 demonstrate the knowledge, communication and relationship management skills required to provide people, families and carers with accurate information that meets their needs before, during and after a range of interventions;

4.4 demonstrate the knowledge and skills required to support people with commonly encountered mental health, behavioural, cognitive and learning challenges, and act as a role model for others in providing high quality nursing interventions to meet people's needs;

4.5 demonstrate the knowledge and skills required to support people with commonly encountered physical health conditions, their medication usage and treatments, and act as a role model for others in providing high quality nursing interventions when meeting people's needs;

4.6 demonstrate the knowledge, skills and ability to act as a role model for others in providing evidence-based nursing care to meet people's needs related to nutrition, hydration and bladder and bowel health;

4.7 demonstrate the knowledge, skills and ability to act as a role model for others in providing evidence-based, person-centred nursing care to meet people's needs related to mobility, hygiene, oral care, wound care and skin integrity;

4.8 demonstrate the knowledge and skills required to identify and initiate appropriate interventions to support people with commonly encountered symptoms including anxiety, confusion, discomfort and pain.

Platform 5: Leading and managing nursing care and working in teams

5.7 demonstrate the ability to monitor and evaluate the quality of care delivered by others in the team and lay carers.

Platform 6: Improving safety and quality of care

6.8 demonstrate an understanding of how to identify, report and critically reflect on near misses, critical incidents, major incidents and serious adverse events in order to learn from them and influence their future practice.

Platform 7: Coordinating care

7.5 understand and recognise the need to respond to the challenges of providing safe, effective and person-centred nursing care for people who have co-morbidities and complex care needs.

Annexe A: Communication and leadership management

2. **Evidence-based, best practice approaches to communication for supporting people of all ages, their families and carers in preventing ill health and in managing their care**

2.1 share information and check understanding about the causes, implications and treatment of a range of common health conditions including anxiety, depression, memory loss, diabetes, dementia, respiratory disease, cardiac disease, neurological disease, cancer, skin problems, immune deficiencies, psychosis, stroke and arthritis;

2.2 use clear language and appropriate, written materials, making reasonable adjustments where appropriate in order to optimise people's understanding of what has caused their health condition and the implications of their care and treatment;

2.8 provide information and explanation to people, families and carers and respond to questions about their treatment and care and possible ways of preventing ill health to enhance understanding.

Annexe B: Nursing procedures

Part 1: Procedures for assessing people's needs for person-centred care

1. Use evidence-based, best practice approaches to take a history, observe, recognise and accurately assess people of all ages.

2. Use evidence-based, best practice approaches to undertake the procedures identified.

Part 2: Procedures for the planning, provision and management of person-centred nursing care

3. Use evidence-based, best practice approaches for meeting needs for care and support with rest, sleep, comfort and the maintenance of dignity, accurately assessing the person's capacity for independence and self-care and initiating appropriate interventions.

4. Use evidence-based, best practice approaches for meeting the needs for care and support with hygiene and the maintenance of skin integrity, accurately assessing the person's capacity for independence and self-care and initiating appropriate interventions.

5. Use evidence-based, best practice approaches for meeting needs for care and support with nutrition and hydration, accurately assessing the person's capacity for independence and self-care and initiating appropriate interventions.

6. Use evidence-based, best practice approaches for meeting needs for care and support with bladder and bowel health, accurately assessing the person's capacity for independence and self-care and initiating appropriate interventions.

7. Use evidence-based, best practice approaches for meeting needs for care and support with mobility and safety, accurately assessing the person's capacity for independence and self-care and initiating appropriate interventions.

8. Use evidence-based, best practice approaches for meeting needs for respiratory care and support, accurately assessing the person's capacity for independence and self-care and initiating appropriate interventions.

9. Use evidence-based, best practice approaches for meeting needs for care and support with the prevention and management of infection, accurately assessing the person's capacity for independence and self-care and initiating appropriate interventions.

10. Use evidence-based, best practice approaches for meeting needs for care and support at the end of life, accurately assessing the person's capacity for independence and self-care and initiating appropriate interventions.

11. Procedural competencies required for best practice, evidence-based medicines administration and optimisation.

Learning features

Learning from reading text is not always easy. Therefore, to provide variety and to assist with the development of independent learning skills and the application of theory to practice, this book contains activities, case studies, scenarios, further reading, useful websites and other materials to enable you to participate in your own learning. You will need to develop your own study skills and 'learn how to learn' to get the best from the material. The book cannot provide all the answers, but instead provides a framework for your learning.

The activities in the book will in particular help you to make sense of, and learn about, the material being presented. Some activities ask you to reflect on aspects of practice, or your experience of it, or the people or situations you encounter. *Reflection* is an essential skill in nursing, and it helps you to understand the world around you and often to identify how things might be improved. Other activities will help you develop key graduate skills such as your ability to *think critically* about a topic in order to challenge received wisdom, or your ability to *research a topic and find appropriate information and evidence,* and to be able to *make decisions* using that evidence in situations that are often difficult and time-pressured.

All the activities require you to take a break from reading the text, think through the issues presented and carry out some independent study, possibly using the internet. Where appropriate, there are sample answers presented at the end of each chapter, and these will help you to understand more fully your own reflections and independent study. Remember, academic study will always require independent work; attending lectures will never be enough to be successful on your programme, and these activities will help to deepen your knowledge and understanding of the issues under scrutiny and give you practice at working on your own.

You might want to think about completing these activities as part of your personal development plan (PDP) or portfolio. After completing the activity write it up in your PDP or portfolio in a section devoted to that particular skill, then look back over time to see how far you are developing. You can also do more of the activities for a key skill that you have identified a weakness in, which will help build your skill and confidence in this area.

This book also contains a glossary to assist you with unfamiliar terms. Glossary terms are in bold in the first instance that they appear.

Developing your knowledge and understanding of pathophysiology and pharmacology, and the ability to apply and integrate these types of knowledge with your professional judgement, can inform your clinical decision-making and, as part of the multi-professional team, deliver safe and patient-centred holistic care. We hope that you enjoy this book and good luck with your studies!

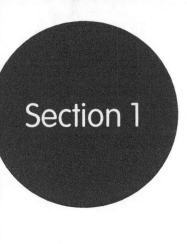

Section 1 Core concepts and key pathophysiological processes

Chapter 1 Introduction to pathophysiology and pharmacology

Chapter aims

After reading this chapter you will be able to:

- explain the terms pathophysiology and pharmacology and their importance to nursing practice;
- explain three key principles of human biology: the levels of biological organisation, homeostasis and cellular communication;
- describe how absorption, distribution, metabolism and excretion affect drug activity;
- describe the general principles of how drugs work in the body;
- explain why some drug interactions occur.

Introduction

Scenario

You are a nursing student on a clinical placement with a practice nurse at a local medical centre. You are observing the nurse during an asthma clinic. The patient, Hannah, is an 11-year-old girl who has recently been diagnosed with asthma. She is attending the clinic for the first time with her mother, Caroline. The nurse explains about asthma to Hannah and answers questions from Caroline. After explaining to Hannah how her blue inhaler will help her to breathe when she feels 'wheezy', the nurse shows Hannah how to use her inhaler correctly. Hannah has been given a peak flow meter which she will use to monitor how well she can blow air out of her lungs. The nurse explains to Hannah and Caroline the importance of monitoring her asthma and how to identify and avoid any trigger factors.

(Continued)

(Continued)

After the consultation, the nurse asks you to reflect on your understanding of asthma, how it is triggered and how the drug treatment works. You are able to explain many of the key points using your knowledge of pathophysiology and how the drug salbutamol from the blue inhaler works. You appreciate that you would like to know more about long-term preventative treatment for asthma which involves the use of a steroid inhaler.

This scenario shows the importance of pathophysiology and pharmacology for enabling effective nursing care. This knowledge will enable you to understand how your patient's treatment works and to be able to monitor this effectively and be aware of any side-effects. Knowledge of pathophysiology and pharmacology is also needed for you to explain the condition and treatments to your patient in a way that they can understand. You will also be in a position to discuss your patient effectively with members of a multi-professional team.

In the first part of this chapter we define the different terms used in pathophysiology to describe a disease or condition. In the second section, we ask you to consider three key principles of human biology: levels of biological organisation; homeostasis; and cellular communication. Using these three principles gives you a framework to help you understand your patient, their disease or condition. The third and final section of this chapter introduces you to the key principles of pharmacology, namely, pharmacodynamics and pharmacokinetics.

Activity 1.1   Reflection

Before continuing with this first chapter, consider what you understand already about pathophysiology and pharmacology. What are these two subjects about? Why are they important for nursing? Write down your initial thoughts and then return to review them at the end of each chapter to see how your understanding is developing.

There is no outline answer because from this activity you will produce a list of your own ideas or observations.

Pathophysiology

Pathophysiology is the study of how a disease affects the functioning of the body. In the scenario above, Hannah has asthma. The pathophysiology of asthma explains how asthma causes breathing difficulties and how this may result in insufficient oxygen reaching the cells.

Pathophysiology contributes significantly to our understanding of the disease a patient may present with. A number of other, closely related concepts are needed to give a full picture of a disease. One of these additional concepts is the cause or aetiology of a disease or condition. We know, for example, that the cause of asthma is complex involving a person's genes, immune response and exposure to environmental factors, such as house dust or pollen that can trigger an attack of asthma (Chapter 9). Many diseases do not have a single cause. Heart disease for example, has many risk factors. The risk factors for heart disease include age, male gender, smoking, high cholesterol and lack of exercise (Chapter 8). Risk factors are factors that cause an increased risk for the disease. Risk factors are worked out by studying populations of individuals with the disease and those without. Further research can then be carried out to determine a mechanism for how the risk factor contributes to the disease. This leads us to another term, pathogenesis, which describes the mechanisms that cause disease.

All diseases involve damage or injury to cells which makes the cells stop functioning correctly or die. Asthma, for example, involves damage to the cells lining the airways from an inflammatory response; heart disease involves damage or even death to the heart muscle cells due to lack of oxygen (**ischaemia**).

The clinical presentation refers to how the disease affects the patient. It includes the signs and symptoms of a disease. Symptoms are how a person experiences their disease; signs are observations that may be made to indicate the presence of disease. As an example, a symptom of asthma is difficulty breathing and a sign would be the nurse's observation of this difficulty. With diabetes, a low blood glucose measurement is a possible sign, whereas thirst and fatigue are symptoms. Throughout this book, we highlight the clinical presentation of disease and relate these to the underlying pathophysiology.

The different terms used above to describe a disease form part of what is referred to as 'the medical model of disease'. The medical model of disease is a scientific, evidence-based framework for analysing disease. The medical model of disease should not be confused with 'a medical model of care'. A medical model of care would be one that solely focuses on treating a patient's disease or managing their symptoms. In today's healthcare system, person-centred care is advocated. A person-centred care approach places the person at the centre of their care and takes account, not only of the best evidence for understanding and managing their disease, but individual patient preferences and the need for holistic care. In person-centred care, health and social care professionals work collaboratively with people who use services. It is coordinated and tailored to the needs of the individual. Person-centred care supports people to develop the knowledge, skills and confidence they need to more effectively manage and make informed decisions about their own health and healthcare (The Health Foundation, 2016). As part of your role delivering holistic person-centred care, the application of pathophysiology and pharmacology will inform your clinical decision-making including your assessment of patients and the planning, intervention and evaluation of patient care. This knowledge will enable you to communicate effectively with the multi-professional team and your patients to promote their health, facilitate early diagnosis, recovery, rehabilitation or to provide palliative and end of life care.

Three key principles of human biology

1. Levels of biological organisation

Figure 1.1 shows the levels of organisation of the human body. You may already know that we can view the human body as a collection of cells organised into clearly defined tissues, and that tissues are the building-blocks of organs. In turn, organs work together to form organ systems. The smallest levels shown in Figure 1.1 are molecules and macromolecular complexes such as the cell membrane. The smallest living unit is the cell.

Activity 1.2   Reflection

Reflect on your current knowledge of the organisation and function of the human body. Start by naming the eleven organ systems of the body. Can you give the function of each system?

Then identify the main component organs of each system and the function of each organ.

Can you name the four tissue types which make up the organs of the body?

The best way to check your answer is using an anatomy and physiology textbook. Recommended textbooks are given in the further reading at the end of the chapter.

In Activity 1.2 you identified the organ systems and individual component organs of each system. Thinking about the structure and function of the human body at the tissue level is more difficult. This is because cells which make up tissues are microscopic. We cannot see directly how they are functioning. By the same reasoning, it is even more challenging to picture how molecules such as hormones, enzymes or drugs work within the body. Drawing diagrams or looking at animations from the internet can help you visualise these interactions. This will greatly enhance your understanding of the topics in this book.

2. Homeostasis

The maintenance of a relatively constant internal environment (homeostasis) is the second biological principle we will look at. Homeostasis ensures the best or 'optimum' conditions for cells to function, as well as delivering the right amount

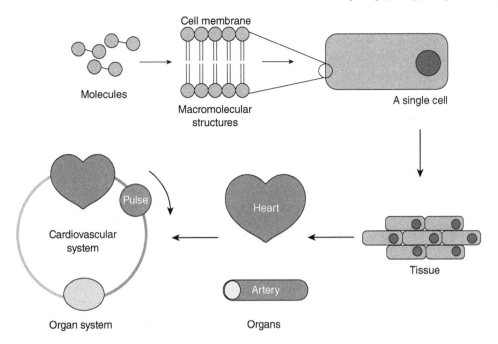

Six levels of organisation of the human body are shown. The smallest is the molecular level which group to form larger macromolecular complexes such as the cell membrane. Macromolecular complexes form cells – the smallest living unit of the body. Cells of a similar type form tissues, such as cardiac muscle cells forming the myocardium, or muscle layer of the heart. Two or more tissues make up an organ, and organs work together to form an organ system, such as the cardiovascular system.

Figure 1.1   The levels of biological organisation

of oxygen and removing waste products, such as carbon dioxide, urea and lactic acid. Other key conditions kept in homeostasis include: body fluid and electrolytes, pH, blood glucose and temperature. To be well, or healthy, our body needs to be in homeostasis. Conversely, a homeostatic imbalance, where one or more conditions have become too high or low, is considered as one definition of illness (Tortora and Derrickson, 2017).

To see how the concept of homeostasis can help in understanding pathophysiology, we can use the example of asthma again. Asthma affects breathing and so reduces **gas exchange** in the lungs. The level of oxygen in the body can drop to a critically low level and the level of carbon dioxide increase to produce a harmful **acidosis**. The body is 'thrown out' of homeostasis with respect to its **acid–base balance** and oxygen levels. This is potentially life-threatening (Chapter 9). Another example is diabetes which involves problems of glucose regulation (Chapter 11). With untreated diabetes, levels of blood glucose can become raised and cause long-term damage. It is beyond the scope of this chapter to review in detail the physiological processes maintaining homeostasis. However, many of the diseases described in this book will affect one or more aspects of homeostasis. For example, Chapter 8 will examine the normal regulation of blood pressure as well as **hypertension**. Chapter 11 will explain the normal regulation of glucose as well as diabetes.

One of the key reasons that homeostasis is so important to health is that cells rely on proteins to function. Proteins are large molecules that fold into particular three-dimensional shapes. The three-dimensional shape of a protein is essential for its optimum function. The shape of a protein is affected by conditions such as temperature and acid–base balance. Any change away from the optimum shape will adversely affect how the protein works. One class of proteins you may have heard of are **enzymes**. Enzymes are biological catalysts that increase the rate of the chemical reactions within the body. The enzymes in the human body work best at 37°C (which is our normal core body temperature). Any changes from this temperature will affect the shape and function of enzymes. Very high temperatures (above 40°C) can destroy completely the shape and function. The enzyme is said to be de-natured (or 'away' from its natural shape). It is vital that all these conditions be kept in homeostasis (Tortora and Derrickson, 2017).

3. Cellular communication

The different organs, tissues and cells must work together to form a fully functioning individual. The working-together of cells, tissues and organs is called integration. Integration requires careful control and co-ordination of the different parts of the body. This in turn requires effective communication between the different cells of the body.

Nearly all cellular communication involves a signalling cell and a target cell which receives the signal. Signalling cells release one or more chemical messengers, or signalling molecules, which act on the target cell. **Neurotransmitters**, **hormones** and **growth factors** are the main signalling molecules used by the body (Figure 1.2). These are recognised by **receptors** on target cells – the signalling molecule and receptor have complementary shapes. Most receptors are cell membrane proteins. Binding of the signalling molecule to the receptor triggers a response by the cell (see 'signal transduction', below).

The difference between types of signalling lies in the distance between signalling and target cells and the means by which the signalling molecule reaches the target cell. We describe three types of signalling: nerve, endocrine and local.

1. *Nerve signalling.* Nerve signalling occurs within the nervous system and is used to regulate muscles and glands. A **neurone** is a single nerve cell that sends a message in the form of a nerve impulse (or **action potential**). Nerve impulses travel very rapidly along the neurone, often over great distances within the body. When the nerve impulse reaches the end of the neurone, signalling molecules called neurotransmitters are released. Neurotransmitter molecules diffuse across a microscopic gap called the **synapse** to reach the target cell. The target cell has neurotransmitter receptors on its surface to receive the signal.

2. *Endocrine signalling.* Signals in the form of hormones are sent round the body in the bloodstream from endocrine glands or tissues to target cells (Figure 1.2). Endocrine signalling is slower than nerve signalling. This is because the circulation is slower to carry the signalling molecule than a nerve impulse which is very rapid.

However, endocrine signals become widespread throughout the body by being distributed in the circulation. A nerve impulse can only reach a limited number of target organs. In this sense, a nerve impulse is more specific.

3. *Local signalling.* Local signalling occurs between cells that are adjacent or very close to each other. This is seen, for example, in the inflammatory response (Chapter 2) and with cancer (Chapter 5). **Inflammatory mediators** are a group of chemical messengers that we will examine in Chapter 2. Although they act locally, some enter the bloodstream and exert their effect at more distance targets. In this sense they act more like hormones.

A signalling molecule will only work if it can cause a response in the target cell. The way in which a cell responds to a signal depends upon the type of signal and the type of cell it is. Each signalling molecule has its own set of target cells in the body on which it can act.

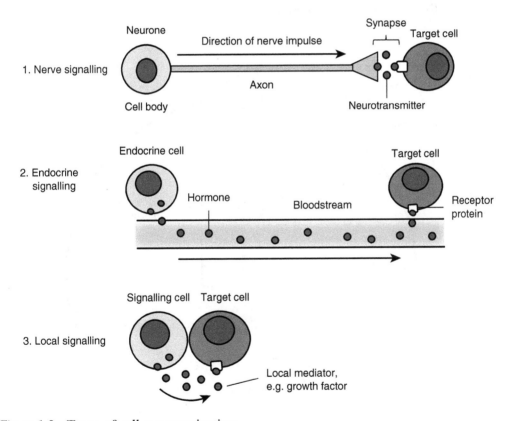

Figure 1.2 Types of cell communication

Many diseases affect cellular communication. A familiar example is type 1 diabetes which is caused by an absence of the signalling molecule insulin. In Chapter 5, you will learn that the uncontrolled growth of cancer cells is a direct consequence of alterations in cell signalling. Many of the newer cancer therapies have been engineered to block the altered signalling pathways of cancer cells. A large number of drugs, in general, work by blocking or enhancing the action of signalling receptors on the surface of cells (as will be described below under 'Pharmacology').

Figure 1.3 shows how the message reaches the inside of the cell in order for a response to be made. This process is known as **signal transduction**. The message is 'transduced' which means carried across the membrane into the cell. The signal is passed on to a number of 'intermediary' proteins within the cell. These act as messengers or 'go-betweens' until a final protein produces a response. In Figure 1.3 the original signal is the hormone adrenaline and the final response inside the cell is the activation of an enzyme that breaks down glycogen to glucose. A commonly used analogy to help understand this is how someone signals their presence at a house using a doorbell (Figure 1.4). The initial signal occurs when the visitor presses the button – this is like the signalling molecule binding to the receptor. The message is converted (transduced) into an electrical signal that causes the doorbell to sound inside the house. Hopefully for the visitor, a final response will be made when the owner hears the bell and goes to open the door.

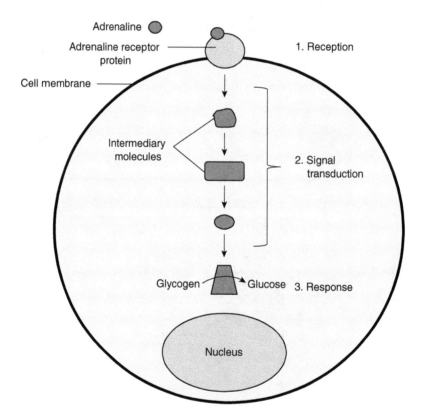

Cell signalling consists of three steps: 1. Reception: in which a signalling molecule binds to a receptor – in this case adrenaline binds to the adrenaline receptor. 2. Signal transduction: in which the signal is conveyed into the cell through a number of intermediary molecules. 3. Response: in which the signal causes the cell's activity to change – in this case the breakdown of glycogen to glucose.

Figure 1.3 Signal transduction using the example of adrenaline acting on a muscle or liver cell causing the breakdown of glycogen into glucose

Cells respond in a variety of ways to a variety of signals. The example in Figure 1.3 has a cell converting glycogen to glucose following a signal from the hormone adrenaline. Smooth muscle cells, for example, may contract; pancreatic cells may secrete insulin; cancer cells may start dividing.

These three principles will be referred to throughout this book in their applications to specific diseases.

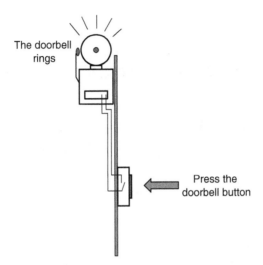

The doorbell rings

Press the doorbell button

When the doorbell button is pressed the signal is changed from one form into another resulting in the bell ringing. The pressing of the button is converted into an electrical signal and then into the sound of the bell. This is an example of signal transduction and enables someone from outside the house to signal to those inside. The door in this example is like the cell membrane and the doorbell button is like the receptor.

Figure 1.4 The doorbell analogy of signal transduction

Pharmacology

Pharmacology is the science that examines the composition, effects and uses of drugs. Before the science of pharmacology started, people had very little idea of how medicines really worked or even if they worked at all. Bold claims were laid down for all sorts of products. At first, pharmacologists concentrated on purified substances from plants, for example digitalis from foxgloves. However, in the twentieth century as knowledge increased of how drugs act, chemical compounds were synthesised in the laboratory to be used as medicines. Two very important concepts are pharmacokinetics and pharmacodynamics. Pharmacokinetics describes how the body processes the drug and pharmacodynamics describes how drugs affect the body.

Pharmacokinetics

When you take a drug your body treats it like an ingested toxin. Pharmacokinetics is the scientific study of how the body processes the drug. Pharmacokinetics is usually broken down into four stages:

1. Absorption of the drug.

2. Distribution of the drug in the different body compartments.

3. Metabolism of the drug.

4. Excretion of the drug.

1. Drug absorption

Activity 1.3   Evidence-based practice and research

Absorption describes the movement of a drug into the blood circulation. Write down all the different routes of administration that can be used to enable a drug to be absorbed. Why do you think there are so many different routes of administration?

An outline answer is provided at the end of the chapter.

Activity 1.3 shows the many ways in which drugs may be administrated to enable their absorption. Following ingestion (the oral route of administration), some of the drug will be absorbed through the stomach lining into the blood. However, for most drugs, absorption will occur in the small intestines. This is because the small intestines are adapted for absorption by having a very large surface area. From the small intestines, the absorbed drug passes directly to the liver. In the liver, some of the drug is chemically altered in a process called **first pass metabolism**. First pass metabolism has a significant impact on how much of a drug is available to exert its effects on the body.

Blood leaving the stomach and small intestines goes directly to the liver via the hepatic portal vein (Figure 1.5). Therefore, any drug taken orally will go first to the liver before it reaches the general (**systemic**) circulation. Some drugs undergo extensive first pass metabolism. This means that a large proportion of the drug is chemically altered during this first passage through the liver and little of the drug may reach the systemic circulation. This is one reason why some drugs cannot be effectively given by the oral route. An example is glyceryl trinitrate which is administered under the tongue (sub-lingual). If it were swallowed it would be almost entirely broken down during its first passage through the liver. The sub-lingual route avoids the first pass metabolism because the drug is directly absorbed into the systemic circulation, diffusing into the blood through tissues under the tongue. Drugs given parenterally (by intravenous, subcutaneous and intramuscular injection) also directly enter the systemic circulation and avoid first pass metabolism in

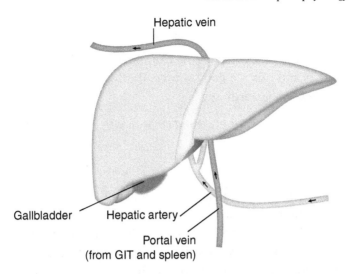

The liver has a dual blood supply. It receives oxygenated blood from the hepatic artery, and blood containing absorbed nutrients from the hepatic portal vein. The hepatic portal vein brings blood from the gastrointestinal tract directly to the liver. Blood is drained from the liver by the hepatic vein.

Figure 1.5   Blood supply to the liver

the liver. Other routes of administration avoiding first pass metabolism include the use of transdermal patches, rectal suppositories and buccal routes (given between gum and cheek).

Other factors affecting absorption

Food and other medicines

Food can affect absorption of certain drugs. Patients need to be informed if they should take their drug on an empty stomach. For example, the antibiotic flucloxacillin (Chapter 3) should be taken before food, as food will affect the amount of drug absorbed. However, the absorption of amoxicillin, another similar (penicillin type) antibiotic, is unaffected by the presence of food in the stomach and does not need to be taken on an empty stomach.

Activity 1.4   Evidence-based practice and research

Mary, a patient in your care, asks you whether or not she should take her drugs with food. She is on Quetiapine modified release (MR) 200 mg at night and fluoxetine 20 mg in the morning. You are aware that the British

(Continued)

(Continued)

National Formulary (BNF) gives the cautionary and advisory labels that need to go on drugs and this is a good source of information. Look these drugs up and advise Mary accordingly.

An outline answer is provided at the end of the chapter.

Sometimes, two drugs may bind to each other making a larger compound that is not well absorbed. An example is alendronic acid and calcium which are both used in the treatment of osteoporosis. It is usually recommended that patients do not take these at the same time of day. If taken together, the calcium binds to the alendronic acid making a very large molecule that is difficult to absorb.

Controlled release drugs

Controlled release drugs often have 'MR', 'SR' or 'LA' attached to their names. Respectively, these stand for modified release, slow release and long-acting. For example, 'Morphgesic SR' is a long-acting form of morphine and SR stands for slow release. These medicines are carefully made (**formulated**) to be released slowly from the GI tract. As a result, the patient is able to take the tablets less frequently which is often more convenient. Morphgesic SR can be taken twice a day whereas morphine tablets or morphine solution might need to be taken every four hours for pain relief. It is important that you are aware of the brand when you are administering a controlled release tablet. Brands are often not interchangeable as they may be formulated differently and have different effects on a patient. In addition, crushing controlled release tablets destroys the slow release mechanism. The patient would receive the whole dose in a non-controlled manner; this may be toxic and the effect of the drug would not be long-acting.

Enteric coated (e.c.) drugs

Some drugs have a special coating that may delay absorption until a different part of the GI tract is reached. This coating may help to protect the stomach from the drug. A well-known example is aspirin e.c. The coating prevents aspirin being absorbed in the stomach which helps protect the stomach from irritation by the aspirin. Crushing enteric-coated drugs is not advisable as this destroys the coating.

Route of administration

As highlighted above, the route of administration will have an impact on first pass metabolism. This is important for some drugs and affects how much ultimately is absorbed into the systemic circulation. In addition, some drugs, for example insulin, are broken down by enzymes in the stomach which will inactivate the drug. This is why these drugs are not administered by the oral route. Sometimes, different routes of administration are used to avoid absorption into the bloodstream altogether in an attempt to reduce side-effects. Examples include inhalers, nose drops and eye drops which are applied directly to the site of action. However, it should be remembered that, despite this local administration, a small amount of the drug will be absorbed.

2. Distribution of the drug

Distribution describes the process of dispersion or dissemination of drugs throughout the fluids and tissues of the body. Drugs are not distributed equally in the different fluids and tissues. Fat-soluble drugs, for example, will concentrate in adipose tissue, and water-soluble drugs in body water. Some parts of the body are less accessible to drugs than others. The nervous tissue of the brain is separated from its blood supply by the **blood–brain barrier**. A number of drugs cannot cross the blood–brain barrier. This helps to explain the difference between sedative antihistamines, such as chlorphenamine, and non-sedative ones, such as cetirizine. Chlorphenamine causes drowsiness by binding to histamine receptors in the brain. By contrast, cetirizine cannot cross the blood–brain barrier to bind to histamine receptors in the brain.

When drugs circulate in the bloodstream, some of the drug binds to proteins in the plasma, whereas some of the drug remains 'free', or unbound in the plasma. The 'bound' drug is effectively inactive as the protein–drug complex is too large to leave the blood capillaries and enter the **tissue fluid** surrounding the body cells. The 'free' drug is small enough to pass through the capillary wall and enter the tissue fluid to exert its effect on the cells. Factors that affect protein binding may affect the amount of drug available to the tissues. Older adults for example may have lower blood albumin. Albumin is a protein in the blood that some drugs bind to extensively. As a result in older adults there may be more 'free' drug available and a lower dose may be needed for the same effect. Some drug interactions occur when one drug affects the protein binding of another as the case study demonstrates.

Case study

Tom, who is stable on warfarin (an anticoagulant), is prescribed sodium valproate as a mood stabiliser. Shortly afterwards he notices that he bleeds and bruises more easily. This happens because the sodium valproate displaces the warfarin that is bound to plasma proteins. This increases the amount of free warfarin available to exert its anticoagulant effect. Close monitoring of blood clotting time is advised if the two drugs are prescribed together.

3. Metabolism

Metabolism comes from a Greek word that means 'to change'. Metabolism of drugs occurs mainly in the liver. We often think of the liver as breaking drugs down and making them inactive but this is too simplistic. Metabolism can reduce activity or create other active metabolites. In some cases metabolism activates drugs (see Evidence summary box). The main purpose of metabolism is to make the drug more water soluble so that it can be excreted from the body by the kidneys.

Evidence summary: Codeine

The Medicines and Healthcare Products Regulatory Agency (MHRA) issued a safety warning about codeine in 2013. They stated that codeine should only be used for acute, moderate pain in children over 12 years and only if other pain killers (analgesics) did not work. This followed cases of children receiving codeine after surgery who developed respiratory depression. Respiratory depression can be a side-effect of morphine. Codeine is a pro-drug. This means it is metabolised in the liver to morphine and this is what is responsible for the **analgesia**. A pro-drug is an inactive precursor that is converted to an active drug by metabolism. It is believed that the affected children were rapid metabolisers of codeine. As a result, these children produced unexpectedly high levels of morphine resulting in respiratory depression. Conversely, some patients are slow metabolisers and benefit little from codeine. This is due to their slow rate of metabolism of codeine into morphine.

There are two phases of metabolism:

Phase 1 metabolism

This is mainly carried out by a large family of enzymes in the liver called cytochrome P450 enzymes which oxidise drugs. There are different kinds of these enzymes and some are quite specific for different drugs. Drug interactions may occur when enzyme activity is altered. Some drugs can increase the activity of specific enzymes. This is known as enzyme induction. By contrast other drugs and some foods can reduce the activity of the enzymes. This is known as enzyme inhibition. An example is the interaction between grapefruit juice and simvastatin. The grapefruit juice reduces the activity of the cytochrome P450 enzyme that metabolises simvastatin. This leads to an increase in simvastatin levels to potentially toxic levels. Another example is the drug interaction between simvastatin and erythromycin (see Chapter 8, Activity 8.2).

Phase 2 metabolism

In phase 2 metabolism, a large ionised molecule is added to the drug. This acts to increase the water solubility of the drug.

Activity 1.5 Evidence-based practice and research

Smoking is an enzyme inducer in that it speeds up the enzymes that usually metabolise the antipsychotic drug olanzapine. What might happen to a smoker on olanzapine who stops smoking?

A suggested answer is provided at the end of the chapter.

Drugs may undergo phase 1 or phase 2 metabolism or both. A drug might also be metabolised by different pathways resulting in many different **metabolites**. Factors that affect the function of the liver, such as disease and ageing, can affect how much of a drug is metabolised. As we have shown in the evidence summary, some people metabolise drugs more quickly than others. This probably reflects differences in their genetic make-up.

The liver is the main site of drug metabolism, but drugs may also be metabolised in the GI tract, the plasma and the lungs. Morphine, for example, is metabolised mainly in the liver but also in the mucosal cells of the small intestine.

4. Excretion (elimination)

Excretion (elimination) refers to the removal of waste products from the body. The kidney is the main organ involved in drug excretion. If you could examine the urine of a patient who is taking drugs, you would find water-soluble drugs and metabolites. Drugs may also be excreted in bile, tears, sweat and breath. In fact, any bodily fluid can contain drugs and their metabolites. Factors that affect kidney function, such as kidney disease and ageing, will affect how efficiently drugs are excreted.

Other important pharmacokinetic concepts

- Bioavailability
- Therapeutic range or therapeutic index
- Half-life
- Peak plasma concentrations.

Bioavailability

Bioavailability is the proportion of the administered dose that reaches the systemic circulation. For intravenous (IV) drugs, it can be assumed to be 100% as the drug is delivered directly into the blood circulation. For oral drugs it can be considerably less. The losses occur in numerous ways. Some of the tablet may not be absorbed from the GI tract and some may be lost during first pass metabolism before reaching systemic circulation. Bioavailability is often expressed as a percentage. For example, the bioavailability of the opioid Oxycodone is 60–87%. This means 60–87% of the orally administered dose reaches the systemic circulation.

Case study

Michael is receiving palliative care. His pain is currently controlled using morphine MST Continus tablets 60 mg twice a day. He is finding it increasingly difficult to swallow and a subcutaneous infusion has been suggested as an alternative route of administration. The equivalent subcutaneous dose of morphine is half the oral dose (British National Formulary [BNF] Palliative Care Guidance), that is 60 mg over 24 hours. This is because the bioavailability of oral morphine is less than morphine given by injection. This difference is largely due to the first pass metabolism of morphine when administered orally.

Sometimes the bioavailability of different brands and **formulations** can be different. For example, the bioavailability of Lanoxin (digoxin) elixir is 75% compared to 63% for Lanoxin tablets. For many drugs this does not matter clinically but, in cases where the drug has a narrow therapeutic index or range, it can be important.

Narrow therapeutic index or range

This describes the difference between the blood levels that need to be reached for a drug to be effective and the level above which the drug is toxic. For many drugs, this range is very wide. For example, with paracetamol, most adult patients need a dose of 1 g to relieve their pain. For drugs with a narrow therapeutic range, including digoxin, gentamycin, vancomycin and lithium, small differences in dose or blood concentration may lead to therapeutic failures or adverse drug reactions. It is often necessary to adjust the dose according to measurement of the actual blood level achieved in the person taking it. Changes in the brand or formulation can result in toxic or sub-therapeutic levels in the blood because of differences in bioavailability.

Plasma half-life

The plasma half-life of a drug is the time it takes for the concentration or amount of the drug in the plasma to reduce by one half. It is a constant for any given drug although a range is often given as some people metabolise and excrete drugs faster than others. Plasma half-life is a useful measure at it can help you to work out how long drugs remain in the body.

Scenario

You are a nurse and one of your patients, Linda, is on Risperidone 4 mg at night for schizophrenia. Her psychiatrist stopped the drug as she was experiencing tremors. She asks you how long it will take for the drug to 'get out of her system'. You ask for advice and learn that Risperidone has an active metabolite with a half-life of 24 hours. It can take 4 to 5 half-lives for a drug to be excreted. You can tell Linda that it might take 4 or 5 days (4–5 × 24 hours) for the Risperidone to be out of her system, but the side-effects should improve every day as, each day, the remaining drug is broken down and excreted.

Peak plasma concentrations

The timing of the peak plasma concentration gives useful information about when drug levels are at their highest in a patient's blood. Some side-effects tend to be most problematic at this time.

Peak concentration and therapeutic range are illustrated in Figure 1.6.

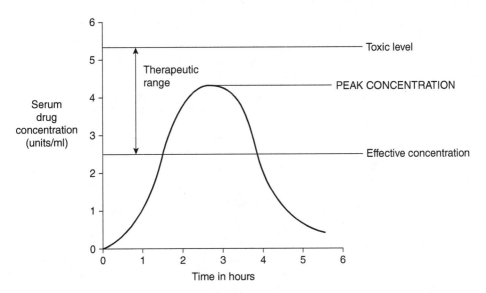

Figure 1.6   Graph showing drug concentration after oral administration of single dose

Pharmacodynamics

Pharmacodynamics, sometimes described as 'what drugs do to the body', is defined as the study of the biochemical and physiological effects of drugs on the body. This includes the mechanism of drug action and the side-effects drugs cause.

In order for a drug to exert an effect, it must first come into contact with, and bind to, the cells of the body it is acting upon. Different drug molecules have different shapes and will only bind to certain proteins in the body. Have you have ever experienced a patient who asked you how a drug knows where to go? For example, 'How does paracetamol know to go to the head and stop a headache?' The drug does not 'know', but will bind to certain binding sites in the body. Most of these binding sites are proteins. As identified earlier in the chapter, there are many different proteins in the body, all with different shapes. The following are common binding sites for drugs: receptors, enzymes and carrier molecules.

Drugs acting at receptors

Many drug receptors are protein molecules on the surface of a cell. As referred to above under 'Cellular communication', signalling molecules bind to these receptors to cause a response in the cell.

The general name for a chemical that binds to a receptor and activates it to produce a response is an **agonist** (Figure 1.7). Many drugs acting at receptors are agonists. For example, adrenaline is an agonist. It binds to beta receptors on heart muscle cells to set off a chain of events which lead to the heart beating faster and more forcefully (Chapters 8 and 9).

Whilst an agonist causes a response, an **antagonist** binds to the receptor but does not cause a response (Figure 1.7). Antagonists block the receptor so that an agonist cannot exert its effect.

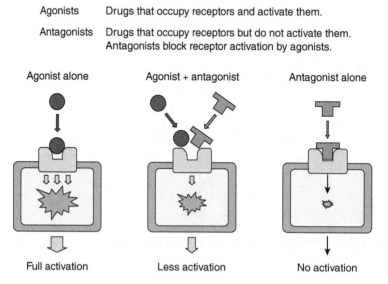

| Agonists | Drugs that occupy receptors and activate them. |
| Antagonists | Drugs that occupy receptors but do not activate them. Antagonists block receptor activation by agonists. |

Agonist alone — Full activation

Agonist + antagonist — Less activation

Antagonist alone — No activation

Figure 1.7 Agonists and antagonists

An example of an antagonist is propranolol, a beta-blocker. Propranolol attaches to the beta receptors on the heart muscle cells preventing adrenaline binding. This consequently prevents the action of adrenaline.

Partial agonists bind to receptors to cause a response, but the response is less than the maximum possible. The opioid buprenorphine is an example of a partial agonist. This makes it a useful drug in the treatment of opioid dependence, where the opioid agonist heroin (also known as diamorphine) is replaced by another agonist, in this case buprenorphine, to prevent withdrawal symptoms. We shall come across many drugs acting as agonists and antagonists in the following chapters.

Drugs acting on enzymes

As mentioned under 'Homeostasis' earlier in the chapter, enzymes are chemicals (usually proteins) that speed up the chemical reactions and keep cells functioning. Drugs that act as enzyme inhibitors bind to the enzyme and decrease its activity (Figure 1.8).

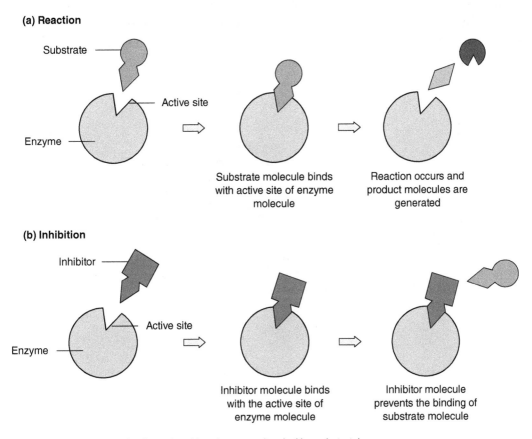

a   Reaction – an enzyme is shown breaking down a molecule (the substrate)
b   Inhibition – a drug can act as an inhibitor by preventing the substrate from binding to the 'active site' of the enzyme

Figure 1.8 Enzyme inhibition

An example of an enzyme inhibitor is the non-steroidal anti-inflammatory drug (NSAID) ibuprofen. Ibuprofen binds to, and inhibits, enzymes called cyclo-oxygenases (COXs). COXs are enzymes that are needed to make a group of inflammatory molecules called prostaglandins. In turn, prostaglandins cause pain and fever (Chapters 2 and 6). Ibuprofen inhibits the COXs and reduces the amount of prostaglandins synthesised. The action of NSAIDS is described more fully in Chapter 6.

Drugs acting on transporters

Transporter proteins are located in the cell membrane. Their function is to transport substances across the cell membrane (Tortora and Derrickson, 2017). An example of a drug acting on transporter proteins are the type of antidepressant drug called selective serotonin reuptake inhibitors (SSRIs). Examples of SSRIs include fluoxetine and citalopram. Between nerve cells there is a gap called a synapse. In order for a message to be carried from one cell to another, a chemical called a neurotransmitter is needed. Serotonin is a type of neurotransmitter. Antidepressant drugs act to increase the level of neurotransmitters in the synapse. SSRIs do this by preventing the reuptake of serotonin from the synapse. This means more serotonin is available for longer to stimulate serotonin receptors on the nerve cell on the other side of the synapse (Figure 1.9). For a fuller explanation of the synapse see Chapter 6.

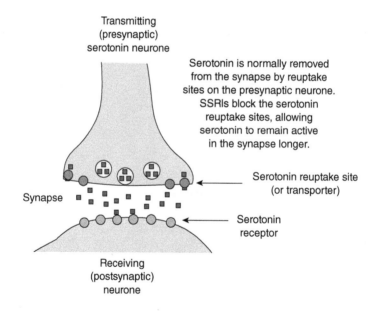

Figure 1.9 Action of selective serotonin reuptake inhibitors at the synapse

Pharmacogenomics

Pharmacogenomics investigates the effects of genetic variation on how people respond to drugs. Our genetic make-up can determine how effective a drug is and whether or not we are likely to get side effects. There are both pharmacokinetic and pharmacodynamics effects. One important example of this are the cytochrome P450 enzymes. As we discussed earlier, these enzymes are involved in the metabolism of drugs by the liver. Our genes determine the types of cytochrome P450 enzymes we make and, in some cases, can determine whether we are 'slow' or 'fast' metabolisers. Genetic variation can also affect transporter proteins and receptors that will influence pharmacodynamics.

Each of us has a unique DNA sequence that makes up our genome. In the future, it is envisaged that each of us could have our complete genome sequenced which may enable 'personalised' medicine. Personalised medicine is a type of medical care that is customised for an individual patient on the basis of genetic make-up. It is already used in the treatment of some kinds of cancer. In this case, the genetic make-up of the cancer is used to target or 'individualise' treatment. This is discussed further in Chapter 5 with respect to cancer treatment.

It is now time to review what you have learned within this chapter by undertaking some multiple choice questions.

Activity 1.6   Multiple choice questions

1. The scientific study of the causes of disease is known as:

   a) Pathophysiology
   b) Pathogenesis
   c) Aetiology
   d) Pharmacology

2. The smallest living unit of the body is the:

   a) Organ system
   b) Organ
   c) Tissue
   d) Cell

3. The working together of cells, tissues, organs is called:

   a) Homeostasis
   b) Integration
   c) Communication
   d) Signal transduction

4. Endocrine signalling involves the release of:

   a) Hormones
   b) Local growth factors
   c) Neurotransmitters
   d) Nerve signals

5. The transmission of a molecular signal from a cell's exterior to its interior is known as:

   a) Nerve signalling
   b) Signal transduction

(Continued)

(Continued)

    c) Endocrine signalling
    d) Signalling pathway

6. Pharmacokinetics is the study of:

    a) The action of drugs on the body
    b) The action of the body on drugs
    c) The production and manufacture of medicines
    d) The study of genetic differences in drug metabolism

7. Which of the following will NOT affect drug absorption?

    a) Plasma albumin concentration
    b) Food
    c) Route of administration
    d) Formulation of medicine

8. The antidepressant fluoxetine can increase the concentration of the antipsychotic clozapine by affecting metabolism by liver enzymes. This is an example of:

    a) Enzyme induction
    b) Enzyme inhibition
    c) Enzyme agonism
    d) Enzyme antagonism

9. What is the definition of plasma half-life?

    a) Half the time it takes to reach therapeutic plasma concentration
    b) The time it takes for half of the drug to be excreted
    c) The time it takes for the plasma concentration of a drug to reduce by half
    d) The time it takes for half of a dose to be absorbed into the plasma

10. A drug which undergoes extensive first pass metabolism will have:

    a) A low bioavailability
    b) A high bioavailability
    c) A low therapeutic range
    d) A high therapeutic range

Chapter summary

In this chapter we have introduced you to the subject of pathophysiology and identified its importance for nursing practice. We discussed the concept of the aetiology of a disease, which is another name for the cause of the disease. Often diseases do not have a single cause but many risk factors. An understanding of the risk factors for a disease is important as some of these can be modified to reduce a person's chance of developing the disease. The idea of risk factors will be important in the subsequent chapters of this book and will help you to give appropriate information of health promotion. The mechanism of pathogenesis of a disease will be an important focus of this book. The pathogenesis, or disease mechanism, can help you to understand the clinical manifestations of a disease, and help you to understand the treatment and management. We revised three principles of human biology: organisation, homeostasis and cellular communication. It is important that you understand these concepts before moving on to the next chapters, where these concepts will be developed to explain specific diseases.

We introduced the two concepts of pharmacology: pharmacodynamics and pharmacokinetics. The science of pharmacology helps us to understand how and why drugs work to alleviate or cure disease (pharmacodynamics). Our bodies also affect the drugs that are taken or administered (pharmacokinetics). This has implications for how medicines are formulated and how kidney and liver impairment may affect metabolism and excretion. Understanding pharmacology can also help explain why patients get certain side-effects, why some drugs interact with each other, and why some patients must avoid certain drugs.

Activities: Brief outline answers

Activity 1.3 Evidence-based practice and research (p22)

There are many routes of administration but some examples are: oral, intravenous, subcutaneous, intramuscular, sub-lingual (under the tongue), buccal (between cheek and gum), topical, rectal, inhaled.

The many different routes can be useful to suit the needs of patients. Unconscious patients or those with swallowing difficulties have alternatives. Routes, other than oral, also avoid first pass metabolism which, in some cases, would break down most of the drug. This would mean that little of the drug would reach the systemic circulation. Sometimes the routes enable the drug to be delivered directly to where it is needed. Inhaled drugs for asthma reach the lungs and less is absorbed into the whole body than if the same drug was given orally.

Activity 1.4 Evidence-based practice and research (pp 23–4)

In the BNF there are numbers that relate to the warning labels given at the start of the Appendix. If a product has the number 23 next to it, this means the pharmacist must put the following on the label: 'Take this medicine when your stomach is empty. This means an hour before food or 2 hours after food'. Quetiapine m/r would need this label. For fluoxetine it is not important. Therefore Mary should take her Quetiapine on an empty stomach, but fluoxetine could be taken with breakfast if that suited the patient.

Activity 1.5 Evidence-based practice and research (p27)

A smoker might need to be on a higher dose of olanzapine as the enzymes that metabolise olanzapine will be speeded up. If the patient stops smoking the enzymes slow back down again.

This would mean olanzapine levels rise. This could lead to toxicity or increased side-effects. You would want to advise the patient of this and that their dose of olanzapine may need to be reduced when they have stopped smoking.

Activity 1.6 Multiple choice questions (pp33–4)

1. The scientific study of the causes of disease is known as:

   c) Aetiology

2. The smallest living unit of the body is the:

   d) Cell

3. The working together of cells, tissues, organs is called:

   b) Integration

4. Endocrine signalling involves the release of:

   a) Hormones

5. The transmission of a molecular signal from a cell's exterior to its interior is known as:

   b) Signal transduction

6. Pharmacokinetics is the study of:

   b) The action of the body on drugs

7. Which of the following will NOT affect drug absorption?

   a) Plasma albumin concentration

8. The antidepressant fluoxetine can increase the concentration of the antipsychotic clozapine by affecting metabolism by liver enzymes. This is an example of:

   b) Enzyme inhibition

9. What is the definition of plasma half-life?

   c) The time it takes for the plasma concentration of a drug to reduce by half

10. A drug which undergoes extensive first pass metabolism will have:

    a) A low bioavailability

Further reading

British National Formulary (BNF) 76 (2018) London: Pharm Press.

The essential practical, evidence-based information for healthcare professionals who prescribe, dispense and administer medicines.

Simonsen, T, Aarbakke, J, Kay, I, Coleman, I, Sinnott, P and Lysaa, R (2006) *Illustrated Pharmacology for Nurses.* London: Hodder Arnold.

A clearly written and well-illustrated pharmacology book aimed at nurses.

Tortora, G and Derrickson, B (2017) *Principles of Anatomy and Physiology* (17th edition). Oxford: Wiley.

A comprehensive and clearly written anatomy and physiology textbook.

Useful websites

http://bnf.org/

Online version of the British National Formulary.

www.medicines.org.uk/

The electronic Medicines Compendium (eMC) contains information about medicines licensed for use in the UK. Summaries of product characteristics (SPC) and patient information leaflets (PILs) are available.

Chapter 2 The inflammatory response

Chapter aims

After reading this chapter you will be able to:

- identify ways in which tissues become damaged;
- explain the key events of the inflammatory response;
- distinguish between acute and chronic inflammation;
- explain the four cardinal signs of inflammation;
- explain the action and potential side-effects of corticosteroids.

Introduction

Case study

Ruby's hand-held food blender was blocked with red cabbage. Carefully picking out the bits by hand, Ruby switched on the rotary blades to help dislodge a particularly large piece. She immediately felt a sharp, stabbing pain and saw blood pouring from her left forefinger. Ruby wrapped a deep gash to her finger in tissue; it bled profusely when pressure was not applied. Ruby felt it wise to call her friend Jane.

By the time Ruby and Jane had reached the emergency department of the nearest hospital, Ruby was feeling faint. Her injured finger was causing a throbbing pain. It looked very red, swollen, and was warm to touch. The nurse assessed, cleaned, closed and bandaged Ruby's deeply cut finger.

Within three months, the wound had healed leaving a small but visible scar. Ruby lost some feeling in her forefinger, but this is expected to return in time. Ruby no longer eats red cabbage.

In the case study Ruby's finger undergoes a typical rapid, inflammatory response to an injury. Ruby immediately felt pain from the gash to her finger and went into mild shock. Over the subsequent minutes, Ruby's injured finger became inflamed. Ruby would clearly have recognised what are known as the four cardinal signs of inflammation: redness, warmth, swelling and pain. Despite the discomfort and pain it causes, the inflammatory response is a vital part of the body's **innate immune response** and wound-healing process.

The inflammatory response is the body's first response to injury or infection. As mentioned above, the inflammatory response forms part of our innate immune response. Before examining the inflammatory response, we identify the main ways in which cells and tissues can become injured.

After examining the causes of tissue injury, we look at the acute inflammatory response. We then examine the signs and symptoms of inflammation. Many of the unpleasant symptoms we feel when we have an illness or injury, such as pain, fever, loss of appetite and fatigue, are due to the inflammatory response. Diseases in which the inflammatory response plays a key part often end with the suffix *-itis*. Examples include: appendicitis, hepatitis, meningitis, pancreatitis and bronchiolitis.

Without an inflammatory response, we would be susceptible to all sorts of infections and damaged tissues would be unlikely to heal. However, in the section on chronic inflammation, we will see that inflammation itself can be a disease mechanism, causing considerable tissue damage, pain and altered function. There are many chronic inflammatory diseases such as Crohn's disease and rheumatoid arthritis, caused by a prolonged inflammatory reaction.

This leads to the final section of the chapter where we introduce an important class of anti-inflammatory drugs: the **corticosteroids**. Specifically, we examine the use and potential side-effects of **glucocorticoid** drugs. The role of another important class of anti-inflammatory drugs, the non-steroidal anti-inflammatory drugs (NSAIDs), is covered in Chapter 6.

Sources of tissue injury

Inflammation is triggered by damage to tissues and/or infection. Perhaps the most common trigger is infection – either bacterial or viral (Chapter 3). There are, however, a number of other ways in which tissues can become injured.

Table 2.1 gives examples of how tissue injury may be caused. In the table, injuries are divided into external and internal causes. External causes include trauma, burns and infection. In these cases, the damaging **stimulus** comes from outside the body. By contrast, internal sources of injury occur due to a disease processes originating within the body. These include: ischaemia, the accumulation of uric acid crystals in synovial joints and exposure of the gastric mucosa to acid.

It can be seen from Table 2.1 that tissue damage is pivotal for understanding a wide range of diseases, many of which will be described further in later chapters of this book.

External causes	Internal causes
Trauma including bone fracture, stabbing, piercing (Chapter 6)	Immune response to self-**antigens** (autoimmunity) (Chapter 4)
Burns	Ischaemia – reduced blood supply to a tissue (Chapter 8)
Extremes of temperature (very hot or very cold)	Hypersensitivity to allergens (Chapter 4)
Infection, e.g. bacterial, viral (Chapter 3)	Accumulation of cholesterol in the walls of arteries (atherosclerosis) (Chapter 8)
Snake venom, bee sting, nettle sting	Tumours – which can compress neighbouring tissues (Chapter 5)
Foreign object, e.g. surgical swab	Exposure of the gastric mucosa to acid, exposure of tissues to digestive enzymes, e.g. from the pancreas (Chapter 10)
Poisons, e.g. cyanide, mercury	Uric acid crystals formed in synovial joints (gout)
Radiation damage, e.g. UV light, radiotherapy (sunburn, this chapter)	Accumulation of protein in nerve cells, e.g. Parkinson's disease (Chapter 12)

Table 2.1 Ways in which tissue injury may occur

Acute inflammation

Ruby's gash to her finger is a typical example of an injury causing an acute inflammatory response. It is important to note that inflammation does not mean infection, even when infection causes inflammation. Infection is caused by a microorganism while inflammation is the body's response to it. Acute inflammation can be defined as the first response to tissue injury, and it is usually short-lived. It involves the local accumulation of fluid, plasma proteins and white blood cells called **neutrophils**.

Whatever the damaging stimulus, the sequence of events of acute inflammation is similar. Figure 2.1 shows the sequence of three main processes that occur in acute inflammation:

1. The release of inflammatory mediators – the release of chemicals such as histamine, from damaged cells, and immune cells, which trigger the vascular and cellular response.
2. A vascular response – the response of the small blood vessels (vasodilation, increased permeability).
3. A cellular response – accumulation of neutrophils from the blood.

We will look at these in turn.

1. Release of inflammatory mediators

Almost within seconds of injury, damaged cells release a 'cocktail' of inflammatory mediators. Table 2.2 shows some of these. Many act as local signalling molecules (Chapter 1) causing **vasodilation**, increased **vascular permeability** and pain. The pro-inflammatory **cytokines** given in Table 2.2 are important in causing systemic symptoms such as fever and malaise.

Bradykinins and prostaglandins are of particular note because they cause pain (Chapter 6).

The table shows that immune cells and platelets are important in producing many inflammatory mediators. In addition, some inflammatory mediators are normal plasma proteins such as clotting factors. These are important for blood clotting in injuries where blood vessels have been damaged. Ruby's injury initially bled profusely until these clotting factors become activated and form a fibrous blood clot.

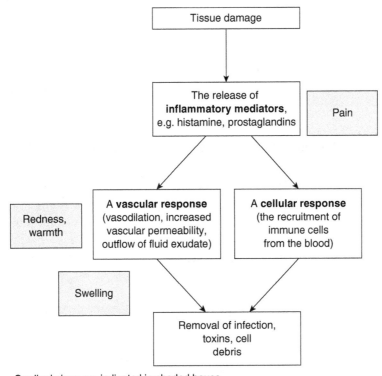

Figure 2.1   Events of acute inflammation

2. The vascular response

Inflamed tissue is red and swollen. This is due to the response of the blood vessels within the damaged tissue. Vasodilation occurs increasing the blood supply to the area. This causes visible redness (erythema) and a feeling of warmth to the touch. There is also a swelling of the tissue, which is due to **oedema**. Oedema is caused when a protein-rich fluid, called an **exudate**, is squeezed out of the blood vessels and accumulates in the tissues. During an inflammatory response, small blood vessels become more porous and leak plasma and plasma proteins. Some of the proteins include **complement**, bradykinins and clotting factors (Table 2.2).

Mediator	Chemical nature	Source	Effect
Histamine	Amine (similar to an amino acid)	Mast cells, platelets	Vasodilation, increased vascular permeability to plasma proteins
Prostaglandins	Lipid-derived	Damaged cells, macrophages, neutrophils	Vasodilation, pain, fever
Leukotrienes	Lipid-derived	Mast cells, eosinophils, basophils	Increased vascular permeability, recruitment of neutrophils
Pro-inflammatory cytokines IL-1, 6, TNF	Proteins	Mast cells, macrophages, lymphocytes	Promote inflammation by: attracting white blood cells called neutrophils and stimulating phagocytosis; they also cause fever, and increase neutrophil production in the bone marrow
Chemokines	Polypeptides	Mast cells, macrophages	Attract neutrophils to the site of inflammation
Complement	Proteins	Plasma (made in the liver)	Kill bacteria, aid phagocytosis
Bradykinins	Proteins	Plasma (made in the liver)	Vasodilation, increased permeability, pain
Clotting factors	Proteins	Plasma (made in the liver)	Blood clotting

Table 2.2 Examples of inflammatory mediators

TNF – tumour necrosis factor; IL – interleukin.

The exudate dilutes any toxins and the plasma proteins it contains help limit infection or blood loss. Complement is a series of plasma proteins which functions primarily to 'complement' the immune response against microorganisms. Complement can trigger an inflammatory response. In the presence of microorganisms complement is activated and can directly destroy bacteria. In addition, clotting factors entering the tissues cause the formation of fibrin – a long fibrous protein, from fibrinogen. Fibrin forms a mesh or matrix around the site of an infection in which the immune cells can function.

The exudate carrying with it bacteria, cell debris and immune cells is drained into nearby lymph vessels. Bacteria, cell debris and immune cells become trapped in the draining lymph node where they activate resident white blood cells called lymphocytes and initiate an **adaptive immune response** (Chapter 4).

3. The cellular response

Immune cells, in particular macrophages, mast cells and neutrophils, play a vital role in inflammation.

Macrophages are found in the tissues and ingest infecting microorganisms. The ability to ingest large particles including microorganisms is called **phagocytosis**. When a macrophage ingests a microorganism the microorganism is usually destroyed – as described below. The ingestion of a microorganism activates the macrophage causing it to secrete a range of pro-inflammatory cytokines, including IL-1, -6 and TNF which promote inflammation (Table 2.2).

A characteristic of acute inflammation is the attraction of neutrophils from the blood to the injured area. The key role of neutrophils in inflammation is phagocytosis. Phagocytosis is shown in Figure 2.2. First, the neutrophil surrounds the microorganism and brings it into the cell in a vesicle called a phagosome. The vesicle fuses with an organelle called a lysosome. The lysosome contains digestive enzymes and highly reactive 'oxygen-species' which kill and digest the microorganism. Bacteria are one of the main targets of phagocytosis for neutrophils. Neutrophils die in the process of phagocytosis. Dead neutrophils, cell debris and bacteria may accumulate as pus (or a 'purulent exudate'). Pus is characteristic of a number of bacterial infections including *Staphylococcus aureus.*

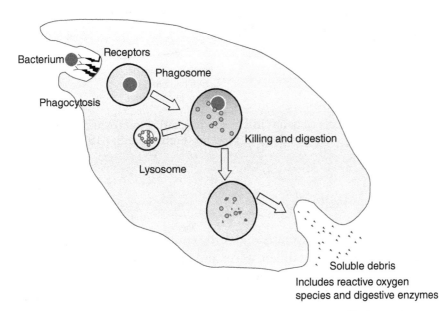

A bacterium binds to receptors on the surface of a macrophage or neutrophil. The cell membrane surrounds the bacterium and brings it into the cell in a vesicle called a phagosome. A cellular organelle called a lysosome fuses with the phagosome. Chemicals from the lysosome start to digest the bacterium. The chemicals include digestive enzymes and reactive oxygen species. Once the bacterium is degraded, the phagosome releases its debris from the cell. This debris includes reactive oxygen species and digestive enzymes which are highly toxic and can cause damage to neighbouring cells and tissues.

Figure 2.2   Phagocytosis

Mast cells play a key part in initiating an inflammatory response through the release of histamine. Mast cells are widely distributed through the tissues of the body. Histamine causes vasodilation and increased vascular permeability. **Allergens,** such as pollen or cat hair, will stimulate mast cells to release histamine in people who are predisposed to allergy. This is the mechanism underlying allergic asthma and anaphylaxis (Chapter 4). Physical pressure to the skin, such as scratching, also releases histamine from mast cells and usually causes minor inflammation.

Figure 2.3 summarises the beneficial effects of acute inflammation.

Complete Activity 2.1 which asks you to explain a case of sunburn.

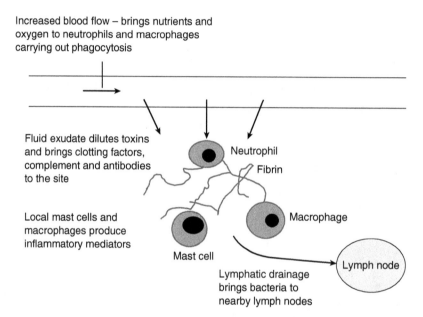

Figure 2.3 Beneficial effects of acute inflammation. Adapted from Bateman and Carr (2009) *Flesh and Bones of Pathology.* Mosby, Elsevier, Figure 3.4.2, p19

Activity 2.1   Reflection

After a day sunbathing, your friend Anne complains of sunburn. Her shoulders are very red, swollen, warm and painful to touch. Using your understanding of acute inflammation, explain Anne's symptoms. Use Tables 2.1 and 2.2 to identify the source of tissue injury, and the main inflammatory mediators responsible for her symptoms.

A suggested answer is provided at the end of the chapter.

Having completed Activity 2.1, you will be in a position to understand many of the clinical features of acute inflammation.

Clinical features of inflammation

Anne's sunburn and Ruby's injured finger illustrate the four cardinal signs of inflammation (redness, warmth, swelling and pain) which are usually localised to the site of injury. There may also be immobility or loss of function of an inflamed limb or tissue.

- Pain – the inflamed area will be painful particularly when touched. Inflammatory mediators, including bradykinins and prostaglandins, stimulate pain fibres and make the area sensitive to touch (Chapter 6).
- Redness – small blood vessels become dilated.
- Swelling – accumulation of fluid (oedema).
- Heat – increased blood flow to the affected area.

The four cardinal signs of acute inflammation are relevant when the affected area is on or very close to the skin. When inflammation occurs deep inside the body only some of the signs may be detectable. Some internal organs or tissue do not contain sensory nerve endings so pain may not be felt. With some types of pneumonia for example, pain is only felt when the inflamed lung tissue stretches the parietal pleura during **inhalation** activating pain fibres in the pleura.

Inflammation can lead to systemic effects such as fever, which is initiated by cytokines that are released into the circulation. Pro-inflammatory cytokines IL-1, -6 and TNF enter the bloodstream and act on the hypothalamus to produce fever (Chapter 3).

A raised white blood cell count can indicate inflammation. Specifically, a raised neutrophil count is often an indication of a bacterial infection. Raised eosinophils can indicate an allergic reaction or infection with a parasitic worm or tick.

Erythrocyte sedimentation rate (ESR), C-reactive protein (CRP) and plasma viscosity are blood tests for inflammation. These are used as non-specific markers of inflammation. These cannot be used to diagnose a particular disease but may be used when an inflammatory disease is suspected, such as rheumatoid arthritis. With chronic inflammatory disease, ESR and CRP can be used to monitor the activity of the disease or the effects of treatments.

Having examined the clinical features of acute inflammation, we now look at the possible outcomes of acute inflammation.

Possible outcomes of acute inflammation

Ideally, an inflammatory response will clear the source of damage (infection or toxin) leaving little tissue damage and minimum scarring. This outcome would be the case after a minor cut or a bee sting. Many microbial infections are completely cleared by an acute inflammatory response without leaving permanent damage.

The outcome of inflammation depends partly on the extent of damage and partly on the type of tissue that is damaged. Scar tissue will form if damage is extensive or if the tissue cannot regenerate itself. Ruby's cut finger left a small scar; the cut extended into the dermis of the skin which cannot regenerate itself. Scarring occurs after damage to the heart following **myocardial infarction** (Chapter 8) and in some cases of pneumonia where lung fibrosis can result.

Another possible consequence of acute inflammation is the formation of an abscess. This is a collection of pus – an exudate containing neutrophils, dead tissue and bacteria. Abscesses can occur anywhere in the body. An abscess may resolve on its own, or if particularly painful may need treatment with antibiotics. An abscess can be drained if it is near the surface such as in the skin or in the gums.

Sometimes the cause of the tissue damage cannot be cleared and inflammation may become chronic. Chronic inflammation is persistent and causes significant tissue damage. Chronic inflammation contributes to the tissue damage in many chronic conditions including atherosclerosis, cancer and Crohn's disease. We now turn to look at the pathophysiology of chronic inflammation.

Chronic inflammation

Chronic inflammation is characterised by its duration and the type of cells that are present in the inflamed tissue. While acute inflammation is characterised by the presence of neutrophils, chronic inflammation is marked by the presence of macrophages and lymphocytes. There is always tissue damage with chronic inflammation and repair processes resulting in scarring.

Chronic inflammation will arise with:

- Persistent infection, where the microorganism has not been removed. An example is *Mycobacterium tuberculosis* which can survive and multiply inside macrophages (Goering et al., 2013).
- Allergic disease, such as asthma and hay fever, where there is continual exposure to the chemical causing the allergy (the allergen).
- Autoimmunity, in which the immune system targets the body's own tissues (Chapter 4).
- Prolonged exposure to potentially toxic agents. Exposure to asbestos and silica can cause chronic inflammation to the lungs, as can cigarette smoking. Cholesterol builds up in the lining of large arteries where it contributes to a chronic inflammatory reaction. This underlies the disease process in atherosclerosis which is the major cause of **ischaemic heart disease** (Chapter 8).

Macrophages accumulate in chronically inflamed tissues and cause tissue damage. As described above, macrophages are capable of phagocytosis of invading microorganisms. Once inside the macrophage, the microorganism is killed and digested by a number of harmful chemicals including reactive oxygen species and digestive enzymes (Figure 2.2). Some of these chemicals are then released by the macrophage and directly damage surrounding tissues. Damaged tissues will eventually be replaced by scar tissue.

Use this information and further research to complete Activity 2.2.

Activity 2.2   Research

You are working as a community nurse with a number of patients with asbestosis. Asbestosis is a chronic lung disease caused by exposure to asbestos in which chronic inflammation plays a key role. Find out how asbestos damages the lungs. You may also be interested in examining the public health measures that are in place to prevent exposure to asbestos.

The following websites may be useful starting points:

www.nhs.uk/Conditions/Asbestosis/Pages/Introduction.aspx/

www.patient.co.uk/doctor/asbestos-related-diseases-pro/

A suggested answer is given at the end of the chapter.

Once you have completed Activity 2.2 you will be in a position to distinguish between acute and chronic inflammation. To help with this, complete Activity 2.3.

Activity 2.3   Reflection

What are the main differences between acute and chronic inflammation? Use the table format below to summarise your answer.

	Acute inflammation	**Chronic inflammation**
Duration		
Onset		
Role (protective/ harmful)		
Main cell types		
Possible outcomes		
Signs/symptoms		
Examples		

A suggested answer is given at the end of the chapter.

Following on from Activity 2.3, we examine the pharmacological treatment of inflammation with corticosteroids.

Corticosteroids

Corticosteroids are one of the main types of drugs used to reduce inflammation. They have both anti-inflammatory and immunosuppressant effects and are used in a wide variety of diseases where inflammation and an overactive immune system are problematic. They are used for example in asthma, eczema, rheumatoid arthritis and ulcerative colitis. Many of these diseases will be visited in more detail in subsequent chapters of this book.

Activity 2.4   Reflection

Fill in the table below to include any corticosteroids you can think of, the route of administration and what they are used for. You may want to use the British National Formulary (2018) or ask a colleague to help you.

Corticosteroid	Route of administration	Condition treated

A suggested answer is given at the end of the chapter.

You may be aware that some corticosteroids are naturally occurring steroid hormones. The cortex of the adrenal gland synthesises and releases two types of corticosteroids: mineralocorticoids and glucocorticoids. Mineralocorticoids regulate extracellular sodium concentrations and extracellular fluid volume. The main mineralocorticoid in the body is aldosterone. Glucocorticoids regulate the body's use of carbohydrates, lipids and proteins and its response to stress. Glucocorticoids also have anti-inflammatory effects (Tortora and Derrickson, 2017).

Glucocorticoids and other steroid hormones are lipid-soluble and can cross the plasma membrane. Once they have entered the cell, they bind to glucocorticoid receptors in the cytoplasm. The receptor–hormone complex then moves into the nucleus where it binds to specific genes. This binding causes some genes to be activated and some to be suppressed. This is turn alters the levels of proteins made by the cell. The main effects of glucocorticoids are metabolic and anti-inflammatory/immunosuppressant:

1. **Metabolic actions:**

   - Stimulation of gluconeogenesis (synthesis of glucose) by the liver.
   - Reduced cellular uptake of blood glucose.
   - Stimulation of fat-breakdown in adipose tissue.
   - Increased breakdown of proteins and mobilisation of amino acids.

2. **Anti-inflammatory/immunosuppressant actions:**

   - Reducing the action and proliferation of a number of immune cells including lymphocytes, macrophages, eosinophils.
   - Inhibiting prostaglandin synthesis.
   - Reduced production of immunoglobulins, IgG and IgA (Chapter 4).
   - Reducing the release of inflammatory mediators, e.g. cytokines.

Cortisol is the body's main glucocorticoid. Figure 2.4 shows how cortisol production is naturally controlled in the body by a negative feedback loop. Cortisol production is regulated by the hypothalamic–pituitary–adrenal cortex (HPA) axis. Inflammation, pain and stress stimulate the hypothalamus to release corticotrophin-releasing factor (CRF). CRF stimulates the pituitary gland to release adrenocorticotropic hormone

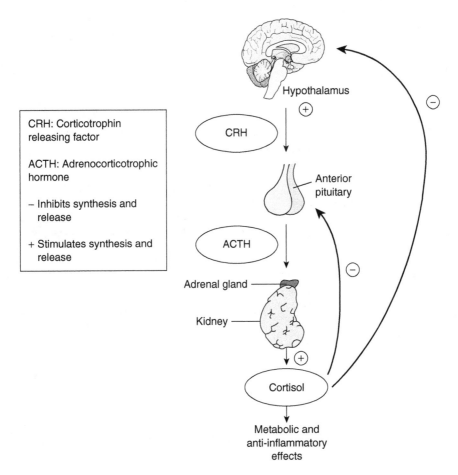

CRH: Corticotrophin releasing factor

ACTH: Adrenocorticotrophic hormone

– Inhibits synthesis and release

+ Stimulates synthesis and release

Figure 2.4 Negative feedback control of cortisol

(ACTH). ACTH stimulates the release of cortisol by the adrenal cortex. Cortisol 'feeds-back' to the hypothalamus and pituitary gland reducing the release of CRF and ACTH. This negative feedback leads to a reduction in cortisol release.

Most synthetic corticosteroid drugs are designed to exploit the immunosuppressive and anti-inflammatory effects of glucocorticoids. One of the reasons there are so many different corticosteroids is that their pharmacokinetics (Chapter 1) are very different. This can influence the route of administration used, which you identified in Activity 2.4. This in turn may dictate which corticosteroid is used. For example, inhaled preparations are used for lung conditions and creams are used for skin conditions.

Corticosteroids are metabolised in the liver and the water-soluble metabolites are excreted by the kidney. Concentrations of corticosteroids can therefore be increased in patients with liver impairment and should be used with caution.

Side-effects and implications for practice

The body's main corticosteroid, cortisol, has very wide ranging effects. It is therefore not surprising that corticosteroids used as drugs have many side-effects. The most important are listed below. Some of these side-effects are very serious and this is the reason we often ask patients to use short courses and keep doses as low as possible. Another way of limiting side-effects is to deliver steroids to the site of action, for example by inhalers, nasal drops and enemas. Even when given by these routes there will still be some systemic absorption and this can lead to side-effects. Side-effects can be such a problem that some people may be asked to carry a steroid treatment card, shown in Figure 2.5. This card is recommended for patients receiving oral, long-term treatment (more than 3 weeks) and/or high doses (NICE, 2017a).

STEROID TREATMENT CARD I am a patient on STEROID treatment which must not be stopped suddenly • If you have been taking this medicine for more than three weeks, the dose should be reduced gradually when you stop taking steroids unless your doctor says otherwise • Read the patient information leaflet given with the medicine	• Always carry this card with you and show it to anyone who treats you (for example a doctor, nurse, pharmacist or dentist). For one year after you stop treatment, you must mention that you have taken steroids. • If you become ill, or if you come into contact with anyone who has an infectious disease, consult your doctor promptly. If you have never had chickenpox, you should avoid close contact with people who have chickenpox or shingles. If you do come into contact with chickenpox, see your doctor urgently. • Make sure that the information on the card is kept up to date.

Figure 2.5 A steroid treatment card

1. **Adrenal suppression:** Corticosteroids used as drugs will inhibit production of the body's own cortisol through negative feedback (Figure 2.4). This is a particular problem when corticosteroids are used in high doses for a long period of time.

In time, the adrenal cortex will reduce in size (atrophy) due to loss of use. If a patient was suddenly to stop their corticosteroid medication, acute adrenal insufficiency would occur due to the lack of cortisol production by the body. This can be life-threatening. The symptoms can include general malaise, lethargy, dizziness, generalised weakness, arthralgia, headaches and emotional lability (Iliopoulou et al., 2013). After stopping a corticosteroid it can take 2–18 months for the adrenal glands to recover.

2. **Immunosuppression:** The immunosuppressant effects of corticosteroids can result in an increased risk of infection, particularly for those on long-term steroids. Research has shown that those on steroid inhalers for chronic obstructive pulmonary disease (COPD) are more likely to get pneumonia (Chapter 9). The steroid treatment card (Figure 2.5) warns people about chickenpox and shingles which are caused by varicella-zoster virus; immunosuppression may lead to a particularly severe infection.

3. **Psychiatric reactions:** Corticosteroids have been reported to cause a wide range of psychiatric effects including nightmares, depression, changeable moods, euphoria, insomnia and psychotic reactions.

4. **Diabetes mellitus:** Corticosteroids can increase the risk of hyperglycaemia. This can lead to type 2 diabetes mellitus in people on long-term steroid use. Corticosteroids should be used with caution for those with a family history of type 2 diabetes. In addition, corticosteroids should also be used with caution in those with pre-existing diabetes as their diabetic control may be worsened. Corticosteroids reduce insulin production in the pancreas and directly increase gluconeogenesis in the liver.

5. **Osteoporosis:** Corticosteroids reduce calcium absorption from the gastrointestinal tract and increase renal calcium excretion. Calcium is needed as the mineral component in bones. Corticosteroids also reduce osteoblast activity; these are the cells which make the matrix of bone tissue. Bone is weakened and becomes porous and fragile (osteoporosis), which in turn can result in bone fractures.

6. **Glaucoma and cataracts:** Both oral and inhaled corticosteroids can affect the eyes causing cataracts. They can also increase the pressure in the eye and cause glaucoma.

7. **Skin thinning:** This is the most common side-effect of topical therapy and is caused because corticosteroids reduce collagen synthesis. Collagen is an important protein which gives the dermis of the skin its structure.

Research summary: Steroid phobia

It is common for patients and parents of children with eczema to underuse corticosteroid creams because of fears of skin thinning and other side-effects. Charman et al. (2000) provided a questionnaire for 200 dermatology outpatients with atopic eczema. They found that 72.5% worried about using topical corticosteroids on their own or their child's skin and 24% were non-compliant as a result. 34.5% worried about skin thinning and 9.5% about side-effects due to systemic absorption. There are four

(Continued)

(Continued)

strengths of steroid in creams: mild, such as hydrocortisone; moderate; potent and very potent – for example dermovate (BNF, 2018). While skin thinning can be a problem with potent steroids it can be minimised by using low potency corticosteroids. Continued use on sensitive skin such as the eyelids and face should be avoided, but elsewhere mild steroid preparations rarely cause problems. It should also be remembered that poorly treated eczema is uncomfortable and can lead to skin thickening (lichenification) and pigmentation due to scratching (Taibjee and Charman, 2009). By understanding the risks and benefits of corticosteroid creams nurses can help patients use their treatments more effectively.

8. **Cushing's syndrome:** Cushing's syndrome (hypercortisolaemia) is a collection of symptoms caused by high cortisol levels. It can occur as an endocrine disorder when the body makes an excess of natural corticosteroids (Kumar et al., 2014). However, high-dose, long-term corticosteroid therapy can also cause Cushing's syndrome. Symptoms include moon face, central obesity, osteoporosis, diabetes mellitus and growth of body hair (hirsuitism).

9. **Peptic ulcers:** As part of their anti-inflammatory effect, corticosteroids reduce prostaglandin synthesis. The stomach usually protects itself from gastric acid by producing mucus. Prostaglandins are needed for mucus production. Prostaglandins also reduce acid secretion in the stomach. If prostaglandin synthesis is reduced the stomach is more susceptible to damage from gastric acid and peptic ulcers can result (Chapter 10).

Activity 2.5   Reflection

Now that we have been through the side-effects of corticosteroids have a look again at the steroid card in Figure 2.5. Imagine talking through the card with a patient. How would you explain to the patient why the steroid card makes the recommendations it does.

A suggested answer is given at the end of the chapter.

Non-steroidal anti-inflammatory drugs (NSAIDs)

This class of drugs exerts its actions by anti-inflammatory effects. These drugs are covered in detail in Chapter 6.

It is now time to review what you have learned within this chapter by undertaking some multiple choice questions.

Activity 2.6   Multiple choice questions

1. The four cardinal signs of inflammation are:
   a) Redness, swelling, oedema, fever
   b) Redness, warmth, malaise, fever
   c) Redness, warmth, swelling, pain
   d) Redness, swelling, pain, fever

2. The following would be considered an *internal* source of tissue damage:
   a) Sunburn
   b) Poisoning
   c) Infection
   d) Ischaemia

3. The first immune cell that will encounter an invading microorganism is likely to be:
   a) Macrophage
   b) Mast cell
   c) Lymphocyte
   d) Neutrophil

4. The following inflammatory mediators contribute to pain:
   a) Pro-inflammatory cytokines IL-1, IL-6, TNF
   b) Prostaglandins and bradykinins
   c) Chemokines
   d) Leukotrienes

5. Plasma proteins leaving the blood and entering an inflamed tissue include all the following except:
   a) Fibrinogen
   b) Complement
   c) Bradykinins
   d) Histamine

6. The main cells involved in chronic inflammation are:
   a) Macrophages and neutrophils
   b) Mast cells and neutrophils
   c) Macrophages and lymphocytes
   d) Lymphocytes and mast cells

(Continued)

(Continued)

7. Chronic inflammation is associated with all of the following except:
   a) Tissue damage
   b) Scarring (fibrosis)
   c) Infiltration of neutrophils
   d) Incomplete resolution

8. A patient has been on 40 mg of prednisolone for two weeks after a severe exacerbation of COPD. It is important for the dose to be reduced slowly:
   a) To reduce withdrawal effects such as anxiety and depression
   b) To reduce the risk of acute adrenal insufficiency
   c) To reduce the risk of contracting measles
   d) All of the above

9. Which of the following statements about the side-effects of corticosteroids is *false?*
   a) They cause hyperglycaemia and should be used with caution in people with diabetes
   b) They cause osteoporosis because they reduce calcium absorption and osteoblast activity
   c) They cause peptic ulcers because they reduce prostaglandin synthesis
   d) They cause skin thickening (lichenification)

10. The following is *not* a major action of the body's main natural glucocorticoid, cortisol:
    a) Increased sodium and water retention
    b) Reduced prostaglandin synthesis
    c) Reduction of bone mineralisation
    d) Stimulation of lipid and protein breakdown

Chapter summary

In this chapter you have learned that inflammatory response is the body's first response to injury or infection. The acute inflammatory response is a carefully mediated response to damaged tissue. It involves four cardinal symptoms: redness, swelling, heat and pain. Long term, however, chronic inflammation causes considerable damage and scarring of tissues. Chronic inflammation causes a number of conditions including asthma, eczema, rheumatoid arthritis and ulcerative colitis. Corticosteroids are a family of anti-inflammatory drugs used in a wide range of inflammatory conditions. Patient information is vital to ensure optimum use of corticosteroids. This is particularly so for patients receiving oral, long-term treatment and/or high doses. Nurses have an important role in monitoring those on long-term corticosteroids and providing accurate, up-to-date patient information.

Activities: Brief outline answers

Activity 2.1 Reflection (p44)

Sunburn is a burn due to over-exposure to ultraviolet light. Ultraviolet damage to the skin cells will trigger an inflammatory reaction. Redness and heat are due to the increased blood supply to the area (erythema). Increased vascular permeability will lead to a fluid exudate leaving the blood vessels and entering the tissues. This causes the swelling. As will be described in Chapter 6 on pain, inflammatory mediators including prostaglandins and bradykinins stimulate and sensitise pain fibres in the skin. Peripheral hyperalgesia (Chapter 6) can cause the area to feel painful to the touch. There is evidence that a molecule called CXCL5 is responsible for the longer-lasting pain of sunburn (Dawes et al., 2011).

Sunburn can happen within 30 minutes of exposure, but most often takes 2 to 6 hours. Sunburn can lead to long-term skin damage and is a risk factor for a type of skin cancer called melanoma.

Activity 2.2 Research (p47)

Asbestos is a family of crystalline hydrated silicates present as microscopic fibres. These fibres are used in building construction because they are long-lasting, durable and fire-resistant. If asbestos fibres are inhaled, the fibres can become trapped in the lungs, often within the alveolar ducts. Alveolar macrophages attempt to remove the fibres by phagocytosis – engulfing and attempting to digest the fibres. The fibres are resistant to digestion by the macrophages. Macrophages release chemicals that trigger inflammation and cause tissue damage (including reactive oxygen species) and pro-inflammatory cytokines. Macrophages also release growth factors which stimulate fibroblasts to replace damaged lung tissue with scar tissue. In the lung this process causes lung fibrosis. When the cause is asbestos the scarring is called asbestosis. It is of note that asbestos exposure is also linked to mesothelioma – a form of lung cancer.

Activity 2.3 Reflection (p47)

	Acute inflammation	Chronic inflammation
Duration	Short-lived (hours to days)	Prolonged (days, months or years)
Onset	Rapid	Usually delayed
Role	Protective	Damaging
Main cell types	Neutrophils	Macrophages and lymphocytes
Possible outcomes	Complete resolution possible or some scarring possible	Replacement of damaged tissues with scarring
Signs/symptoms	Prominent local and systemic	Less prominent
Examples	Appendicitis, bacterial pneumonia, allergy, sepsis, sprained ankle, wasp sting, common cold	Crohn's disease, rheumatoid arthritis, asthma, systemic lupus erythematosus, multiple sclerosis, asbestosis

Activity 2.4 Reflection (p48)

Examples of corticosteroids include:

Corticosteroid	Route of administration	Condition treated
Beclomethasone	Inhalation	Asthma and COPD
Dexamethasone	Oral	Cerebral oedema, nausea and vomiting in cancer
Hydrocortisone	Topical	Eczema, psoriasis
Hydrocortisone	Parenteral (injection)	Anaphylaxis
Prednisolone	Oral	Exacerbation of COPD
Prednisolone	Rectal	Ulcerative colitis

Activity 2.5 Reflection (p52)

Steroids should not be stopped suddenly, but slowly withdrawn because of adrenal suppression. The immune system might be impaired and some infections can be particularly severe, for example chickenpox. Further recommendations are given in the clinical knowledge summary for corticosteroids (NICE, 2017a).

Activity 2.6 Multiple choice questions (pp53–4)

1. The four cardinal signs of inflammation are:

   c)   Redness, warmth, swelling, pain

2. The following would be considered an *internal* source of tissue damage:

   d)   Ischaemia

3. The first immune cell that will encounter an invading microorganism is likely to be:

   a)   Macrophage

4. The following inflammatory mediators contribute to pain:

   b)   Prostaglandins and bradykinins

5. Plasma proteins leaving the blood and entering an inflamed tissue include all the following except:

   d)   Histamine

6. The main cells involved in chronic inflammation are:

   c)   Macrophages and lymphocytes

7. Chronic inflammation is associated with all of the following except:

   c)   Infiltration of neutrophils

8. A patient has been on 40 mg of prednisolone for two weeks after a severe exacerbation of COPD. It is important for the dose to be reduced slowly:

   b)   To reduce the risk of acute adrenal insufficiency

9. Which of the following statements about the side-effects of corticosteroids is *false*?

   d)   They cause skin thickening (lichenification)

10. The following is *not* a major action of the body's main natural glucocorticoid, cortisol:

    a)   Increased sodium and water retention

Further reading

Kumar, V, Abbas, A, Fausto, N and Mitchell, R (2014) *Robbins Basic Pathology* (9th edition). Philadelphia: Saunders Elsevier.

A comprehensive and detailed textbook on pathology. Chapter 1 gives details on cell injury. Chapter 2 on acute and chronic inflammation is particularly relevant.

Simonsen, T, Aarbakke, J, Kay, I, Coleman, I, Sinnott, P and Lysaa, R (2006) *Illustrated Pharmacology for Nurses*. London: Hodder Arnold.

A clearly written and well-illustrated pharmacology book aimed at nurses.

Useful websites

http://cks.nice.org.uk/corticosteroids-oral/

Clinical knowledge summary on oral corticosteroids by the National Institute for Health and Care Excellence.

www.youtube.com/watch?v=DU2YoRINYzw/

Immunosuppressant drugs – glucocorticoids. A clear and detailed illustration of the immuno-suppressant effects of corticosteroids.

Chapter 3　Infection

Chapter aims

After reading this chapter you will be able to:

- describe the main types of microorganism important for human health;
- explain the difference between pathogenic and commensal microorganisms;
- explain the chain of infection and how it may be broken;
- relate the signs and symptoms of infection to the underlying pathophysiology of infection;
- explain how the main anti-microbial drugs work and their main side-effects;
- demonstrate awareness of antibiotic resistance and the steps that can be taken to reduce the risk of antibiotic resistance developing.

Introduction

Imagine a world in which it is too dangerous to go into hospital for surgery and just cutting your finger could result in death. It seems ridiculous yet according to the World Health Organization (WHO) the threat from bacterial infection due to increasing resistance to antibiotics is making this a real possibility (WHO, 2015).

In this chapter we examine four of the main types of microorganisms important to human health and give examples of the infectious diseases they cause. The microorganisms we have included are: viruses, fungi, protozoa and bacteria. We will examine how microorganisms are passed on in 'the chain of infection' and how this chain may be broken. We then look at the general signs and symptoms of infection and how these are caused. We will consider the drugs used to treat the different types of infections and the side-effects of these. Finally, we will examine how antibiotic resistance occurs and what steps you can take to reduce antibiotic resistance developing.

Infection

Statistics from the World Health Organization for 2000–2016 place infectious diseases among the top ten causes of death worldwide (WHO, 2018). These infections include lower respiratory tract infections, diarrhoeal diseases and tuberculosis. In low income countries lower respiratory tract infections and diarrhoeal diseases are the top two causes of death. In high income countries, such as the United Kingdom, people predominantly die of chronic diseases, such as cardiovascular disease, cancer and dementia. However, lower respiratory tract infections remain a leading cause of death.

Infectious diseases are caused by microorganisms including bacteria, viruses and fungi. Disease-causing microorganisms are said to be **pathogenic**. A microorganism that causes disease is called a **pathogen**. Infection arises when a microorganism enters the body, resists the innate defences, and invades the tissues. The most common sites of infection are the respiratory and gastrointestinal tracts. The skin can be a site of entry – usually when it is disrupted, for example by a wound. Another important site of entry is the genitourinary tract. Pathogens can spread from person to person, directly or indirectly, or from animals to humans in what is called a **zoonotic** disease. *Salmonella* food poisoning is a classic example of a zoonotic disease, originating from contaminated food, often poultry.

Not all infections with pathogenic microorganisms cause symptoms. An infection is said to be **subclinical** if it produces no symptoms. Infection will result in disease and clinical symptoms if the infection causes tissue injury. Some microorganisms such as viruses cause direct damage to cells because they multiply inside our cells. Many viruses then spread by rupturing or 'bursting' the cell and spreading through the tissues or bloodstream (see below under 'Viruses'). Some bacteria produce toxins which kill or damage cells and tissues. An example is *Vibrio cholera*. This microorganism produces a toxin that damages the gastrointestinal tract leading to severe diarrhoea. However, our immune response and inflammatory responses to invading pathogens can cause additional tissue damage.

The microbiome

In a healthy person, the internal tissues are normally free of microorganisms. The skin and parts of the body connected to the external environment (for example, the mouth, nose, intestinal and genitourinary tracts) become colonised by microbial species soon after birth. These organisms make up what is called the microbiome. The microorganisms making up the microbiome are commensal, which means they live harmlessly in or on the body. The microbiome prevents more pathogenic microorganisms colonising and infecting us. The microbiome includes some fungi, viruses and protozoa but is mainly made up from bacteria (Goering et al., 2013). The microbiome can contain pathogenic species. For example, *E. coli* bacteria usually live harmlessly in the gastrointestinal tract but can cause urinary tract infections (UTIs) if they enter the urinary system. Wounds may become infected by microorganisms from the skin microbiome. **Immunocompromised** people (those with a weakened immune response) are particularly susceptible to infections and these infections often originate from the microbiome.

Activity 3.1   Reflection

Identify five infectious diseases. For each disease write down whether it is caused by a virus, bacteria, fungi or protozoa. Name the microorganism that causes the disease.

Examples are given at the end of the chapter. As you proceed through the chapter, compare your choices with the infectious diseases discussed.

Activity 3.1 will have enabled you to connect five infectious diseases with the type and name of the pathogen responsible. We now examine four main types of microorganisms that can cause disease in humans.

Bacteria

Bacteria are **prokaryotic** organisms. Prokaryote means 'lacking a nucleus' (Figure 3.1). Bacteria are all single-celled organisms, and although they do not have a nucleus, they do have genetic material in the form of DNA (deoxyribonucleic acid). Bacteria have their own cellular 'machinery' to grow and reproduce. This cellular machinery includes enzymes, and **ribosomes** needed to manufacture proteins. By contrast, **eukaryotic** cells, which includes all human cells, have a more complex structure. Human cells have a cell **nucleus** and other **organelles**, such as lysosomes (Chapter 2). The cellular machinery of human cells is different from that of bacteria. The difference in cellular machinery of human and bacterial cells enables the effective use of antibacterials. When we take antibacterial drugs, orally for example, the drugs circulate throughout the body. However, antibacterial drugs target the bacteria's unique cellular components and machinery without affecting the cellular components of our own cells. This helps reduce the number of side-effects. Antibacterial drugs are explained further later in the chapter.

Bacteria are free-living organisms. 'Free-living' means that bacteria can live independently of the human body (or any other host organism). Most bacteria do not cause human disease but approximately 50 pathogenic species of bacteria exist. As mentioned under 'The microbiome', pathogenic species of bacteria may live harmlessly as part of the microbiome of the skin, mouth or intestines. Disease may occur if they invade our body tissues to cause damage. Some clinically common bacteria are identified in Table 3.1.

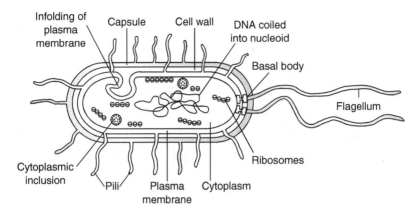

Figure 3.1 A bacterium

Name of bacterium	Disease expression
Staphylococcus aureus	Skin infections, pneumonia, sepsis, endocarditis
Clostridium difficile	Diarrhoea, pseudomembranous colitis
Klebsiella pneumoniae	Pneumonia
Escherichia coli	Diarrhoea, urinary tract infections, respiratory disease, sepsis
Pseudomonas aeruginosa	Sepsis, wound and burn infections
Bacteroides fragilis	Gastrointestinal upset
Mycobacterium tuberculosis	Tuberculosis

Table 3.1 Selected human bacterial diseases

Table 3.1 shows that the same bacterial species may be responsible for more than one type of 'disease expression'. The disease expression refers to the nature of the disease caused (for example, skin infection or respiratory disease), and depends on the part of the body that is infected.

Viruses

Viruses are one of the simplest types of microorganism. Viruses are smaller and simpler than cells. Viruses are not free-living and need to infect our cells to multiply. Viruses are descried as 'intracellular parasites'.

Figure 3.2 shows the structure of the human immunodeficiency virus. The simplest viruses are particles made of a protein 'coat' or capsid, containing the genetic material. The genetic material can be RNA (ribonucleic acid), or DNA (deoxyribonucleic acid), depending on the type of virus. Some virus particles are more complex and have an envelope surrounding the capsid. For example, HIV and influenza virus are more complex viruses with envelopes. The envelope comes from the host cell membrane as the virus particles are release. The envelope contains viral envelope proteins which are needed for cell infection, and are also important targets of the host immune response (Chapter 4). Virus particles are called virions.

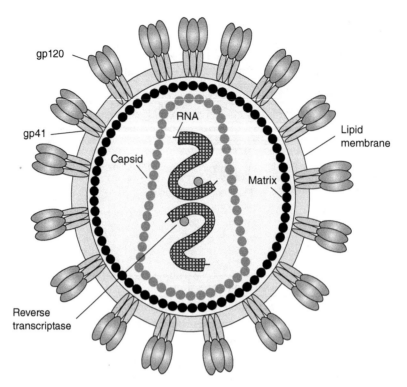

Figure 3.2　The structure of HIV-1

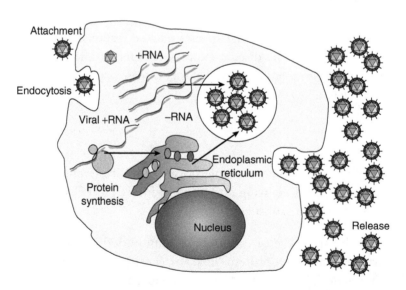

A single virus particle is shown to attach to the host cell membrane. This will result in the virus particle being brought into the cell by a process called endocytosis. Once inside the cell cytoplasm, the virus's genetic material, which in this case is made of a single molecule of RNA (ribonucleic acid), is copied many times. At the same time this genetic material is used to make the proteins making up the virus particle. The proteins are manufactured using the host cell machinery. The virus proteins and genetic material are then brought together to make many thousands of new viruses. These are released from the cell.

Figure 3.3　Virus replication within a host cell

Viruses lack the cellular 'machinery' (such as ribosomes) needed to convert their genetic material into new virus particles. Viruses are therefore reliant on a host cell which they infect in order to make more copies of themselves ('replicate'). This makes antiviral therapy difficult to develop as any antiviral agent that stops viral replication will also affect the host cell function. Antiviral therapy is considered later in the chapter. The virus life cycle is shown in Figure 3.3.

Viruses show 'host cell specificity'. This means that they can only usually infect one cell type. Virus infection involves attachment of the virus particle to a cell membrane receptor on the host cell. This interaction needs a specific protein on the surface of the virus particle and a target receptor on the host cell. Only those host cells with the 'matching' receptor for the virus surface protein can be infected. For example, HIV uses the virus membrane protein gp120 (Figure 3.2) to infect white blood cells which have a target receptor called CD4. This restricts HIV to infecting only cells with the CD4 receptor on the surface. These cells include T helper lymphocytes and macrophages (Chapter 4). Influenza virus uses the sialic acid receptor which is found on lung epithelial cells and the upper respiratory tract.

Some examples of clinically important viruses are given in Table 3.2.

Viral pathogen	Disease expression
Herpes simplex type 1	'Cold sores'
Herpes simplex virus type 2	Genital herpes
Human papilloma virus 6, 11, 16, 18	Warty growths, cervical carcinoma
Hepatitis B virus	Hepatitis
Rhinovirus	Upper respiratory tract infections
Varicella-zoster virus	Chickenpox, shingles
Norovirus	Acute gastroenteritis
Human immunodeficiency virus	Acquired immunodeficiency disease (AIDS)

Table 3.2   Selected human viral diseases

Fungi

Most fungi are multicellular organisms. Not all fungi are considered to be microorganisms. Many fungi grow as thread-like filaments. Other well-known types include single-celled yeast and mushrooms. Fungi are free-living organisms and are important ecologically for breaking down dead plant material. Pathogenic fungi invade tissues and cause damage by releasing digestive enzymes.

Examples of clinically important fungi that cause disease are given in Table 3.3.

Diseases associated with fungal infections are mostly seen in those with compromised immune systems. For example, patients on oral steroids (Chapter 2) or people with a pre-existing disease may have weakened immunity. Many fungi cause opportunistic infections. These are infections that occur more frequently in those with weakened immune systems. People with healthy immune systems do not usually develop disease when exposed to these pathogens. Oral thrush (candidiasis) is a common side-effect of chemotherapy. Opportunistic infections are the common cause of death for those people with AIDS (Chapter 4).

Fungal pathogen	Disease expression
Candida albicans	Thrush
Aspergillus fumigatus	Lung infection in immunocompromised patients
Trichophyton interdigitale	Athlete's foot
Pneumocystis jirovecii	Pneumonia in immunocompromised patients

Table 3.3 Selected human fungal diseases

Protozoa

Protozoa are single-celled animals. Many are free-living but some are important parasites of humans. Some free-living species infect humans as opportunistic infections if the person's immune system is weakened.

Examples of clinically important protozoa are shown in Table 3.4.

Protozoan pathogen	Disease expression
Cryptosporidia parvum	Cryptosporidiosis
Giardia lamblia	Giardiasis
Toxoplasma gondii	Toxoplasmosis
Entamoeba histolytica	Amoebic dysentery
Plasmodium vivax	Malaria

Table 3.4 Selected human protozoan diseases

The chain of infection

The chain of infection (Figure 3.4) illustrates the stages needed for microorganisms to be passed on from one individual to another and cause disease. Prevention of infection is one of the most important roles of nurses and other healthcare professionals. By being aware of each potential link in the chain, infection may be reduced or eliminated within the clinical setting.

Terms used in the chain of infection are given in Table 3.5.

For example: methicillin-resistant *Staphylococcus aureus* (MRSA) is an example of an organism. A reservoir might be a person who is either colonised or infected with MRSA. The portal of exit might be contaminated body fluids such as wound exudate from an infected wound. Mode of transmission might be hands or contaminated equipment. The portal of entry in this case would be by a wound that another person has. That person is the susceptible host. From this scenario we can see that handwashing could break this chain at more than one point.

For further information on the chain of infection, please see the further reading section at the end of this chapter.

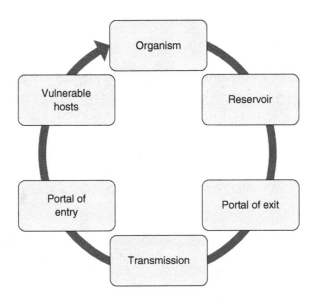

Figure 3.4   Chain of infection

Term	Description	Examples
Organism	The pathogenic microorganism	*E. coli, C. difficile,* MRSA (meticillin-resistant *Staphylococcus aureus*)
Reservoir	Source of the infection	A patient/health professional, animal, equipment, food, water
Portal of exit	How the microorganism leaves the body of the host	Faeces, urine, aerosols, droplets from respiratory tract (coughing/sneezing), vomit, blood, wound drainage
Transmission	How the microorganism is passed on	Direct contact, airborne
Portal of entry	How the microorganism enters the body	Break to the skin (wound), injection, needle-stick injury, scalpel, animal bite, catheter, mucous membranes
Vulnerable hosts	The person who becomes infected	Any susceptible person, elderly, pre-existing disease, immunocompromised

Table 3.5   Terms used in the chain of infection

In the next section we will look more closely at bacterial infection.

Bacterial infection

Scenario

You are the staff nurse on duty when George is admitted to the ward. He is a 72-year-old man who lives alone at home. He is confused and disorientated on admission and has a respiratory rate of 35 breaths per minute. He has a temperature of 38°C and has been expectorating ('coughing up') yellow sputum. He is diagnosed with probable community acquired pneumonia. Sputum samples are taken and empirical antibiotic treatment with amoxicillin is started.

In this scenario, George's symptoms and history have led to a diagnosis of community acquired pneumonia. A 'best-guess' approach is used to consider which microorganism may have caused the infection. Then an antibiotic is selected which is most likely to be effective. This is known as empirical antibiotic therapy. In clinical practice, it is not possible to wait for the results from the sputum sample to confirm the bacteria as this can take some time. However, a sputum sample has been sent for microbiology to confirm the causative bacteria. We will consider how microbiologists use the sputum sample to identify the bacteria.

Microbiologists have a range of tests they can use to identify which bacteria are causing the disease. They might prepare a sample of the sputum and look at this under the microscope to identify the bacteria. Many bacteria can, however, appear very similar. Special stains can help with the identification. A common stain which is used is the Gram stain. Bacteria are described as either Gram-positive or Gram-negative. Gram-positive bacteria take up the stain and appear purple under the microscope. Gram-negative organisms are not stained. In general, Gram-positive bacteria have a simpler cell wall structure than Gram-negative bacteria. This may mean that antibiotics are more able to penetrate and destroy Gram-positive bacteria. The shape and colour of the bacteria can also give vital clues. *Staphylococcus aureus*, for example, is round (coccus = round) and golden in colour (aureus = golden). The microbiologist may also identify the conditions the bacteria need in order to grow. Some grow well with no oxygen (called anaerobic bacteria) while others require oxygen (aerobic bacteria). Some are described as facultative anaerobes. This means that they prefer oxygen but can grow without it. Identifying the bacteria which are causing the disease is very important as different bacteria will be sensitive to different antibacterial drugs. Microbiologists can also test this directly by testing whether the bacteria grow in the presence of certain antibiotics.

The bacteria which could be causing George's community acquired pneumonia are shown in Table 3.6.

In George's case, the microbiology report identified *Streptococcus pneumoniae* and that the bacterium is sensitive to amoxicillin, confirming that the antibiotic choice was appropriate.

Bacterium	Gram staining	Oxygen needs	Shape
Streptococcus pneumoniae	G +ve	Anaerobic but tolerates oxygen	Cocci (round shape)
Haemophylis influenza	G –ve	Facultative anaerobe	Rod shaped
Staphylococcus aureus	G +ve	Facultative anaerobe	Cocci (round shape)
Klebsiella pneumoniae	G –ve	Facultative anaerobe	Rod shaped

Table 3.6   Properties of bacteria associated with community acquired pneumonia

G +ve: Gram-positive; G –ve: Gram-negative.

General signs and symptoms of microbial infection

In the scenario, we can see that George was exhibiting some signs of a bacterial lung infection, for example rapid respiration, cough, yellow sputum and a high temperature (pyrexia).

Many of the signs and symptoms of infection are due to the body's immune response to the infection. Pyrexia is caused when our temperature control centre, the hypothalamus in the midbrain, is reset to a higher than normal temperature, which in humans is 37°C. This occurs when chemicals called prostaglandins and pro-inflammatory cytokines are released from immune cells as part of the inflammatory response (Chapter 2). Metabolism is increased and tissue oxygen requirements increase resulting in increased respiratory rate. The advantages of pyrexia are unclear as it consumes energy at a time when a person is often eating little. It is thought that higher temperatures might stop some microorganisms multiplying as quickly. Higher temperatures may also stimulate the immune system and tissue repair. In most cases the pyrexia does not need treatment and the temperature will return to normal. Some microorganisms, however, may cause a rise in temperature above 41.5°C. This is considered a medical emergency. The pro-inflammatory cytokines which cause fever, also cause general malaise, weakness and loss of appetite associated with infection.

The course of an illness can be divided into different stages (Table 3.7) which help to explain the pattern of symptoms shown by a patient.

Invading microorganisms can cause tissue injury through a variety of mechanisms. For example, HIV causes the destruction of CD4-positive T lymphocytes during its active replication phase (Chapter 4). CD4-positive lymphocytes are vital for our immune system to work properly. HIV-infection may eventually lead to immunodeficiency.

Stage	Description
Incubation period	Pathogen begins to replicate but symptoms not noticeable.
Prodromal phase	Initial appearance of symptoms but these may be vague and non-specific, for example malaise, fatigue.
Acute stage	Maximum impact of infection. Symptoms are obvious and usually specific for sites of infection.
Convalescent period	Infection is contained and is progressively eliminated.
Resolution	Pathogen is eliminated from the body. No further symptoms.

Table 3.7 Stages of illness

Some microorganisms damage our cells by producing toxins. An example of this is *Vibrio cholera*, the bacterium which results in cholera. *V. cholera* infects the gut and releases a toxin causing severe watery diarrhoea. The toxin is classified as an exotoxin. This means a toxin that is released from the bacterial cells. By contrast, an endotoxin is part of the cell wall of Gram-negative bacteria. It is only released if the bacterial cell disintegrates. At low levels endotoxins are useful and activate our innate immune system. However, at high levels, the immune response to the endotoxin can lead to sepsis (see below, under 'sepsis'). Many microorganisms cause damage indirectly by activating the body's immune system. The immune system responds by killing infected cells. For example, the immune response to hepatitis B virus results in destruction of liver cells through a type IV hypersensitivity response (Chapter 4). The long-term complication of hepatitis B infection can be cirrhosis of the liver or liver cancer.

Pharmacological management of infections

Antimicrobial drugs

An antimicrobial is a substance which kills or inhibits the growth of microorganisms. The British National Formulary (BNF) groups these according to which type of microorganism is killed and lists: antibacterials, antifungals, antivirals and antiprotozoal drugs. In general, antibimicrobials work by exploiting differences between human cells and those of the microorganism. If the antimicrobial was not selective in this way it would kill human cells as well as killing the microorganism.

Antibacterial drugs

Antibacterial drugs are used to combat infections caused by bacteria. They will not kill viruses. Antibacterial drugs are sometimes referred to as antibiotics. Antibacterial drugs can be classified in different ways. A common way to group them is by chemical structure. Penicillins, for example, all have a similar chemical structure called a beta lactam ring. Groups of antibiotics may share certain features including the way they work, side-effects and any contraindications they may have. They may also kill similar bacteria, although this is not always the case. Activity 3.2 will give you an overview of some of the important groups of antibiotics and the names of drugs that belong to each group.

Activity 3.2   Research

Using the table format below, list one or two drugs for each group of antibacterial drugs. Use the British National Formulary to help you. You should be able to access paper copies from the ward or library. An electronic version is also available for NHS staff.

Antibacterial group	Name of individual antibacterials
Example: Cephalosporin	Example: Cefaclor, Cefalexin
Penicillins	
Macrolides	
Quinolones	
Tetracyclines	

Suggested answers are found at the end of the chapter.

Now that you are more familiar with the different antibacterial groups, we will look more closely at how these drugs act to treat infections.

Some antibacterial drugs kill bacteria. These are known as **bactericidal** antibiotics. Examples include penicillins and aminoglycosides. Other antibacterial drugs do not kill the bacteria outright but prevent bacteria replicating. These are known as **bacteriostatic** antibiotics. Examples include tetracyclines. The bacteriostatic action helps the body's immune system kill the bacteria.

Narrow spectrum antibiotic drugs kill only very specific bacteria. By contrast, **broad spectrum** antibiotics kill a wide variety of bacteria. Examples of broad spectrum antibiotics include erythromycin, ciprofloxacin and doxycycline. A broad spectrum antibiotic is useful when the cause of infection is unknown. Unfortunately, they tend also to kill bacteria comprising the gut microbiome. The possible consequences of this are illustrated in the scenario below.

Clostridium difficile is a Gram-positive bacterium. It can persist in the environment for a long time as it produces tough spores which are resistant to alcohol based cleaning agents. It is found in the gastrointestinal tract of about 5% of the population where it usually causes minimal harm. However, in Edward's case in the scenario below, treatment with the broad spectrum antibiotic ciprofloxacin disrupted his normal gastrointestinal bacteria (microbiome). As a result, *C. difficile* was able to grow without competition from other bacteria. *C. difficile* can lead to **pseudomembranous colitis** as it produces toxins which inflame the bowel. Although still a problem in hospitals, infection control procedures and more careful use of antibiotics have reduced the incidence of *C. difficile* infections.

Mechanism of action of antibacterial drugs

Antibacterial drugs work in different ways and we can divide them up according to their mechanism of action.

1. **Antibacterials that disrupt cell wall synthesis:** Examples of antibacterial drugs that disrupt cell wall synthesis are penicillins, cephalosporins, carbapenems and monobactams. The bacterial cell wall is made of a substance called peptidoglycan which forms a protective mesh. The antibacterial drugs interfere with the synthesis of peptidoglycans and, as a result, the cell wall is weakened. In the absence of a rigid cell wall, water enters the bacterial cell by osmosis, causing it to swell, burst and die.

2. **Antibiotics that affect bacterial protein synthesis:** Antibacterial drugs that affect bacterial protein synthesis are tetracyclines, chloramphenicol, macrolides and aminoglycosides. Bacterial proteins are manufactured within the bacterial cell using cellular 'machinery' called ribosomes (Figure 3.1). Antibacterial drugs that affect bacterial protein synthesis bind to the bacterial ribosomes and prevent bacteria from making proteins. This stops the bacteria growing or multiplying.

3. **Antibacterial drugs that inhibit bacterial DNA synthesis:** Antibacterial drugs that inhibit bacterial DNA synthesis include quinolones. DNA synthesis is vital for bacterial cell replication.

4. **Antibacterial drugs that affect folic acid synthesis:** Antibacterial drugs that affect folic acid synthesis include Trimethoprim. Bacteria need to manufacture their own folic acid to survive. Some antibacterial drugs interfere with this folic acid synthesis and kill bacteria.

Side-effects and clinical implications of antibacterial drugs

Many antibacterial drugs cause gastrointestinal upset as a side-effect leading to symptoms of nausea, vomiting and diarrhoea. This is often because the antibacterial has damaged the natural gut bacteria (microbiome). This was seen in the scenario with Edward, above.

Drug allergies

Many people report that they are allergic to antibiotics. It is important to understand the symptoms that lead to this belief. Some people may have experienced feeling sick which would not be a true allergic reaction. Symptoms such as rashes, difficulty breathing, and swelling, are more indicative of allergy. If a person is truly allergic to an antibacterial it may make their infection much more difficult to treat. Penicillins are especially prone to causing allergies. If patients are allergic to one type of penicillin, for example amoxicillin, they are likely to be allergic to all of them, for example flucloxacillin and penicillin V. This is because they all have the same beta lactam ring which causes the allergy. They may also be allergic to cephalosporins but these can be used as alternatives if people are monitored. A patient with a penicillin allergy would have to be given an alternative from a different group. For example, patients allergic to penicillins are often offered the macrolide erythromycin instead.

Activity 3.3   Decision-making

A patient on your ward has a drug chart which states that they are allergic to penicillin. The following antibiotic is written up for the patient: Co-amoxiclav 500 mg three times a day. Would this be safe to give?

An outline answer is available at the end of the chapter.

Some antibacterial drugs are more toxic and cause more side-effects than others. Aminoglycosides, such as gentamicin for example, are toxic to the kidney and ear. The dose and blood levels need to be closely monitored to prevent toxicity. The full range of side-effects caused by antibiotics can be found in the BNF or the summary of product characteristics for each antibiotic.

Choosing antibiotics

Scenario

Josie is a 30-year-old woman who attends your nurse-led clinic appointment. She describes increasing urinary frequency over the last couple of days and a burning

(Continued)

(Continued)

sensation on passing urine. She has also felt tired and a bit flu-like since yesterday. She has no drug allergies and is on no other medication. You carry out a mid-stream urinalysis test. This tests positive for nitrite and leucocyte esterase. You suspect a lower urinary tract infection. Josie is prescribed a three-day supply of Trimethoprim tablets 200 mg twice a day.

In order to treat infection an antibiotic has to be chosen which is likely to kill the infective organism. As we can see from the scenario, a diagnosis has been made according to symptoms and the results of the urinalysis test. As the infection is mild, no attempt has been made to identify the microorganism causing the disease and a best-guess has been made as to what the likely microorganism is. You may remember that the same 'best-guess' occurred with Edward. Activity 3.4 should give you an insight into how empirical antibiotic therapy is chosen.

Activity 3.4   Critical thinking

Do you think that Trimethoprim, at this dose and for this length of time, was an appropriate choice of antibacterial therapy for this urinary tract infection? The BNF contains a summary of antibacterial therapy which you might find useful.

A suggested answer is given at the end of the chapter.

Although the BNF gives a useful quick reference guide it is important to be aware of where this information comes from and to be able to compare it to other sources of information. Public Health England have issued a guideline 'Management of infection guidance for primary care for consultation and local adaptation'. It can be accessed from Public Health England's website. A link is provided at the end of the chapter.

You may want to research the evidence for treatment of urinary tract infections and compare the guidance with that in the BNF. NICE also has guidance relating to many different types of infection. Local hospitals often have their own antibacterial policies which take into account local patterns of resistance. We will look at resistance later in the chapter.

Antifungals

Fungi are eukaryotic and therefore have more similarity to human cells than bacteria. Ensuring antifungals are selective (which means they kill only fungi and not human cells as well) can be a challenge as many of the targets used by antibacterial drugs do not exist in fungi. Penicillins, for example, would not kill fungi as fungi do not contain peptidoglycans in their cell walls. Luckily, although both human cells and fungi have cell membranes they are slightly different. Antifungal agents act by damaging the cell membrane of fungi. The two most commonly used groups of antifungals are 'Triazole' antifungals and 'Imidazole' antifungals. The name relates to their chemical structure. Some antifungals are available as oral or parenteral formulations but many are also used topically to treat localised infections, for example, clotrimazole cream for vaginal thrush.

Side-effects and implications for practice

Like antibacterial drugs, common side-effects include gastrointestinal disturbance. Many antifungal agents are toxic to the liver and should be used with care or avoided in patients with liver problems.

Antifungals often interact with other drugs. This is because they inhibit specific enzymes in the liver which are involved in the metabolism of other drugs (Chapter 1). So, for example, a patient on simvastatin should not be given ketoconazole at the same time because the levels of simvastatin could rise leading to toxic side-effects.

Antivirals

Viruses can be very difficult to kill as they are such simple structures and offer few targets for killing agents. Immunisation with a vaccine is often our best defence against viruses (Chapter 4). However there are some very useful antiviral agents. Aciclovir was one of the first effective antivirals to be developed. It is effective against herpes simplex, which causes cold sores and genital infections. It is also effective against varicella-zoster, which causes shingles and chickenpox. Aciclovir is actually a pro-drug (Chapter 1) and is activated by an enzyme in the virus. This is what makes the drug selective. The active form of aciclovir prevents DNA replication and inhibits this process for viral DNA more effectively than for human DNA. Viruses are therefore prevented from reproducing. Other useful antiviral agents include those used for the treatment of HIV but these are outside the scope of this book.

Antimicrobial resistance

Resistance is the ability of a microorganism to resist the effects of an antimicrobial drug. It is becoming a serious global health concern. In 2013 the Chief Medical Officer said that 'Antibiotic resistance poses a catastrophic threat' and went on to explain that if we do not act now we could be at risk of dying from ordinary infections we now think of as treatable. Some microorganisms are naturally resistant to some antimicrobials; this is known as innate resistance. We cannot kill a virus with an antibacterial agent such as penicillin, for example. Knowing which microorganism is causing the infection helps us choose the right antimicrobial and should mean this kind of resistance is not generally a problem. In other cases microorganisms evolve and become resistant to antimicrobials that previously treated the infection they caused. It is this second type of resistance which is the most troubling. Although resistance can occur to many antimicrobials, we will concentrate here on resistance to antibacterials, the drugs that treat bacterial infections, as this is causing the greatest concern. The more that antibacterials are used, the more likely resistant organisms are to emerge. The resistant organisms go on to infect other people and may become widespread in the population.

Scenario

You are a nurse working on a surgical ward. Your patient, Nisa, is going for hip replacement surgery. She had a screen for meticillin resistant *Staphylococcus aureus* (MRSA) earlier and was found to be positive for this bacterium. As a result, you have been asked to ensure that she receives mupirocin nasal ointment and chlorhexidine body wash and shampoo. This will help to reduce the amounts of MRSA present and thereby reduce the risk of infection by MRSA during surgery. If Nisa was infected during surgery, the treatment would be much more complicated than for non-resistant strains of *Staphylococcus aureus*. This is because MRSA is resistant to the antibacterial agent flucloxacillin. This antibacterial would therefore not cure the infection. More toxic antibacterials such as vancomycin might be needed instead.

Mechanisms of resistance

Bacteria reproduce by binary fission – that is, dividing into two. This is an example of asexual reproduction which, in biology, means without the mixing of genes. One parent therefore gives rise to two identical daughter cells. However, in order to survive in a world with a changing environment, which may include one with the new challenge of antibacterial therapy, bacteria need to mutate, which means they need to change genetically. Spontaneous mutations may occur in a bacteria's genetic make-up as it reproduces. *E. coli*, for example, can replicate itself every 20 minutes. This means that in 7 hours one bacterium can generate over two million bacteria. If a mutation means the bacteria is more able to survive the antibacterial than other bacteria this will quickly be passed on. However, in reality, if an appropriate antibacterial is taken properly the body's immune system will usually mop these resistant bacteria up. The most important way that resistance is passed on is when bacteria pass genes to each other via a process called conjugation (see Figure 3.5). Bacteria have one main chromosome but also contain separate pieces of DNA called plasmids. These plasmids often contain genes for antibacterial resistance. Two bacteria join together using sex pili and pass plasmids from one bacterium to another. The genes that are passed on in the plasmid now enable the bacteria to counteract the antibacterial. Bacterial conjugation enables bacterial antibacterial resistance to spread very rapidly through bacterial populations. The mechanisms bacteria use to counteract antibacterials are outlined below:

- Bacteria may produce enzymes that inactivate the antibacterial.
- Bacteria may actively remove the antibacterial from themselves.
- Bacteria may alter the binding site that the antibacterial usually adheres to so that it no longer 'sticks'.
- Bacteria may begin using different metabolic pathways to those that are being inhibited by the antibacterial.

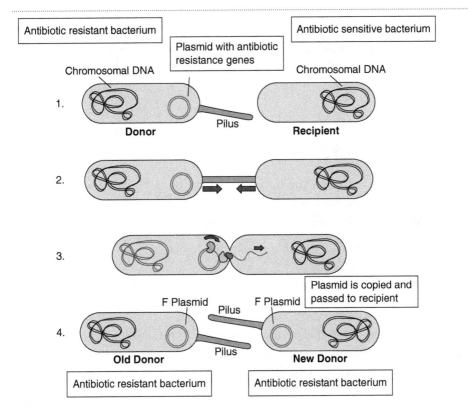

Antibiotic resistance genes are often carried on circular pieces of DNA called plasmids. A donor bacterial cell joins with a recipient bacterial cell through the pilus. The plasmid is copied and passed on to the recipient cell. Both the donor and recipient cell now have a copy of the plasmid. This process can continue with other bacterial cells and antibiotic resistance genes can be passed on very rapidly through the bacterial population.

Figure 3.5 Conjugation

Overcoming antibacterial resistance

Resistance is a global issue and needs to be tackled with different approaches. New antimicrobial agents need to be developed which microorganisms are not yet resistant to. However, there has been a decline in the development of new antimicrobials as they are expensive to research and are held in reserve for serious infections which means relatively little money is spent buying them. Countries also need to tighten control of antibacterial supplies so they are not used for inappropriate infections. Healthcare professionals also have a role to play. The more that antimicrobials are used the faster resistance develops. If infection prevention and control is improved, the need for antimicrobials in the healthcare setting can be reduced. Correct use of antimicrobials is also important. Advice from experts such as microbiologists is important for choosing the correct drug. Narrow spectrum antibacterials are preferable to broad spectrum which was illustrated by the *Clostridium difficile* case study. Patient education is important. Patients should be encouraged not to seek antibacterials for viral infections. It has been shown that people are satisfied to receive reassurance and accurate explanations about their condition compared to antibacterials they do not need (Britten, 1995). The TARGET antibacterials toolkit produced by the Royal College of General Practitioners and others has some useful resources and leaflets for patients. The website can be found at the end of the chapter.

Activity 3.5   Reflection

List interventions that you have carried out or observed others carrying out which help to prevent the spread of antimicrobial resistance. For each think about how this helps to combat resistance.

A suggested answer is given at the end of the chapter.

Having reviewed the general signs and symptoms of infection and the pharmacological management of infections, we turn to examine sepsis which is one of the most important concerns in healthcare today (NICE, 2016).

Sepsis

Sepsis is defined as 'life-threatening organ dysfunction caused by a dysregulated host response to infection' (Singer et al., 2016). This rather technical definition tells us that sepsis is a life-threatening response to infection. Sepsis is estimated to affect 31.5 million people worldwide every year and cause an estimated 5.3 million deaths each year.

Our understanding of sepsis has changed over the years, and its definition has been updated a number of times. The current definition is The Third International Consensus Definitions for Sepsis and Septic Shock (Sepsis-3; Singer et al., 2016). As sepsis is such an important concern in healthcare today, it is worth examining this definition. How sepsis is understood in the healthcare setting affects its recognition and prompt treatment. The box below examines the Sepsis-3 definition.

Sepsis-3

Our understanding of sepsis has evolved over the years. The 1991 and 2001 consensus definitions were based upon the 'systemic inflammatory response syndrome' (Balk, 2014). The systemic inflammatory response syndrome (SIRS) is a widespread (systemic) inflammatory response that can follow a diverse group of injuries. The injuries include not only infection, but trauma, burns, and pancreatitis and other injuries. Within the SIRS framework, sepsis was defined as 'SIRS with documented or suspected infection'. There were two further categories within a sepsis continuum: severe sepsis and septic shock – of increasing severity.

The Sepsis-3 definition was developed to reflect advances in our understanding of the pathogenesis of sepsis (Singer et al., 2016). In particular, the Sepsis-3 definition focuses on the central role of infection in sepsis. Singer et al. (2016) argue that this is an important development of the previous central focus on the systemic inflammatory response, SIRS. The stronger emphasis on infection, it is argued, helps focus treatment on prompt antimicrobial therapy (see below under 'Treatment of sepsis'). Sepsis is clearly more complex than the original 'systemic inflammatory response with infection' suggests. There is often an anti-inflammatory response, especially in the late stages of sepsis that can make patients susceptible to further infection. There are metabolic dysfunctions which affect cellular respiration and cell function. These advances in the understanding of sepsis pathogenesis have important implications for sepsis management and the development of new treatments.

The Sepsis-3 definition has produced different criteria for recognition of sepsis than the older SIRS criteria. There is ongoing debate about the most appropriate criteria for recognition of sepsis in clinical practice. For example, the British Medical Journal Best Practice: Sepsis in Adults (2018) notes that 'these changes have prompted much debate and the 1991 definitions remain in widespread clinical use while the controversies are resolved'.

Having examined the Sespis-3 definition of sepsis in the box above, we will now look at the most common causes of sepsis, the risk factors for sepsis and the pathophysiology of sepsis.

The most common causative agents of sepsis are bacteria – either Gram-negative or Gram-positive. Fungal infections can also cause sepsis. However, the causative agent of sepsis is only isolated and identified in around half of all cases. Of those cases in which the agent has been identified, common agents are Gram-positive *Staphylococcus aureus*, Gram-negative *Escherichia coli* and *Pseudomonas* spp. Common fungal agents include *Candida* spp. and *Aspergillus* spp. In the UK, sepsis is the most common direct cause of maternal death. In the 6-week postnatal period, group A *Streptococci* are the most common causative agent. Many causes of sepsis in the community setting are likely to be from the patient's microbiome and are described as **endogenous** (or 'from within').

NICE (2016d) provides guidelines for early recognition, diagnosis and treatment of sepsis. The guidelines state: 'Think "could this be sepsis?" if a person presents with signs or symptoms that indicate possible infection'. Assessment includes a person's risk of infection, and in a face-to-face assessment includes assessing temperature, heart rate, respiratory rate, blood pressure, level of consciousness and oxygen saturation. The details of risk stratification tools can be found within NICE (2016d).

Knowledge of risk factors for sepsis are pivotal in early recognition (NICE, 2016d). Table 3.8 lists some of the main risk factors for sepsis.

Risk factor
Underlying malignancy
Age > 65 years
Haemodialysis
Alcoholism
Diabetes mellitus
Recent surgery or other invasive procedures
Breached skin integrity
Indwelling lines or catheters
Intravenous drug use
Pregnancy or recent pregnancy

Table 3.8   Key risk factors for sepsis

As can be seen from Table 3.8, many risk factors involve a pre-existing medical condition, such as a malignancy, alcoholism or diabetes. These may be associated with a weakened immune system and a greater susceptibility to infection. Other risk factors include breached skin integrity and indwelling lines or catheters. These again increase the risk of infection.

The common sites of infection in sepsis include the respiratory tract, the bloodstream, the abdomen, the skin and urinary tract. However, infection at any site in the body can potentially lead to sepsis. To help with the recognition and management of sepsis, an understanding of the pathophysiology of sepsis is essential. We turn to describing this below, building from the Sepsis-3 consensus definition.

Pathophysiology of sepsis

Sepsis-3 defines sepsis as a dysregulated host response to infection which can lead to life-threatening organ dysfunction. 'Dysregulation' refers to impairment of normal regulatory responses. In sepsis, the dysregulated host response to infection has components which will be explained shortly. These responses are often described as the 'sepsis cascade' and can occur very rapidly in some patients, in some cases over a period of hours. Multi-organ failure can result and possible death.

Figure 3.6 shows the main components of the 'dysregulated host response' to infection that are found in sepsis. Many of these responses have been described in Chapter 2 within the sections on acute inflammation. In an acute inflammatory response, the responses were noted as being localised, well-regulated and offering a protective effect. By following the description below, you will see the contrast between a well-located and well-regulated response and the 'dysregulated' response which constitutes part of the host response in sepsis. This, in turn, can cause widespread life-threatening organ dysfunction.

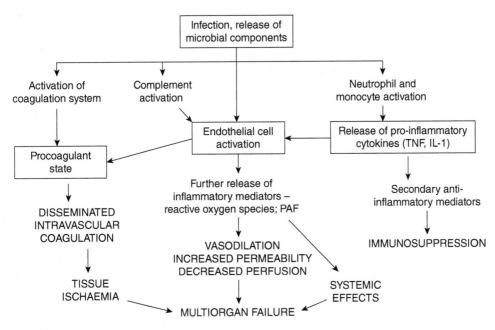

Figure 3.6   Pathophysiology of sepsis. PAF, platelet activating factor; TNF, tumour necrosis factor; IL-1, interleukin-1. Adapted from Mitchell et al., 2016.

An infection and/or the presence of microbial products from disrupted bacterial cells causes a widespread host response. Part of this host response includes activation of:

- innate immune cells – especially white blood cells called neutrophils and monocytes;
- the complement system (a set of plasma proteins which help fight infection);
- the coagulation system (another set of plasma proteins which lead to blood clotting);
- the endothelial cells (these cells make up the 'endothelium' or inner lining of the blood vessels).

These responses result in the widespread release of 'pro-inflammatory cytokines' and other mediators of inflammation (Chapter 2). Pro-inflammatory mediators and complement components cause further endothelial activation and further activation of immune cells. The activated immune cells and the endothelium continue to produce mediators of inflammation. These include IL-6, IL-8, nitric oxide, platelet activating factor, and reactive oxygen species. There is a counter-balancing production of anti-inflammatory mediators, which paradoxically, may lead to immunosuppression.

The activation of the endothelium is key to understanding the progression to low blood pressure (hypotension) and organ failure in sepsis. Activation of the endothelium results in widespread vasodilation, and an increased permeability of blood vessel walls. Increased vascular permeability causes excessive fluid loss from the vascular compartment (from the circulation) and a reduced blood volume. Vasodilation and reduced blood volume together reduce blood pressure (hypotension) and may lead to reduced tissue perfusion, potentially leading to organ failure.

Activation of the endothelium also activates the coagulation system in the blood. A 'procoagulant state' may be reached in which microthrombi (small 'blood clots') form in small blood vessels. This is known as disseminated intravascular coagulation (DIC) and can lead to tissue ischaemia.

The inflammatory mediators also cause systemic effects including fever. There is evidence that mediators and reactive oxygen species directly affect cell metabolism. This includes a reduction in contractility of the myocardial cells of the heart. Sepsis is also characterised by insulin resistance and hyperglycaemia. This has been attributed to the production of stress hormones glucagon, adrenaline and cortisol.

Multi-organ failure may result. This is due to the multiple impacts of hypotension, oedema, and disseminated intravascular coagulation. There are direct metabolic effects from inflammatory mediators and cytokines, leading to anaerobic metabolism and cell dysfunction. In many cases the lungs are the first organs affected. This manifests as acute respiratory distress syndrome and acute lung injury. There is often cardiovascular instability and deteriorating renal function. Acute kidney injury can result (Chapter 14).

The magnitude of a patient's response and hence the outcome and severity of sepsis depends upon a range of factors: the virulence of the infecting microorganism, the host's immune status and other co-morbidities (Mitchell et al., 2016). The nature and level of mediators and cytokines released has a significant effect.

Treatment of sepsis

As we have seen sepsis is a complicated condition. Early recognition and treatment is vital for the patient. Treatment guidelines suggest that a range of interventions are needed to stop a patient deteriorating. One bundle of therapies is known as the 'sepsis six bundle'. This has been shown to improve patient outcomes (Daniels et al., 2011). These interventions are:

1. **Administer oxygen:** Oxygen should be given to all patients with sepsis. In sepsis oxygen saturation of the tissues falls. This is because blood pressure is reduced leading to hypoperfusion of tissues. In addition, leaky capillaries lead to oedema which means oxygen must diffuse further to reach tissues. Small blood clots can occur in the capillaries which reduces oxygen delivery.

2. **Take blood cultures:** This should be done before antibiotic therapy is started where possible. Blood cultures help to identify the causative pathogen and antibiotics can be adjusted accordingly.

3. **Give IV antibiotics:** Sepsis is usually triggered by a bacterial infection and it is important that the infection is treated as soon as possible. Intravenous antibacterial drugs should be given within one hour of a sepsis diagnosis (NICE, 2016d). At the beginning it may not be clear which bacteria is causing the infection. Broad-spectrum antibacterial drugs are therefore often prescribed as they kill a wide variety of bacteria. The exact antibacterial prescribed will vary depending on local resistance patterns and the likely causative pathogen. It is also important that any potential sources of infection, such as urinary catheters, are removed.

4. **Give intravenous (IV) fluids:** During sepsis a patient's blood pressure may fall leading to reduced tissue perfusion. Intravenous fluid replacement such as Hartmann's solution would be given. Fluid replacement increases the circulating volume and restores blood pressure.

5. **Check serial lactate levels:** High lactate levels indicate anaerobic metabolism due to reduced tissue perfusion; this means the patient is in shock. Monitoring lactate helps to show how effective oxygen therapy and IV fluids are.

6. **Monitor hourly urine output:** Urine output falls when renal perfusion is reduced. This is a useful way of monitoring cardiac output which again helps to monitor response to treatment.

It is now time to review what you have learned within this chapter by undertaking some multiple choice questions.

Activity 3.6   Multiple choice questions

1. What is the definition of a commensal microorganism?
   a) A microorganism that causes disease
   b) A microorganism that is transmitted from animal to human
   c) A microorganism that usually lives harmlessly on our bodies
   d) A microorganism that needs other microorganisms to survive

(Continued)

(Continued)

2. For each of the following state whether the answer is TRUE or FALSE.

   a) *Candida albicans* is a bacterium
   b) Hepatitis B is a virus
   c) *Toxoplasma gondii* is a protozoan
   d) *Escherichia coli* is a fungus

3. Bacteria are prokaryotic cells and differ from human, eukaryotic cells because:

   a) They have no nucleus
   b) They have no DNA
   c) They have no cell wall
   d) They have no ribosomes

4. Symptoms of infection can be caused by

   a) Our immune system
   b) Toxins produced by microorganisms
   c) The death of invaded human cells
   d) All of the above

5. Which of the following statements about *Clostridium difficile* is TRUE?

   a) It is a type of virus which infects the gastrointestinal tract
   b) It is one of the leading causes of pneumonia
   c) It can occur after the use of broad spectrum antibiotics
   d) It is spread by droplets which are inhaled by patients

6. If a patient is allergic to penicillin which of the following antimicrobial drugs can they take? Answer TRUE or FALSE for each drug.

   a) Flucloxacillin
   b) Trimethoprim
   c) Co-amoxiclav
   d) Fluconazole

7. Which of the following is NOT an example of how an antibacterial agent works?

   a) Inhibition of cell wall synthesis
   b) Inhibition of mitochondrial respiration
   c) Disruption of protein synthesis
   d) Inhibition of DNA synthesis

8. For each of the following statements about antimicrobials state whether the answer is TRUE or FALSE.

   a) Aciclovir is an antiviral agent
   b) Clotrimazole is an antibacterial agent

c) Oxytetracycline is an antifungal agent

d) Metronidazole is an antibacterial agent

9. As part of a strategy to combat antibiotic resistance, patients may be given a leaflet explaining why they are not being given an antibiotic and explaining how long symptoms of their illness might last. A cough usually lasts:

a) 4 days

b) 7 days

c) 14 days

d) 21 days

10. Which of the following are useful strategies for preventing antibiotic resistance? Mark each answer as TRUE or FALSE.

a) Using broad spectrum antibiotics where possible

b) Preventing infections by good hygiene

c) Ensuring doses of antibiotics are not missed

d) Ensuring courses of antibiotics continue for at least two weeks

Chapter summary

There are many different types of microorganisms but many live harmlessly in the environment and on our body. Microorganisms include bacteria, viruses, protozoa and fungi. However sometimes microorganisms are pathogenic and cause diseases. The body has many defences against disease, but infectious diseases can still be lethal. Different medicines have been developed to fight infections. These usually work by exploiting differences between human cells and the cells of the invading microorganism. Resistance to antimicrobial agents is an increasing problem. Microorganisms are constantly evolving different ways to survive the antimicrobials that we design to kill them. If we do not use the antibacterials we have very carefully and invent new ones, then we could one day be faced with dying from simple infections. Understanding the importance of correct antibacterial choice and administration can help nurses prevent resistance spreading. The cycle of infection can be used to identify infection control measures nurses can undertake to prevent infections in the first place.

Sepsis is a life-threatening response to infection and is an important concern in healthcare today. Early recognition and management of sepsis are essential. Sepsis results from complex poorly regulated host responses to infections. It can lead to septic shock, multi-organ failure and death.

Activities: Brief outline answers

Activity 3.1 Reflection (p60)

List five infectious diseases. For each disease write down whether it is caused by a virus, bacteria, fungi or protozoa. If you can, name the microorganism that causes the disease.

There are many examples you could have used – here are a few:

The common cold is caused by a virus. The name of the virus is *rhinovirus*.

Meningitis can be caused by bacteria, viruses or fungi. Bacteria causing meningitis include *Neisseria meningitidis* and *Streptococcus pneumoniae*. Viruses causing meningitis include enteroviruses and mumps virus. *Cryptococcus neoformans* is a fungus that can cause meningitis.

Activity 3.2 Research (p69)

For each of the groups of antibacterials list one or two medicines that belong to this group. Use the BNF to help you.

Antibacterial group	Name of individual antibacterials
Example: Cephalosporin	Cefaclor, cefalexin
Penicillins	Amoxicillin, flucloxacillin
Macrolides	Erythromycin, clarithromycin
Quinolones	Ciprofloxacin, moxifloxacin
Tetracyclines	Doxycycline, oxytetracycline

Activity 3.3 Decision-making (p71)

A patient on the ward has a drug chart which states they are allergic to penicillin. The following antibiotic is written up for the patient. Co-amoxiclav 500 mg three times a day. Would this be safe to give?

No. Co-amoxiclav consists of clavulanic acid and amoxicillin. Amoxicillin is a penicillin and could cause an allergic reaction in this patient.

Activity 3.4 Critical thinking (p72)

Trimethoprim is an appropriate choice. A three-day course may be enough for women with uncomplicated infections.

Activity 3.5 Reflection (p76)

List interventions that you have carried out or observed others carrying out which help to prevent the spread of antimicrobial resistance.

There are many examples you could give. These might include ensuring correct dose, route frequency, not missing doses, keeping to administration times for antibiotics on drug charts. These all help to kill microorganisms most effectively and prevent resistant organisms occurring. You may have seen pharmacists checking charts and querying doses, times, frequencies. You may have seen prescribers referring to guidelines, local policies or microbiologists. You may have had to ensure samples were sent to labs quickly to allow early identification of microorganisms. Washing your hands after seeing each patient prevents the spread of infections and hence the need for antimicrobials. Explaining to patients how to take their antimicrobials or educating them about what antibiotics can and cannot treat is also useful. Involvement in antimicrobial audits is another example.

Activity 3.6 Multiple choice questions (pp81–3)

1. What is the definition of a commensal microorganism?

   c) A microorganism that usually lives harmlessly on our bodies

2. For each of the following state whether the answer is TRUE or FALSE.

   a) *Candida albicans* is a bacterium   False

   b) Hepatitis B is a virus   True

   c) *Toxoplasma gondii* is a protozoan   True

   d) *Escherichia coli* is a fungus   False

3. Bacteria are prokaryotic cells and differ from human, eukaryotic cells because:

   a) They have no nucleus

4. Symptoms of infection can be caused by:

   d) All of the above

5. Which of the following statements about *Clostridium difficile* is TRUE?

   c) It can occur after the use of broad spectrum antibiotics

6. If a patient is allergic to penicillin which of the following antimicrobial drugs can they take? Answer TRUE or FALSE for each drug.

   a) Flucloxacillin   False

   b) Trimethoprim   True

   c) Co-amoxiclav   False

   d) Fluconazole   True

7. Which of the following is NOT an example of how an antibacterial agent works:

   b) Inhibition of mitochondrial respiration

8. For each of the following statements about antimicrobials state whether the answer is TRUE or FALSE.

   a) Aciclovir is an antiviral agent   True

   b) Clotrimazole is an antibacterial agent   False

   c) Oxytetracycline is an antifungal agent   False

   d) Metronidazole is an antibacterial agent   True

9. As part of a strategy to combat antibiotic resistance, patients may be given a leaflet explaining why they are not being given an antibiotic and explaining how long symptoms of their illness might last. A cough usually lasts:

   d) 21 days

10. Which of the following are useful strategies for preventing antibiotic resistance? Mark each answer as TRUE or FALSE.

   a) Using broad spectrum antibiotics where possible   False

   b) Preventing infections by good hygiene   True

   c) Ensuring doses of antibiotics are not missed   True

   d) Ensuring courses of antibiotics continue for at least two weeks   False

Further reading

Appelbaum, PC (2007) Microbiology of antibiotic resistance in *Staphylococcus aureus. Clinical Infectious Diseases,* 45 (Supplement 3): S165–70. Available at: **http://cid.oxfordjournals.org/content/45/Supplement_3/S165.full/**

Goering, R, Dockrell, H, Zuckerman, M, Roitt, I and Chiodini, P (2018) *Mims' Medical Microbiology* (6th edition). Oxford: Elsevier.

A very accessible textbook on medical microbiology.

Gotts, and Matthay, M (2016) Sepsis: pathophysiology and clinical management. *BMJ,* 353: i1585. Available at: **www.bmj.com/content/353/bmj.i1585/**

This is a comprehensive review of sepsis.

Health Protection Agency (2009) *MRSA Screening and Suppression: Quick Reference Guide for Consultation and Local Adaptation.* Available at: **www.gov.uk/government/uploads/system/uploads/attachment_data/file/330793/MRSA_screening_and_supression_primary_care_guidance.pdf/**

Public Health England (2013) *Primary Care Guidance: Diagnosing and Managing Infections.* Available at: **www.gov.uk/government/collections/primary-care-guidance-diagnosing-and-managing-/**

Public Health England (2017) Clostridium difficile: *Guidance, Data and Analysis.* Available at: **www.gov.uk/government/collections/clostridium-difficile-guidance-data-and-analysis/**

Royal College of General Practitioners, Public Health England and The Antimicrobial Stewardship in Primary Care. TARGET antibiotic toolkit. Available at: **www.rcgp.org.uk/TARGETantibiotics/**

Useful websites

For further information on drugs, their uses, side-effects and patient information leaflets:

www.medicines.org.uk/

Summary of product characteristics.

www.earthlife.net/prokaryotes/welcome.html

Website for more information on microorganisms.

https://sepsistrust.org/professional-resources/education-resources/

Educational resources from the UK Sepsis Trust.

Chapter 4 The adaptive immune response

Chapter aims

After reading this chapter you will be able to:

- identify the key components and targets of the adaptive immune response;
- explain how antigens are recognised by B and T lymphocytes to stimulate an immune response;
- explain the functions of B and T lymphocytes in fighting infections;
- outline the nature and functions of monoclonal antibody therapy;
- explain the role of hypersensitivity reactions with special reference to type 1 hypersensitivity and autoimmune diseases;
- explain how immunodeficiency can arise and outline infection with the human immunodeficiency virus.

Introduction

The human body is constantly engaged in a bitter internal war against vast armies of microscopic enemies . . . Thankfully for us, we are equipped with an internal defence mechanism designed to combat these threats . . . [whose] purpose is remarkably simple: to recognize, disable and dispose of all intruders – and then to remember them, in case they return at a later date.

(The Immune System: In Defence of Our Lives.
Nobelprize.org. Nobel Media AB, 2014)

The quote above provides a vivid image of an army fighting a dangerous enemy. This is a common image of the immune system. It serves to remind us of the vital importance of the immune system and its remarkable ability to distinguish invading 'enemies' from healthy body cells. Without an immune system we would soon die of infection or cancer. There are occasions, however, when the immune system 'over-reacts' and ends up causing damage to our own cells and tissues. The protective and potentially harmful effects of the immune system are the subject of this chapter.

This chapter follows on from Chapter 2 where we examined the inflammatory response and Chapter 3 which looked at infection. The inflammatory response forms part of the **innate immune response**. The innate immune response forms part of the first line of defence against invading microorganisms. While many potentially harmful infections will be eliminated by the innate immune response, some infections take longer to control and eradicate. In these cases, a second line of defence is needed. This second line of defence is called the adaptive immune response. The adaptive immune response is the subject of this chapter.

In this chapter we start by examining the components of the adaptive immune system and describe how they work together to provide effective defence against infection. We then look at ways in which an inappropriate or 'hypersensitive' adaptive immune response causes harm. This is followed by examining **immunodeficiency** which occurs when the immune system is not strong enough to fight infections. We illustrate this with a section on HIV (human immunodeficiency virus) infection. In the last section, we look at how molecules called monoclonal antibodies are being used to provide effective treatments for cancer and autoimmune diseases.

The innate and adaptive immune responses

As noted above, the innate immune system forms part of the first line of defence against infection. This first line of defence also includes barriers to infection such as the skin and mucous membranes. Mucous membranes, or mucosa, line the open body cavities which include the respiratory and gastrointestinal tracts. These tracts are, in effect, open (or connected) to the outside world. Due to being connected to the outside mucosa are a major target of infection by microorganisms (Chapter 3).

The innate immune system includes the phagocytic cells we introduced in Chapter 2. These include macrophages and neutrophils. Macrophages are strategically located around the body especially at mucosal surfaces in order to engulf and destroy invading pathogens. An initial infection will activate the acute inflammatory response (Chapter 2). The inflammatory response is a carefully co-ordinated part of the innate immune response.

Innate means 'born with'. With respect to the immune system, innate refers to that part of the immune system that remains essentially the same throughout our lifetime. Despite the huge variety of microorganisms we are exposed to during our lifetime, the innate response is more or less the same against each microbe; it does not change or adapt in anyway. For these reasons, the innate immune response is also called the non-adaptive or non-specific immune response.

If the innate immune response fails to clear an infection, within about four days the adaptive immune response will come into action and provides a second line of defence.

The adaptive response is carried out by a type of white blood cell called lymphocytes. The adaptive immune response is more specific than the innate response and should be able to clear the infection. The adaptive response develops over our lifetime with each new infection. It is known as the acquired or specific immune response.

Cells of the immune system

There is a wide-range of immune cells which make up the cellular components of the immune responses. White blood cells (leukocytes) are key immune cells (Figure 4.1). Other immune cells include macrophages, mast cells and dendritic cells. All immune cells are made in the bone marrow from stem cells called **hematopoietic stem cells** (Janeway and Murphy, 2012). A stem cell is a cell that continues to divide throughout our lifetime. Two daughter cells result from cell division; one of these remains as a stem cell capable of further cell division. The second daughter cell develops into a mature, differentiated cell. In the case of the hematopoietic stem cell, the mature cell will be one of the blood cells (a white blood cell, a red blood cell or a platelet).

Once mature, immune cells leave the bone marrow and circulate in the blood. Some immune cells then leave the blood and enter the tissues (for example, macrophages). Lymphocytes circulate in the blood and in the lymphatic system, and some (B cells) return to the bone marrow when 'activated'.

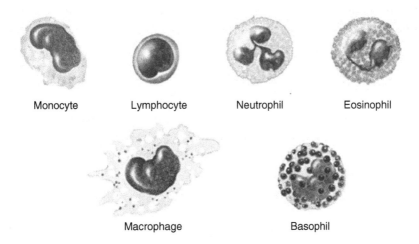

| Monocyte | Lymphocyte | Neutrophil | Eosinophil |

| Macrophage | Basophil |

Figure 4.1   White blood cells and a macrophage

The list below gives the main types of immune cells:

Macrophages are a mature form of monocytes that have migrated into the tissues. Macrophages are present in almost all tissues of the body. Macrophages play a role in both the innate and adaptive immune responses. They are phagocytic and secrete cytokines which trigger inflammation and activate other immune cells. Macrophages also clear dead cells and cell debris in their role in healing damaged tissues.

However, macrophages produce much of the tissue damage occurring in chronic inflammation.

Monocytes are a minor component of the white blood cell count. Monocytes quickly enter the tissues of the body where they develop into macrophages.

Neutrophils are a major component of the white blood cell count. Their role is in innate immunity where they play a key role in acute inflammation. Neutrophils are recruited from the blood to the site of infection and are phagocytic.

Basophils and eosinophils defend against parasitic worms and ticks which are too large to be engulfed by neutrophils or macrophages. They are involved in allergy. They form only a minor component of the white blood cell count.

Mast cells are found in many tissues of the body, especially just beneath epithelial surfaces of the skin and mucosa. Like basophils and eosinophils, mast cells have a role in immunity against parasites. They contain granules of histamine. Mast cells are involved in acute inflammation and allergy.

Lymphocytes are responsible for the adaptive immune response. There are two main types of lymphocytes: B and T cells. There is also a lymphocyte called natural killer cells (NK cells) which responds to virally infected cells and tumour cells. Lymphocytes originate in the bone marrow. B lymphocytes mature in the bone marrow and on reaching maturity are released into the blood. T lymphocytes mature in the thymus gland during childhood and are then released into the blood. These cells are mature but naïve. This means that they have yet to encounter antigens. Antigens are molecules, usually fragments of invading microorganisms, which B and T cells recognise and respond to as part of the adaptive immune response.

All mature lymphocytes circulate in both the blood and the lymphatic system. Lymphocytes are present in high numbers in lymph nodes and lymphatic tissues where they are exposed to foreign molecules and are activated.

Dendritic cells are present in the tissues and lymph nodes. Dendritic cells 'display' or 'present' fragments of the microorganisms on their surface. This display helps to activate T cells. As noted above, fragments of a microorganism are antigens, and for this reason dendritic cells are called antigen-presenting cells.

Langerhans cells are specialised antigen-presenting cells found in the skin.

The role of these immune cells will be described more fully in the various sections of this chapter.

In addition to the cells of the immune system, it is important to be aware of a very important family of signalling molecules associated with the immune response – the cytokines. We introduced pro-inflammatory cytokines in Chapter 2 (The inflammatory response) where they helped mediate both the local and systemic effects of inflammation. In Chapter 3 (Infection) we noted that both pro-inflammatory and anti-inflammatory cytokines had a pivotal role in the pathophysiology of sepsis. Cytokines are small protein molecules released by a variety of cells, especially immune cells. They act as signalling molecules in cell-to-cell communication and help regulate the cellular responses to inflammation and the immune response. Examples of cytokines include: the interleukins, interferons, and tumour necrosis factor. They generally act locally to affect the cells near them but can act on more distant parts of the body.

The lymphatic system

The lymphatic system plays a key role in the adaptive immune system. The lymphatic system is a network of lymph nodes, lymphatic organs and lymphatic vessels. It works alongside the circulatory system to regulate the circulation of body fluids. The lymphatic vessels carry lymph, a clear fluid derived from the blood plasma. Tissue (**interstitial**) fluid is formed as water and soluble components of the plasma are squeezed out of capillaries. The lymphatic capillaries drain tissue fluid from the tissues and eventually return it to the blood circulation. Cell debris and microorganisms will also be drained into the lymphatic vessels and taken to local lymph nodes (Figure 2.3; Chapter 2). The lymph nodes are where the adaptive immune response is stimulated.

Antigens: the targets of the adaptive immune system

An antigen is a molecule which can bind specifically to an antibody. The name comes from '**anti**body **gen**erator' – a substance that will generate antibodies. More broadly the term antigen refers to a molecule that will be recognised by the adaptive immune system.

We will look at three types of antigen:

- foreign antigens
- tumour antigens
- self-antigens.

Figure 4.2 shows a virus particle and a bacterium with antigens exposed on their surface. Most antigens are proteins. Surface proteins of microorganisms are key antigens targeted by the adaptive immune response. These are examples of foreign antigens, which are antigens that come from outside our body. In reality, bacteria, viruses and other pathogens will have many different antigens on their surface, not just the single type shown in Figure 4.2. Foreign antigens can also come from internal fragments of digested microorganisms.

Figure 4.2 also shows a tumour cell with tumour antigens on its surface. Tumour antigens are proteins on tumour cells which stimulate an immune response. Some tumour antigens have been developed for diagnostic tests to identify tumour cells (Chapter 5). Tumour antigens are also under intense research as targets for cancer therapy and can be used to monitor the response to cancer treatment.

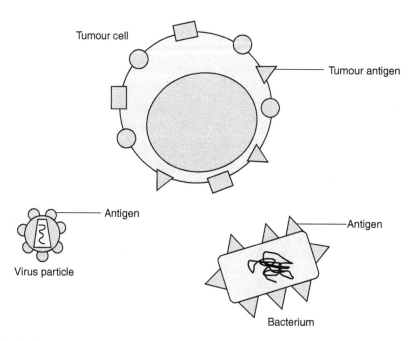

Figure 4.2 Antigens on the surface of a tumour cell, virus particle and bacterium

We do not normally mount an immune response against our own cells. Our cells are covered in many antigens which are capable of stimulating an immune response. This can be seen in blood transfusion and organ donations in which the antigens on the donor cells must match those of the recipient's cells. If the antigens do not match sufficiently an immune response will occur leading to organ rejection or a transfusion reaction.

Our own immune systems are tolerant to our own antigens. The antigens which coat our own cells are called self-antigens. Breakdown in this tolerance creates an auto-immune response and an autoimmune disease. Tolerance is partly brought about by the destruction of T cells that can recognise self-antigens. Those T cells that can recognise self-antigens are called autoreactive. During their development in the thymus autoreactive T cells are destroyed. There is, in addition, a means of making auto-reactive B cells inactive and unable to mount an immune response against self-antigens. This is believed to occur by special regulatory T cells which act to 'silence' or suppress autoreactive B cells and any autoreactive T cells that escaped being destroyed in the thymus. Autoimmune reactions occur when this tolerance is some-how broken. The breakdown of tolerance occurs in autoimmune disorders and the immune system begins to attack self-antigens. Towards the end of this chapter (under 'Autoimmune diseases') we describe autoimmune diseases further and give a scenario of Sheila who has rheumatoid arthritis.

Activity 4.1   Evidence-based practice and research

Estimates indicate that 30–35% of the population will suffer from an allergic reaction during their lifetime. This makes allergy a common complaint. Allergy involves an immune response to an allergen.

Allergens are a type of antigen that triggers an allergic reaction. Allergens are normally harmless environmental substances. In those who are allergic, allergens can trigger a number of harmful allergic reactions. Depending on which part of the body is affected, symptoms of allergy can range from a runny nose, sneezing, itchy red eyes, nausea, vomiting, diarrhoea, asthma and anaphylaxis. We look more closely at this under 'Hypersensitivity', below.

Find out what the most common allergens are. You can do this by simply surveying the people you know, or by looking on the internet. Distinguish allergy from what is known as *intolerance*, e.g. lactose intolerance.

A suggested answer is given at the end of the chapter.

Allergens, examined in Activity 4.1 above, and antigens in general trigger the adaptive immune response. In the next section we look more closely at the distinctive properties of the adaptive immune response.

Properties of the adaptive immune response

The adaptive immune response has three unique properties:

* antigen specificity
* diversity
* memory.

We will explain these properties using the B cell which produces antibodies. The principles apply to the T cells as well.

Each B cell recognises an antigen through a special receptor on its surface (Figure 4.3A). Each B cell has a slightly different shaped receptor on its surface and will recognise a different antigen. The recognition works because the antigen has a complementary shape to the receptor. Each B cell is said to be specific for one antigen.

It is estimated that there are 20,000 different B and T cells in the blood. In other words, there is a huge diversity of B or T cells. This diversity is so great that it is estimated that we have sufficient B cells to recognise all the possible microorganisms that might ever infect us. On infection, antigens from any given microorganism will activate only a small proportion of the total B cell population.

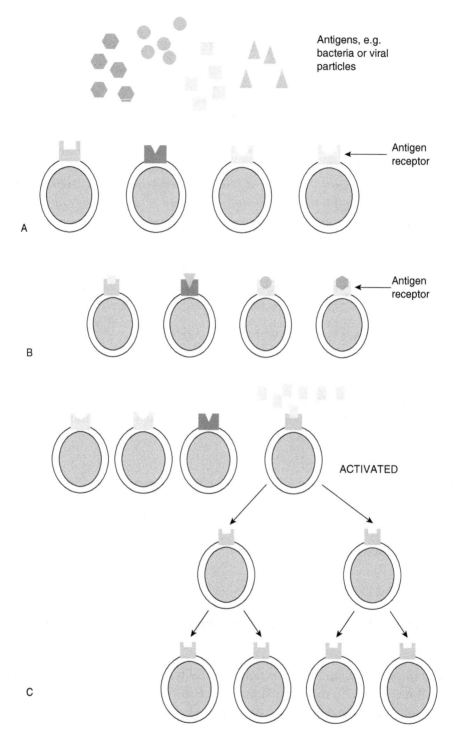

A. Four B cells are shown, each with a different-shaped antigen receptor. Four collections of different-shaped antigens are also shown. These may be different types of microorganism, or different strains of the same microorganism.
B. Each B cell in the blood or lymph recognises a different-shaped antigen. Each B cell is said to be specific for a single antigen.
C. When a foreign antigen enters the body (squares), the B cell that recognises the antigen becomes activated. It starts to divide rapidly producing a clone of identical cells. This process is called clonal selection.

Figure 4.3 Antigen recognition by B cells and clonal selection

Figure 4.3 shows what happens when a B cell recognises and binds to an antigen. The B cell becomes activated and divides to produce many more copies. A population of identical cells is produced called a **clone**. B cells with the receptors that recognise the antigen are 'selected' by the antigen: only those B cells which recognise the antigen are activated and divide to form a clone. This is known as clonal selection (Figure 4.3C). In this way, a clone of B cells capable of recognising and destroying the antigen is produced.

Of the activated clone of B cells most mature into plasma cells which secrete antibodies. A small proportion of the clone remains inside the lymph node as memory cells. Memory cells stay in the lymph node for your lifetime. Should the same microbe infect you a second time, the memory cells become activated very quickly. They reproduce rapidly to form a population of cells capable of destroying the microbe before it has time to establish an infection and cause symptoms. Memory is the basis of **immunity** to an infection you have recovered from once already in your lifetime and the basis of vaccination (covered below under 'Active/passive immunity').

Activity 4.2   Evidence-based practice and research

In your role as a practice nurse at a medical centre you administer influenza vaccinations. David, a 78-year-old patient, would like to know why he needs a different influenza vaccine every year. Find out the answer to David's question. Use the recommended websites at the end of this chapter from Public Health England's Green Book on vaccination.

A suggested answer is given at the end of this chapter.

Activity 4.2 involved research into the influenza vaccine. Natural infection and vaccination stimulate the immune responses made by B cells and T cells. The B and T cell responses are known as the two 'arms' of the adaptive immune response and these are described next.

The B cell response (the antibody-mediated immune response)

As noted above, when a foreign antigen enters the body, those B cells that recognise the antigen are activated by clonal selection. Most B cells need help from a type of T cell called a T helper cell in order to become activated. This help is described under 'the cell-mediated response' below. Activated B cells rapidly divide to produce a population (clone) of B cells. Most of these will mature into antibody-producing plasma cells. A small number develop into memory cells and remain long term in the lymph nodes. The plasma cells migrate to the bone marrow where they secrete antibodies which will target the foreign antigens.

The main role of the B cell response is to counter bacterial infections. Most bacteria multiply within our tissues but remain outside our cells (Chapter 3). This makes bacteria a key target for antibodies which neutralise or destroy them. Antibodies can also neutralise virus particles present in body fluids – but cannot enter cells and therefore cannot attack the virus particles being manufactured within cells.

Antibody structure and function

Figure 4.4 shows a single antibody molecule. Each antibody has a unique antigen-binding site and binds specifically to one antigen. There are five different classes of antibody in humans. Antibodies of the same class have the same overall structure and are referred to as **immunoglobulins (Ig)**. The five classes are: IgA, IgM, IgG, IgD, IgE. Each immunoglobulin class has a different function and makes up a different percentage of the total immunoglobulins made. The functions of the different immunoglobulin classes are given in Table 4.1 below.

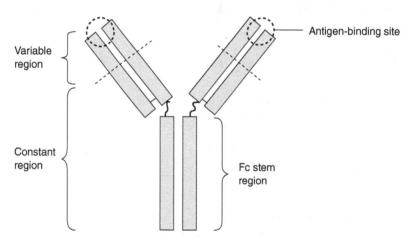

This is an example of an IgG antibody. The antibody has two identical antigen-binding sites. Antibodies of class IgG differ in the variable region but are identical in the constant region. Fc = constant fragment

Figure 4.4 An antibody molecule

Antibodies work in three main ways to neutralise and destroy pathogens and toxins:

1. *Neutralisation:* antibodies coat the pathogen and prevent it from interacting with the host cell surface.

2. *Opsonisation:* antibodies that coat the pathogen enhance phagocytosis. (Antibodies coating the pathogen make the pathogen more easily recognised by the **phagocyte**.) This process of enhancing phagocytosis is called opsonisation.

3. *Complement fixation:* antibodies coating the pathogen activate the complement system of blood proteins (Chapter 2). Complement can directly kill the pathogen.

Antibody class	Percentage of total	Function
IgA	13	Present in mucous membranes and in body secretions, e.g. saliva, tears, sweat, where it plays an important role in destroying microorganisms attempting to invade mucous membranes
IgD	18	Acts as the antigen receptor on the surface of B cells
IgE	< 1	Involved in immunity against parasitic worms and in allergy. Binds to allergens and causes histamine release from mast cells and basophils
IgG	70	The main antibody involved in antibody mediated immunity. Can cross the placenta to give passive immunity to the foetus
IgM	6	Involved in the early stages of antibody-mediated immunity before sufficient IgG is made

Table 4.1   The five immunoglobulin classes

Antibodies and blood tests

Antibodies present in serum can provide useful diagnostic markers. For example, total serum immunoglobulin levels (the levels of all classes of immunoglobulins) may be measured in suspected immunodeficiency, or in suspected myeloma (which is a cancer of immunoglobulin-secreting plasma cells). It is also possible to test for antibodies specific for a particular antigen or set of antigens. This is used for example to monitor hepatitis B vaccination. Pregnant mothers are tested for antibodies against rubella virus to check their immunity. Specific antibody tests are also used to diagnose HIV infection and for Epstein–Barr virus (EBV). Auto-antibodies (antibodies against self-antigens) are used to evaluate various autoimmune diseases such as rheumatoid arthritis, systemic lupus erythematosus and autoimmune thyroid diseases.

Monoclonal antibody therapy

Monoclonal antibodies are antibodies that are made by a single B cell clone. Each type of monoclonal antibody is identical and will bind to a single antigen. Monoclonal antibodies have been developed over the past two decades for treating cancer patients (Chapter 5). Monoclonal antibody therapy is being extended for other conditions and, in particular, for hypersensitivity and autoimmune disorders. Monoclonal antibodies are given the suffix -*mab* which stands for monoclonal antibody. Key examples include: trastuzumab, infliximab and bevacizumab.

Monoclonal antibody therapy is often referred to as biological or 'targeted' therapy because the antibody targets a single protein (or antigen). In cancer treatment, monoclonal antibodies have been developed to target specific tumour antigens. The monoclonal antibody works by binding to the tumour antigen on the surface of the tumour cell. The antibody 'marks' the tumour cell for destruction by the patient's own immune system. The body's own macrophages, natural killer cells or CTLs will recognise the monoclonal antibody and destroy the tumour cell.

Monoclonal antibodies have also been developed to target cytokines and growth factors. One example of this is bevacizumab which targets vascular endothelial growth factor (VEGF). VEGF is produced by tumour cells and causes the development of a blood supply to the tumour. Bevacizumab binds to secreted VEGF preventing it binding to its target receptor on nearby blood vessels. It in effect 'mops up' the VEGF.

Infliximab is a monoclonal antibody that targets the pro-inflammatory cytokine tumour necrosis factor (TNF). This has been used to counter the chronic inflammation associated with autoimmune disorders including rheumatoid arthritis and psoriasis.

The cell-mediated immune response

The cell-mediated arm of the adaptive immune response is carried out by T cells. There are several different types of T cells. In this section, we will look at the role of two of these: the cytotoxic T cell (CTL) and the T helper cell (Th cell). T helper cells express a surface protein called CD4, so they are often referred to as CD4$^+$ T cells. Cytotoxic T cells express a different surface protein called CD8 and are referred to as CD8$^+$ T cells.

The main role of CTLs is to destroy virus-infected cells. This enables the elimination of virus-infected body cells. Th cells help activate both B cells and CTLs.

To understand the role of both the CTL and the Th cell we need to look at the role of another type of immune cell: the antigen-presenting cells (APCs). On infection, which is most likely to be through a breach in the skin or through attachment to a mucosal membrane, invading microorganisms are engulfed by an antigen-presenting cell. The antigen-presenting cells then move to the local lymph node, and 'present' the antigen to naïve T cells. The most important antigen-presenting cells are macrophages and dendritic cells. Macrophages and dendritic cells are located throughout the body; they are found in high numbers in the skin and mucous membranes and in lymphatic tissue and lymph nodes. Langerhans cells are specialised dendritic cells found in the skin.

Antigen-presenting cells engulf antigens by phagocytosis. The antigen is processed inside the cell where it is broken up into fragments. The fragments are then 'displayed' on the cell surface of the antigen-presenting cell. CD4$^+$ T cells or CD8$^+$ T cells recognise the antigen fragment. This specific recognition activates the T cells which start to divide rapidly by clonal selection (Figure 4.5).

The stimulation of T helper and CTLs by antigen-presenting cells occurs inside the lymph nodes – usually those near to the site of infection. This can be experienced as swelling and possibly tenderness of the lymph nodes.

Activated T helper cells then activate specific B cells (shown below in Figure 4.5). The T cell interacts with a B cell and secretes cytokines which activate B cells to become plasma cells.

Activated CTLs leave the lymph nodes and travel to the sites of virus-infected body cells. Virus-infected body cells display fragments of viral antigens through cell surface

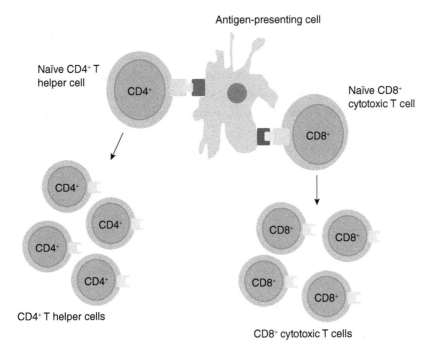

Figure 4.5 Antigen-presenting cells activate CD4 or CD8 T cells

receptors. This allows virus-infected body cells to 'indicate' to the immune system that they are infected. This recognition causes the CTL to release cytotoxic molecules which kill the infected cell. This ensures the destruction of virus-infected cells and is a key part of the elimination of and immunity to viral infections.

Active/passive immunity

Immunity refers to the ability to resist a particular infection or toxin through the action of the immune response. There are two types of immunity: active and passive.

Active immunity develops when someone is exposed to the actual disease-causing microorganism or to a vaccine. Active immunity involves the stimulation of the adaptive immune response. Active immunity is said to be *natural* when acquired through infection. Active immunity is *vaccine-induced* when acquired through vaccination. Active immunity involves the development of immunological memory and provides protection against future exposure to the pathogen. Protection is usually long-lasting, and sometimes lifelong. We have described (under 'Properties of the adaptive immune response') how, during the activation of the adaptive immune response, B and T cells that recognise the antigen undergo clonal expansion. Most of the B and T cells formed from clonal expansion go on to fight the infection. However, a small proportion of the activated B and T cells become memory cells. Memory cells can remain in the body for many years. If we are exposed a second time to the same antigen later in life, these memory cells become quickly activated and are able to eliminate the antigen before it becomes established and causes disease. Figure 4.6 shows the primary and secondary immune responses to an antigen. Vaccination works by introducing microbial antigens into the person being vaccinated, inducing a primary response. There are various ways to introduce microbial antigens from a particular microorganism without causing disease. For example, the vaccine may contain a killed or harmless form of the microorganism. An effective vaccine will be one which stimulates the production of memory cells. We will then have vaccine-induced immunity for as long as the memory cells remain in the body.

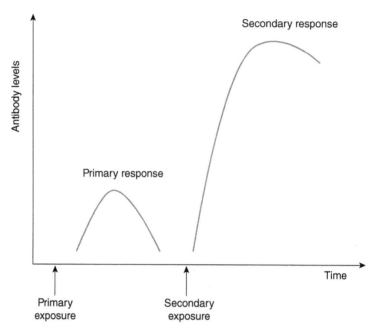

Figure 4.6 The primary and secondary immune response. The figure shows the levels of antibody in the plasma following the first (or primary exposure) to an antigen, followed by a later second exposure to the same antigen. The secondary response is considerably stronger than the primary response and occurs more rapidly after exposure to the antigen (the curve has a steeper slope and reaches much higher level of antibodies). The primary and secondary response is the basis of active vaccination whereby vaccination represents the primary exposure to the antigen (in harmless form). The secondary reaction should ensure the elimination of any subsequent exposure to the same antigen.

Activity 4.3   Evidence-based practice and research

Vaccination has proved to be one of the most successful public health tools to protect against infectious diseases (Goering et al., 2013). Vaccines work by 'priming' the adaptive immune response to the antigens of a particular microbe. Someone who has been given a vaccine will on first contact with the microbe produce a rapid and effective immune response against it through the action of B and T memory cells. It is beyond the scope of this chapter to describe in detail the types of vaccines that are in current use.

Find out the current vaccination schedule in the UK.

There is no suggested answer for this question as it is a piece of research. However, the Public Health England Green Book websites given at the end of the chapter will be a good place to start.

Passive immunity occurs when a person is given antibodies against a pathogen or bacterial toxin. Immunoglobulin preparations can be given following exposure to certain infections. The aim is to give immediate protection against the disease. For example, following suspected infection with hepatitis B or rabies, human hepatitis B immunoglobulin or human rabies immunoglobulin may be given to prevent establishment of infection.

Passive immunity will work immediately whereas active immunity takes days or weeks to develop. Passive immunity, however, only lasts a few weeks or months until the immunoglobulins disappear. The adaptive immune response is not activated in passive immunity and there will be no immunological memory.

A baby has passive immunity when it is born through acquiring maternal antibodies through the placenta. During the last three months of pregnancy maternal antibodies (of type IgG) reach the foetus by crossing the placenta. In addition, breast milk contains some antibodies which will also contribute to the baby's passive immunity. Maternal antibodies last several months.

Maternal antibodies provide vital protection against infections in the newborn baby. A newborn baby's immune system is present but immature. At this stage in life the baby's immune system is naïve. As a result the baby's immune system needs to generate a full immune response to every pathogen; there is no immunological memory to mount a rapid defence against a pathogen. This can take around 10 days. Maternal antibodies are therefore important in protecting from infection following the first 10 days of an infection. It is of note that babies are particularly susceptible to infection by polysaccharide encapsulated bacteria because they produce only low levels of IgG. These bacteria include meningococcal and pneumococcal infections which can cause meningitis.

Vaccination against some pathogens can be given at birth, but others need to be given later. The timing of a vaccination depends upon the age at which the baby can mount an immune response against the vaccine as well as the age-specific risk of disease.

Activity 4.4   Reflection

Using your understanding of immunity, explain why infants pick up more infections at 6 months than at 2 months, and why children's infection rate declines as they get older.

A suggested answer is given at the end of the chapter.

Following Activity 4.4, we look next at when the immune system produces harm or 'hypersensitivity'.

Hypersensitivity

Hypersensitivity reactions are 'excessive' immune responses that cause tissue damage. An individual who has been exposed to an antigen and has mounted an immune response against the antigen is said to be sensitised. The term hypersensitivity means that the sensitised individual produces an excessive and damaging immune response to the antigen.

Hypersensitivity may occur to different types of antigens:

- Normally harmless environmental antigens. These are referred to as allergens which were identified in Activity 4.1 above.
- Antigens from microbes. The immune response to microbial antigens may elicit a hypersensitivity reaction. Glomerular nephritis and rheumatic heart disease can result from hypersensitivity to infection with *Streptococcus* bacteria.
- Self-antigens. Hypersensitivity reactions against our own antigens produce autoimmune disorders. Examples include: rheumatoid arthritis, systemic lupus erythematosus (SLE), Graves' disease, psoriasis, Crohn's disease, ulcerative colitis.

There are four types of hypersensitivity reaction:

Type I (immediate) hypersensitivity is caused by the production of immunoglobulin class E (IgE) antibody which binds to mast cells. These are allergic reactions and are the commonest type of hypersensitivity. Examples include: food allergy, asthma, anaphylaxis, urticaria.

Type II (antibody-mediated) hypersensitivity is caused by binding of antibody (IgG or IgM) to an antigen which is attached to the surface of a body cell. The binding of antibody causes the cell to be destroyed by complement or a phagocyte. An example of this is a blood (haemolytic) transfusion reaction. Here the recipient's antibodies react with antigens on the red blood cells of an incompatible donor. This results in the destruction of the donor red blood cells.

Type III (immune complex) hypersensitivity is caused by the formation of an immune complex (antigen with antibody bound to it) which lodges in a tissue and triggers an inflammatory response. This results in considerable tissue damage. Antigens may be from microorganisms or self-antigens. Type III hypersensitivity can produce a range of problems depending upon where the immune complex lodges. Examples include: vasculitis (immune complexes lodge in the small blood vessels of the skin), arthritis (within the joints), glomerulonephritis (kidneys).

Type IV (delayed) hypersensitivity is caused by reactions mediated by T helper cells. The reaction is 'delayed' in that it occurs around 48–72 hours after exposure. This distinguishes delayed hypersensitivity from type I (immediate) hypersensitivity reactions which occur within minutes. The mechanism of delayed hypersensitivity is a normal immune response to microbial infection. Its undesirable effects include contact dermatitis, type 1 diabetes, hepatitis B infection and graft rejection.

Activity 4.5   Research

Blood transfusions are used in a range of healthcare situations where they can be a life-saving measure. These include: to replace blood lost during major surgery, childbirth or accident; to treat blood disorders such as thalassaemia and sickle cell anaemia; or as part of the treatment of those with haematological malignancies.

Blood given in a transfusion must be compatible with the donor or a transfusion reaction will occur. Find out about the ABO blood group system. Donor and recipient blood must be compatible to avoid a transfusion reaction. Find out which blood types are compatible and why. Ensure you can explain this in terms of blood group antigens and antibodies. Identify the blood type called the 'universal donor' and the type known as the 'universal recipient'.

Use the recommended reading at the end of the chapter.

A suggested answer is given at the end of the chapter.

Blood transfusion reactions which you researched in Activity 4.5 are an example of type II (antibody-mediated) hypersensitivity reactions. Next we will look more closely at allergy (type I hypersensitivity), which is the most common type of hypersensitivity.

Allergy (type I hypersensitivity)

Type 1 (immediate) hypersensitivity reactions (Figure 4.7) are better known as allergy. These include skin reactions such as urticaria (or hives), hay fever, food allergies and as a component of the inflammatory response in asthma. The clinical manifestations of allergy depend upon the site of exposure to the allergen and the degree of previous exposure. Examples are shown in Table 4.2 below.

Name of condition	Site of antigen exposure	Symptoms
Urticaria	Skin	Raised, itchy rash usually short-lived. Generally clears after six weeks. May be the first symptom of more serious anaphylaxis
Hay fever (allergic rhinitis)	Nasal cavity, sinuses	Runny nose, sneezing
Food allergy	Digestive system	Diarrhoea
Asthma (atopic forms)	Lungs	Wheezing, cough, chest tightness, shortness of breath

(Continued)

Table 4.2   (Continued)

Name of condition	Site of antigen exposure	Symptoms
Anaphylaxis	Systemic, injected wasp venom, injected penicillin	Urticaria, difficulty breathing, abdominal cramps, vomiting, systemic vasodilation and drop in blood pressure. May result in circulatory collapse and death

Table 4.2   Examples of allergic reactions

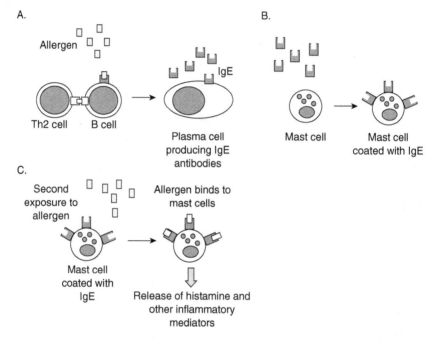

A: On first exposure to an allergen, B cells specific for the allergen will be stimulated to develop into antibody-secreting plasma cells. The type of antibodies produced by the plasma cells is IgE. The production of IgE antibodies specific for an allergen is the basis of type I hypersensitivity or atopy. T helper cells of type 2 are required for the production of IgE antibodies by plasma cells (Janeway and Murphy, 2012).

B. The IgE antibodies bind to mast cells. The mast cells are now 'primed' to respond to a second exposure to the same allergen.

C. On second exposure to the allergen, the allergen binds to the IgE on the surface of the mast sites. This triggers the mast cells to release histamine and other inflammatory mediators which initiate the allergic response. The allergic response may be local or systemic depending upon allergen exposure (Table 4.2).

Figure 4.7   Development of type 1 hypersensitivity (allergy)

Type 1 hypersensitivity reactions occur within minutes of exposure to an allergen to which the individual has previously been sensitised. Individuals susceptible to allergy are said to be atopic. This means that they are likely to develop antibodies of immuno-globulin class E (IgE) when exposed to an allergen. Both genetic and environmental factors are required to make an individual atopic, that is, susceptible to producing high levels of IgE. Many allergens are harmless environmental chemicals such as dust mites, animal dander, pollen and peanuts.

Type 1 hypersensitivity reactions start with a sensitisation phase when the allergen is first encountered as shown in Figure 4.7. The allergen may enter the body by inhalation, ingestion or injection. During the sensitisation phase, in the presence of a subtype of Th cells called Th1 cells, B cells specific for the allergen become activated and secrete IgE. The IgE then coats mast cells. Mast cells are located in most tissues of the body and contain granules of the inflammatory mediator histamine (Chapter 2). Mast cells coated in IgE are said to be sensitised.

Sensitised individuals with a previous exposure to the allergen develop an immediate hypersensitivity reaction when exposed a second time to the allergen. On second exposure, the allergen binds to the IgE coating the mast cells. This occurs at the site of entry of the allergen. The allergen links together two IgE molecules on the mast cells. When this happens, the mast cells are stimulated to release histamine and other inflammatory mediators, including prostaglandins. Histamine causes vasodilation, increased vascular permeability and increased secretion of mucus. Cytokines and chemokines attract neutrophils and eosinophils. This can lead to further damage and inflammation.

The role of allergy is described in relation to asthma in Chapter 9.

Type 1 hypersensitivity is said to be 'Th2 cell-driven'. Th2 cells are a subset of Th cells (along with Th2 and Th17), which secrete the cytokines Il-4, Il-5 and Il-13. Il-4 induces B cells to undergo an immunoglobulin 'class switch' which means that the B cells switch from producing class IgG immunoglobulins to producing immunoglobulins of class IgE (i.e. IgE antibodies). As we have seen, IgE antibodies play a key role in type 1 hypersensitivity reactions by coating (or sensitising) mast cells and thereby making the mast cells 'primed' to recognise and respond to any further exposure to the same allergen. In addition, it is known that IL-5 causes the activation of eosinophils and their migration into the lung (Chapter 9, on asthma). The Th2 response is usually made in response to infection with parasitic worms and ticks which remain extracellular (Endo et al., 2014). The Th2 response, as we have seen, causes the B cells to produce IgE antibodies and also stimulates mast cells and eosinophils. In type 1 hypersensitivity, the Th2 driven response is not to parasitic worms but to allergens. The question arises as to why people with allergy make a Th2 cell-driven IgE response to allergens. In addition, there is the related question of why allergy is increasingly common worldwide. Activity 4.6 below asks you to find out more about one of the recent hypotheses that has been proposed to account for these phenomena.

Activity 4.6   Research

Allergy is becoming increasingly more common and is more prevalent in developed countries than in developing countries. This would suggest that an environmental factor is causing this increase. A number of possibilities

(Continued)

(Continued)

including changes in diet, increases in pollution and allergen levels have been suggested. The 'hygiene hypothesis' is one idea suggested to account for the increase and has evidence to support it. The hygiene hypothesis suggests that children growing up in modern households may no longer be exposed to a range of infections needed to develop a well-regulated immune system. As a result, these children's immune systems may be more likely to react inappropriately to common allergens.

Find out more about the 'hygiene hypothesis' and the evidence in favour of it and the evidence against it. The hygiene hypothesis has been reported by the media to suggest that modern hygiene standards are detrimental to health. What advice should we give to worried parents?

As this is for your own research, no answer is given at the end of the chapter.

Having examined type 1 hypersensitivity in some detail, we turn to examine autoimmune diseases. Autoimmune diseases are also mediated by hypersensitivity reactions but in contrast to allergy, the hypersensitivity response in autoimmunity is to self-antigens.

Autoimmune diseases

Case study

Sheila (aged 55 years) has been living with arthritis for 30 years. She was always very active and enjoyed samba classes at her local sports centre. In her twenties, Shelia noticed that the joints in her hands felt stiff, especially first thing the morning. After a few months, her knees became swollen and she felt extremely tired most of the time. She was unable to move well in her samba classes which she gave up and spent much time at home sitting or in bed. Following a visit to her GP, Sheila was referred to a rheumatologist where a diagnosis of rheumatoid arthritis was made. Her condition is now controlled with anti-inflammatory medication. Sheila reports the importance of 'getting back to her life' and has taken up swimming and has returned to her samba classes.

Sheila in the above case study was diagnosed with rheumatoid arthritis in her twenties. Rheumatoid arthritis is one of the most common autoimmune disorders. Rheumatoid arthritis mainly affects the joints but can affect other parts of the body. Autoimmune diseases affect around 8% of the population.

Table 4.3 gives examples of the most common autoimmune disorders. As can be seen autoimmune diseases can affect most organs or tissues of the body. They are significantly more frequent in women than men: it is estimated that over three quarters of those with an autoimmune disease are women. This suggests a role for sex hormones in the development of autoimmune diseases.

Autoimmune diseases occur when an excessive and inappropriate inflammatory reaction occurs against self-antigens. Examples of autoimmune diseases and the tissue or organ damaged are given in Table 4.3. However, some autoimmune disorders result in damage of more than one organ (e.g. arthritis, SLE).

Name of autoimmune disease	Target tissue/organ
Type 1 diabetes	β cells of the Islets of Langerhans in the pancreas (Chapter 11)
Graves' disease	Thyroid (hyperthyroidism)
Hashimoto's disease	Thyroid (hypothyroidism)
Inflammatory bowel disease	GI tract (Chapter 10)
Multiple sclerosis	Nerve fibres (myelin sheath) in central nervous system
Rheumatoid arthritis	Synovial joint
Psoriasis	Skin
Systemic lupus erythematosus (SLE)	Affects many organs and tissues, or the whole body

Table 4.3   Examples of autoimmune diseases

Autoimmune diseases result from a breakdown in tolerance. Self-tolerance refers to the state in which the immune system does not recognise self-antigens. Under normal circumstances, T cells that recognise self-antigens are destroyed in the thymus gland. There are, in addition, other mechanisms to inactivate self-reactive T and B cells.

Both genetic factors and environmental causes are indicated as risk factors in the breakdown of immunological self-tolerance in autoimmune diseases. Genetic risk has been found in many autoimmune diseases to be linked to specific immune response genes called human leucocyte antigens (HLA) (Janeway and Murphy, 2012). Environmental factors, including diet and exposure to toxins and pathogens, further increase the chances of autoimmunity developing.

The mechanism by which immune damage occurs is through hypersensitivity. For example, rheumatoid arthritis involves the autoimmune damage to the synovial joints. There is widespread inflammation of the joints. An as yet unidentified self-antigen stimulates T cells. Both CD8[+] and CD4[+] T cells are found in the joints where they contribute to a prolonged chronic inflammatory response. This causes pain and swelling as well as destruction of cartilage and bone. The ongoing immune response leads to high levels of cytokines released into the bloodstream. These can cause mild temperature, feelings of malaise and fatigue.

Autoimmune diseases cannot be cured, but symptoms can be greatly relieved through a range of medications. Pain killers such as NSAIDs (Chapter 6) can help reduce pain, steroids (Chapter 2) can be used to suppress the immune system and chemotherapy (Chapter 5) at low dose can be used. Anti-TNF medication, such as infliximab (see under 'Monoclonal antibody therapy', above), can be used to reduce inflammation in rheumatoid arthritis and psoriasis.

Immunodeficiency

Immunodeficiency occurs when the immune system is unable to fight infections. Immunodeficiency diseases are classified as primary or secondary. Primary immunodeficiency diseases are usually due to rare genetic mutations. There are around 200 different types of genetic diseases causing primary immunodeficiency. Primary immunodeficiency may affect the innate immune system (e.g. affecting complement or neutrophils) or the adaptive immune systems (affecting the B or T cell arms). Secondary immunodeficiency arises as complications of other conditions. These include: viral infections (e.g. HIV, cytomegalovirus, rubella); malignancy; extremes of age (prematurity or old age); poor nutrition and starvation; chronic disease (e.g. chronic renal disease) and immunosuppressive drugs (e.g. cancer chemotherapy).

The main clinical feature of immunodeficiency disease is recurrent infection. This refers to two major infections in one year, infection with an unusual organism (e.g. fungal – *Aspergillus*, *Pneumocystis*) or at an unusual site (e.g. liver abscess, osteomyelitis (bone)). Primary immunodeficiency diseases usually present between 6 months to two years of age.

AIDS (acquired immunodeficiency syndrome) is a secondary immunodeficiency disease caused by infection with the human immunodeficiency virus (HIV). HIV/AIDS has worldwide importance for healthcare and is described briefly below.

HIV infection

Infection with the human immunodeficiency virus (HIV) can lead to the acquired immunodeficiency syndrome (AIDS). It is estimated that 35 million people were living with HIV in 2013. The majority of these were in low and middle income countries. Of all infectious diseases, HIV has caused the most deaths worldwide, estimated at 39 million in total.

HIV is transmitted through sexual contact, transfusion with infected blood, or injection with a needle that has infected blood in it. It can also be transmitted from mother-to-child during pregnancy, childbirth and breastfeeding. In sexual transmission, HIV first infects a dendritic cell on the body's mucosal membranes. The dendritic cell transports the virus to CD4$^+$ T cells (T helper cells) in the lymph nodes. The virus replicates within CD4$^+$ T cells and this results in the death of the cell. Infection causes a slow depletion in CD4$^+$ T cells. HIV therefore progressively weakens the immune system causing immunodeficiency.

If the number of CD4$^+$ T lymphocytes falls to below 200 cells mm^3 the individual is said to have progressed to AIDS. At this stage, opportunistic infections occur, such as *Pneumocystis carinii* pneumonia and fungal infections (candidiasis) of the mouth and lungs. Certain cancers and lymphomas are common, such as Kaposi's sarcoma. Tuberculosis is the most common cause of death among HIV-infected people in Africa.

Today, antiretroviral infection (ART) is so effective that HIV positive people can enjoy a normal lifespan and may never progress to AIDS. ART can also prevent transmission of HIV (WHO, 2014a). However, in low to middle income countries just over one-third (36%) of those living with HIV have access to ART.

It is now time to review what you have learned within this chapter by undertaking some multiple choice questions.

Activity 4.7   Multiple choice questions

1. The first line of defence which changes very little during our lifetime is called:

    a) Adaptive immune response
    b) Innate immune response
    c) Passive immunity
    d) Active immunity

2. White blood cells responsible for adaptive immunity:

    a) Neutrophils
    b) Monocytes
    c) Lymphocytes
    d) Eosinophils

3. A molecule that will stimulate the adaptive immune response:

    a) Antibody
    b) Antigen
    c) Pathogen
    d) Immunoglobulin

4. Immunity gained by acquiring 'ready-made' antibodies:

    a) Specific
    b) Active
    c) Innate
    d) Passive

5. Deficiencies in the cell-mediated immune response will lead particularly to infections by:

    a) Bacteria
    b) Protozoa

(Continued)

(Continued)

    c) Viruses

    d) Fungi

6. This property of the adaptive immune response is the basis of immunity to previously encountered infections:

    a) Specificity

    b) Diversity

    c) Tolerance

    d) Memory

7. The major antibody class involved in the adaptive immune response is:

    a) IgA

    b) IgD

    c) IgE

    d) IgG

8. The type of immunoglobulin produced in high amounts in those with allergy:

    a) IgA

    b) IgD

    c) IgE

    d) IgM

9. Autoimmunity arises following a breakdown in 'self-_____'

    a) Specificity

    b) Tolerance

    c) Memory

    d) Immunity

10. The main target of HIV infection:

    a) CD4$^+$ T cell

    b) Neutrophil

    c) CD8$^+$ T cell

    d) B cell

Chapter summary

In this chapter we have focused on adaptive immune response in health and its role in immune-related diseases. We have highlighted important types of antigens which are the target of the adaptive immune system. We have looked at the antibody – and cellular – arms of the adaptive immune response. We introduced monoclonal antibody therapy which is revolutionising cancer therapy and therapy for many hypersensitivity and autoimmune disorders. We have looked at the ways in which the immune system can 'over-react' to cause hypersensitivity – which include allergies and autoimmune diseases. This was followed by examining immunodeficiency which occurs with a weakened immune system. This was illustrated with a section on HIV infection.

Activities: Brief outline answers

Activity 4.1 Evidence-based practice and research (p93)

Common allergens include: pollen, dust mites, fish, shellfish and nuts. Intolerance is an adverse reaction to a substance, often a type of food or medication, but one which shows no evidence of involvement of the immune system.

Activity 4.2 Evidence-based practice and research (p95)

Through your research to answer this activity, you should be able to describe and understand the implications of 'antigenic drift' of influenza virus type A for vaccination. Specifically, as a practice nurse administering influenza A vaccinations, you will be able to inform David that he needs a new vaccine every year because influenza virus shows antigenic drift. Antigenic drift refers to the small changes the main influenza antigens undergo during its life cycle. Influenza A is a virus which replicates using host cells (Chapter 3). During virus replication within the patient's cells, it undergoes small changes, or mutations, in two of the proteins on the surface of the influenza A virus particles. These proteins are called haemagglutinin and neuraminidase. These two proteins are the main target of the adaptive immune response, stimulated by vaccination. The small changes in these two surface proteins alter the shape of the two proteins in such a way that they will not be recognised by the antibodies produced by an earlier vaccine. These small changes in the surface proteins are the antigenic drift. Antigenic drift shown by influenza A means that every year, David and other members of the population who are recommended influenza A vaccination need to be given a new vaccine. The new vaccine will contain the 'latest' versions of the surface proteins haemagglutinin and neuraminidase. David's immune system needs to produce antibodies effective to the current influenza A virus.

Activity 4.4 Reflection (p101)

Infants pick up more infections at 6 months than at 2 months, because at 2 months the maternal antibodies which crossed the placenta during pregnancy are still circulating in the infant. These will provide some passive immunity. At 6 months many of these antibodies will have disappeared from the circulation, predisposing the infant to more infections. Children's infection rate declines as they get older as their active immunity builds up from the infections they have been exposed to from birth onwards.

Activity 4.5 Research (p103)

With the ABO blood type system, individuals are of one of four types: A; B; AB; or O. Your blood type depends upon which antigens are present on the surface of your red blood cells (antigen A, B or both). Type A blood group have antigen A on their surface; type B have antigen B; type AB have both antigens A and B; but type O have neither A or B antigens (table below). The type of antigens present on your red blood cell determines which antibodies (anti-A, anti-B, both or neither) you have in your serum. Type A individuals have anti-B antibodies in the serum; type B individuals have anti-A antibodies; type AB individuals have no anti-ABO antibodies; and type O individuals have both anti-A and anti-B antibodies in the serum.

In blood transfusions, the antibodies in the serum of the recipient must not react with the donor blood cells. So, for example, type A individuals with anti-B antibodies (antisera) cannot receive blood from a type B or type AB donor. The recipient's anti-B antisera would recognise the type B antigens on the surface of the donor cells and a type II incompatibility reaction would arise.

ABO blood groups				
Antigen (on RBC)	Antigen A	Antigen B	Antigens A + B	Neither A or B
Antibody (in plasma)	Anti-B antibody	Anti-A antibody	Neither antibody	Both antibodies
Blood type	**Type A** Cannot have B or AB blood Can have A or O blood	**Type B** Cannot have A or AB blood Can have B or O blood	**Type AB** Can have any type of blood Is the universal recipient	**Type O** Can only have O blood Is the universal donor

Activity 4.7 Multiple choice questions (pp109–10)

1. The first line of defence which changes very little during our lifetime is called:

   b) Innate immune response

2. White blood cells responsible for adaptive immunity:

   c) Lymphocytes

3. A molecule that will stimulate the adaptive immune response:

   b) Antigen

4. Immunity gained by acquiring 'ready-made' antibodies:

   d) Passive

5. Deficiencies in the cell-mediated immune response will lead particularly to infections by:

   c) Viruses

6. This property of the adaptive immune response is the basis of immunity to previously encountered infections:

   d) Memory

7. The major antibody class involved in the adaptive immune response is:

   d) IgG

8. The type of immunoglobulin produced in high amounts in those with allergy:

   c) IgE

9. Autoimmunity arises following a breakdown in 'self-_____'

    b) Tolerance

10. The main target of HIV infection:

    a) CD4⁺ T cell

Further reading

Janeway, C and Murphy, K (2012) *Janeway's Immunobiology* (8th edition). London: Taylor and Francis.

This is a comprehensive immunology textbook.

Georing, R and Mims, C (2013) *Mim's Medical Microbiology* (5th edition). Oxford: Elsevier/ Saunders.

This is a microbiology book with a very clear account of 'host defences' against infection.

Websites

www.gov.uk/government/uploads/system/uploads/attachment_data/file/144249/Green-Book-Chapter-1.pdf/

Immunity and how vaccines work: the Green Book, chapter 1. Part of Immunisation against infectious disease from Public Health England. Provides a useful introduction to immunity and how vaccines work.

www.gov.uk/government/uploads/system/uploads/attachment_data/file/365793/Green_Book_Chapter_19_v6_0.pdf/

Influenza: the Green Book, chapter 19. Provides influenza information for health professionals.

http://highered.mheducation.com/sites/0072495855/student_view0/chapter24/animation__the_immune_response.html

This education site provides very clear animations on the immune system.

www.piduk.org/

Website of Primary Immunodeficiency UK (PID UK) – an organisation supporting individuals and families affected by a primary immunodeficiency in the UK.

www.tht.org.uk/myhiv/HIV-and-you/Simple-science/Stages-of-hiv-infection/

Information about HIV/AIDS from the Terrence Higgins website.

Chapter 5   Cancer

Chapter aims

....

After reading this chapter you will be able to:

- describe what cancer is and how cancer cells differ from normal cells;
- explain the role of proto-oncogenes and tumour suppressor genes in abnormal cell growth;
- describe the hallmarks of cancer;
- describe how cancer cells are graded and how cancers are staged to guide the selection of cancer treatment;
- explain the pharmacological treatment options available for cancer.

Introduction

One in two people born after 1960 in the UK will be diagnosed with some form of cancer during their lifetime.

(Ahmad et al., 2015)

Cancer is a group of diseases characterised by unregulated cell growth, invasion and spread of cells from the site of origin, or primary site, to other sites in the body (Pecorino, 2012). Cancer starts when one cell grows and multiplies in an uncontrolled way. This leads to a lump or tumour. If not treated, the primary tumour, which is where the cancer starts, can cause problems in the following ways:

- Invading nearby healthy tissues and compressing local structures, blocking ducts and vessels.
- Causing pressure on other body structures.
- Spreading, or metastasising, to other parts of the body through the lymphatic system or bloodstream.

- Altered hormone production – cancer cells that would normally produce a hormone can begin to produce an excess of the hormone in an unregulated way. In contrast, a cancer cell that would not normally produce a hormone may start to produce a protein that mimics the action of a hormone. For example, some cancer cells produce a protein that acts like parathyroid hormone. This protein causes the bone to release calcium into the blood and can lead to hypercalcaemia.

Cancer is the second commonest cause of death in the UK. Most deaths occur from the effects of the tumour metastasising to other parts of the body.

There are over 200 different types of cancer because there are over 200 different types of cells making up the body. Lifetime risk for cancer has increased in recent years due to our longer life expectancy. More people are living into older age which is when most cancers are diagnosed. Scientists, health professionals, cancer charities, politicians and the public have many questions about cancer biology, detection, diagnosis, causes and strategies for prevention, treatment and support, some of which we will discuss here.

In this chapter, we begin by explaining some common terms used to describe cancer. We will also identify the four common cancers in the UK. Next, we discuss the risk factors and the strategies used for prevention and early detection of cancer. The process of carcinogenesis, where normal cells become cancer cells, is described. This will include a discussion of the genes involved and how mutations in these genes lead to the formation of a tumour. The process of grading and staging cancer is explained before the final section which focuses on cancer treatment. As you will see, understanding the process of carcinogenesis has helped in the development of new targeted therapies for cancer treatment.

Definitions

The following definitions are important for your reading and understanding of cancer in this chapter.

Neoplasm: a 'new growth' of cells or an abnormal mass of tissue. Neoplasm is a more accurate word for tumour (which literally means a 'swelling').

Benign: a benign tumour, or neoplasm, is one that does not invade neighbouring tissue or spread to other parts of the body. Benign tumours are not usually harmful but they can cause problems if they compress nearby structures such as blood vessels or nerves. Some benign tumours secrete large amounts of hormones that may disrupt normal homeostasis.

Malignant: a malignant neoplasm is one that is capable of invasion of neighbouring tissues and spreading to other parts of the body.

Cancer: this refers to any malignant neoplasm.

Nomenclature

Over 200 different types of cancer have been classified. Different cancers arise from different cell types making up the tissues of the body. The different types of cancer have different causes (aetiology), patterns of growth and sites of metastases that influence how cancers present, are detected and treated. In clinical practice, a variety of technical names are used to distinguish the many different types of cancers:

- *Carcinoma* refers to malignant tumours of epithelial origin. Around 85% of cancers are epithelial arising from epithelial tissues that cover external and internal body surfaces. Carcinoma of the lung, breast, prostate and colon are the most common cancers of this type in the UK.
- *Adenocarcinoma* is a cancer arising from glandular epithelial cells.
- *Sarcomas* are cancers arising from cells found in the supporting tissues of the body such as bone, cartilage, fat, connective tissue and muscle. These arise from tissues of mesenchymal origin – embryonic connective tissue that differentiates into haematopoietic and connective tissue.
- *Leukaemia and lymphoma* are cancers known as haematological malignancies arising from cells of the blood and bone marrow.

Common cancers

In adults, four cancers – breast, lung, bowel and prostate – account for more than half of cancer incidence. In women, since the 1970s, breast and lung cancers have had the biggest impact on lifetime risk. The increase in breast cancer has been related to lifestyle changes such as women having fewer children later, and breast screening detecting more cancers. The increase in lung cancer rates is thought to reflect smoking patterns in previous decades.

In men, the biggest impact on lifetime risk has been from prostate and bowel cancer. Much of the increase in the incidence of prostate cancer has been due to better detection. Prostate Specific Antigen (PSA) testing is a relatively new test for prostate cancers. PSA is a tumour marker – an antigen that can be found in the blood. We discuss PSA in the section on tumour markers. The increase in bowel cancer rates may be related to an increase in red meat consumption and obesity.

Cancer in children (0–14 years) is relatively rare accounting for less than 1% of all cancers. Cancer Research UK (CRUK) identify that about 1600 children are diagnosed with cancer each year. This is approximately 30 children every week. Leukaemia is the most commonly diagnosed cancer in children. Other common cancers include brain, central nervous system (CNS), intracranial tumours and lymphomas. Together, these cancer types account for more than two-thirds of all cancers diagnosed in children. Whilst the incidence of childhood cancer has increased by more than 40% since the 1960s in the UK, the five-year survival for children's cancer has more than doubled. For every ten children diagnosed with cancer, more than eight now survive for five years or more compared with fewer than three in ten in the 1960s (CRUK, 2018a). As with adults, a child's risk of developing cancer depends on many factors including age, genetics and other risk factors including some potentially avoidable lifestyle factors. We now discuss risk factors in more detail.

Risk factors for cancer

Activity 5.1 Evidence-based practice and research

Usually, it is not possible to know exactly why one person develops cancer. Research has identified some of the risk factors that may increase a person's chances of developing cancer. Some risk factors cannot be avoided, such as inherited genetic changes and ageing, but other lifestyle factors can be modifiable.

Research the risk factors associated with cancer and list these.

As this is a research activity, there is no model answer. Compare your list with the factors discussed in this section of the chapter.

Cancer is caused by damage to specific genes. Factors in our environment or lifestyle can damage DNA, the genetic material. This damage builds up over time and can lead to cancers developing in adulthood.

The main risk factors for cancer are summarised in Table 5.1.

Most cancers develop from genetic changes in a single cell that happen during our lifetime. Faults that arise in the genes are called mutations. Mutations occur during the normal process of cell division. The older we are, for example, the more cell divisions our cells will have made. Similarly, the constant replacement of cells in some tissues, such as the GI tract (Chapter 10), means there is an increased chance for mutations to occur. In addition, certain chemicals we are exposed to, called carcinogens, can increase the chance of cells developing mutations causing cancer. These factors make it more likely that we will develop cancer as we age as any mutations that have occurred accumulate and are passed onto daughter cells. The specific genes are discussed in the 'Genes and cancer' section. Genetic changes affect a limited population of cells (the primary tumour). These mutations are not passed on to our children.

Cancer prevention strategies focus on taking action to lower the risk of developing cancer. This is called primary prevention and aims to stop cancer developing. Actions include maintaining a healthy lifestyle and reducing our exposure to known carcinogens. It is estimated that more than 40% of cancer cases could be prevented by adopting the lifestyle changes that reduce exposure to the risk factors identified in Table 5.1.

Risk factor	
Age, lifestyle and diet	**Age** – 63% of people who develop cancer are over the age of 65 years.
	Smoking – the single biggest avoidable cause of cancer. About 1 in 5 cancers are related to smoking, increasing the risk of cancers of the mouth, lung, bladder and bowel. Passive smoking, breathing in other people's smoke, is also identified as increasing risk of developing cancer.
	Weight/diet – being overweight increases the risk of several cancers including cancer of the pancreas, bowel, uterus and breast. Reducing weight can help to reduce this risk. A healthy diet, limiting intake of red meat and processed meat, and increasing intake of fruit and vegetables can reduce risk.
	Alcohol – increases the risk of cancers of the mouth, throat and oesophagus. The more alcohol consumed the more the risk increases.
	Physical activity – lack of physical exercise has been associated with increased risk of developing cancers of the bowel, uterus, lung and breast.
	Ultraviolet (UV) UVA/B exposure – the body uses UVB from sunlight to make vitamin D which is important for bone health, but over-exposure of the skin to UVB and UVA rays from the sun, or from use of a sunbed which results in reddening or burning of the skin, can increase risk of skin cancers.
Occupational and environmental factors	Substances in the environment or workplace have been identified as risk factors including:
	Asbestos – can lead to mesothelioma.
	Natural radiation – the **sun** is one environmental contributor to cancer development. **Radon**, a naturally occurring gas, has been linked to the development of lung cancer.
Viruses and bacteria	Cancer is not infectious and cannot be caught from someone. A number of viruses are, however, thought to influence the development of cancer by causing genetic changes in cells including:
	Human papilloma virus (HPV) – increases risk of cervical cancer, head and neck cancer, anal cancer and cancer of the vulva.
	Hepatitis B and C – increases risk of liver cancer.
	Human immunodeficiency virus (HIV) – can increase risk of lymphoma or sarcoma.
	Epstein–Barr virus – linked to types of lymphoma.
	H. pylori bacterial infection – associated with the development of stomach cancer (Chapter 10).
Lowered immunity	Some types of cancer, lymphomas and certain types of skin cancer are more likely to occur in people with a lowered or poor immune response. This may include people who have had an organ transplant and are taking immunosuppressant drugs to prevent organ rejection.
Family history	All cancers develop because something has gone wrong with one or more genes in a cell. It is important to understand the difference between cancers occurring due to genes you were born with and cancers due to a gene change in a cell that has happened during your lifetime. Some people inherit faulty genes from their parents that give them a higher risk of developing certain cancers.
	For example, inheriting a faulty copy of the BRCA genes is linked with breast, ovarian and prostate cancers. The proportion of cancers caused by inherited faulty genes is small with about 3% of breast cancers due to an inherited faulty gene.

Table 5.1 Risk factors for cancer (adapted from CRUK)

The goal of secondary cancer prevention strategies is to detect and treat 'precancerous' cells or early, asymptomatic, cancer. National cancer screening programmes are part of this cancer prevention strategy.

Activity 5.2 Evidence-based practice and research

As a nurse, you will be involved in advising people about reducing their risk of developing cancer and also providing information and support to people participating in the national cancer screening programmes.

National cancer screening programmes include bowel, breast and cervical cancer screening. Details about screening are available at the CRUK website: **www.cancerresearchuk.org/about-cancer/screening**. You should review this, and other relevant websites, to complete the box below relating to the target population, the tests involved and the benefits of screening.

Screening for:	Target population	Tests involved	Benefits of screening
Cervical			
Breast			
Bowel			

You might also investigate the screening available on request for prostate cancer. Prostate cancer screening is not part of the UK screening programme.

As this is a research activity, there is no model answer.

Cell biology

In this section, having identified some risk factors for cancer, we will discuss carcinogenesis. Carcinogenesis is the process by which normal cells are transformed into cancer cells. The process involves a progression of changes at the genetic and cellular level that enable the cell to acquire certain properties, or hallmarks, which result in unregulated cell division and, for some cells, the capability to invade and metastasise to other parts of the body (Figure 5.1). Figure 5.1 uses the growth of a colorectal cancer to illustrate tumour growth and progression. Table 5.2 summarises the hallmarks of cancer described by Hanahan and Weinburg (2000, 2011). The hallmarks provide a framework for understanding the diversity of cancers. In 2000, six hallmarks were described to explain the progressive evolution of normal cells to acquire the traits that enable them to become cancer cells during the multistep development of tumours. In 2011, two 'emerging' hallmark capabilities and two 'enabling' characteristics were added. The hallmarks are pivotal for our understanding of cancer and the cancer treatment. Table 5.2 introduces some complex cell and molecular biology that will be explained in the subsequent sections.

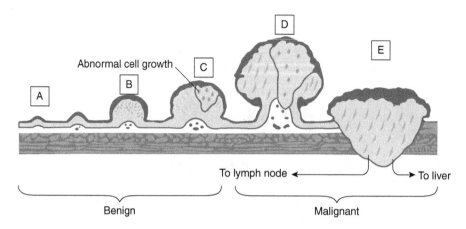

A Single cell within a mucosal gland acquires gene mutations.
B The abnormal cell proliferates to produce a clone of cells populating one gland.
C Further proliferation results in populations of cells starting to over-grow, called hyperplasia, to form a non-invasive polyp (adenoma) protruding from the mucosal surface.
D The transformed cells become invasive as a result of acquiring further genetic changes; the cells are dysplastic (look irregular) and the growth is described as a carcinoma.
E The cancer cells invade blood vessels and lymphatics, and are carried to the liver and lymph nodes to form secondary tumours (metastases).

Figure 5.1 Biology of tumour growth

Hallmark	Description
1. **Cell division in the absence of growth stimulatory signals**	• Normal cells carefully control the production and release of growth promoting signals which signal a cell to enter into and progress through the cell cycle (G_1 of cell cycle). This control ensures homeostasis of cell number, maintenance of tissue architecture and function. You will remember from Chapter 1 that growth factors bind to receptors on the cell surface and work through signal transduction pathways to regulate progression through the cell cycle.
	• Cancer cells 'deregulate' these growth-promoting signals and become independent of external growth stimulation signals.
	• Acquired mutations in key genes (called proto-oncogenes) can 'short-circuit' growth factor pathways leading to unregulated cell division.
	• The mutations in these key genes may lead cancer cells to: (i) produce growth factors to which they can respond (autocrine stimulation). They are independent of, and are not dependent on, the normal external growth factor (paracrine) signalling produced by neighbouring cells for promoting cell division; (ii) produce increased number of receptors at the cell surface making the cell hyper-responsive to the usual circulating levels of growth factor; (iii) develop signal transduction pathways within the cell which are permanently active in the absence of external growth factor stimulation at the cell surface receptor.

2. Evading growth suppressors	• In addition to Hallmark 1, cancer cells must also overcome processes which normally negatively regulate (stop) cell proliferation – these are inhibitory signals which normally limit growth and proliferation of cells (most cells of the body are not dividing).
	• Normally, tumour suppressor genes produce proteins that limit cell growth and proliferation. These proteins regulate processes that can signal a cell to proliferate, undergo repair of damage to DNA, or signal cell death (apoptosis see 3).
	• Acquired mutations in these tumour suppressor genes interfere with these inhibitory pathways that are critical gatekeepers of cell cycle proliferation. Cancer cells do not respond to the growth inhibitory signals permitting persistent cell proliferation.
3. Evading apoptosis – programmed cell death	• Normal cells are signalled to die (apoptosis), often in response to DNA damage and chromosomal abnormalities that cannot be repaired. Apoptosis is, therefore, normally a barrier to the development of cancer. The cell is disassembled and consumed by its neighboring cells and phagocytic cells.
	• Cancer cells evade apoptotic signals. This hallmark results from mutation and loss of function of a tumour suppressor gene called TP53 and other proteins that normally signal apoptosis, and enables cancer cells to survive and proliferate passing on damaged DNA to daughter cells.
4. Enabling replicative immortality	• Normal cells have a finite number of cell divisions after which they become senescent (cease to divide).
	• The 'cellular counting device', which regulates the number of cell divisions a cell undergoes, is the shortening of chromosomal ends (telomeres) that occurs after every round of DNA replication. This counting device limits the replication potential of normal cells, and with apoptosis, is one of the two barriers to cell proliferation.
	• Cancer cells are able to maintain the length of their telomeres. Telomerase, an enzyme normally absent in cells, has been found at high levels in cancer cells and acts to add telomeres to the end of chromosomes. This prevents the progressive telomere loss which would normally cause cell senescence or apoptosis.
	• Altered regulation of telomere maintenance results in unlimited replicative potential of a cell.
5. Inducing angiogenesis	• Normal cells depend on blood vessels to supply oxygen and nutrients, and remove metabolic wastes and carbon dioxide.
	• The development of the normal vascular structure occurs during embryogenesis and becomes generally quiescent in adults except during wound healing or during the female reproductive cycle.
	• In cancer, an 'angiogenic switch' is activated increasing the expression of genes such as VEGF (vascular endothelial growth factor).
	• Cancer cells can induce angiogenesis, the growth of new blood vessels, needed for tumour survival and expansion.

(Continued)

Table 5.2   (Continued)

6. Activating invasion and metastasis	• Normal cells maintain their location in the body and generally do not migrate. This is due to cell-to-cell adhesion molecules that enable cells to hold their shape and their attachment to other cells and the extracellular matrix. • Cancer cells may acquire the capacity to move to other parts of the body and develop secondary tumours (this is the major source of cancer deaths). This may result from downregulation or mutations that result in the inactivation of genes which produce the cell-to-cell adhesion molecules. • Invasion and metastasis have been described as a sequence of discrete steps called the invasion-metastasis cascade. The cascade involves a succession of cell changes – beginning with local invasion, intravasation of cancer cells into the blood and lymphatic systems, transit through the blood and lymphatic systems, followed by escape of cancer cells into distant tissues to form metastatic lesions, and tumours.
Enabling characteristics: **7. Genetic instability in cancer cells** **8. Inflammatory state of premalignant and malignant tumours**	The hallmarks above are acquired functional capabilities that enable cancer cells to survive, proliferate and disseminate. These capabilities are possible by 2 enabling characteristics: • Genomic instability of cancer cells – random mutations which occur, accumulate and confer advantage on cancer cells – enabling their growth and dominance in the tissue environment. • Inflammation that is driven by cells of the immune system can contribute to the hallmark capabilities by providing molecules to the tumour environment including growth factors which promote cell proliferation, angiogenesis, invasion and metastasis.
Emerging hallmarks: **9. Capability to modify cell metabolism to support tumour proliferation** **10. Cancer cell evasion of immunological destruction**	Two emerging hallmarks have been proposed subject to further study: • Modification of cell metabolism to support continuous cell growth and proliferation. • Evasion of cancer cells from attack and destruction by T and B lymphocytes, macrophages and natural killer cells (see Chapter 4).

Table 5.2   The hallmarks of cancer (adapted from Hanahan and Weinberg, 2000, 2011)

To understand cancer and to develop new treatments, scientists are examining closely these hallmarks and the underlying genetic changes (mutations) involved. As we will discuss in 'Treating cancer' many new cancer drugs target the pathways producing one or more of the hallmarks. To understand these pathways, we have to look closely at cell division and how it is normally regulated.

The cell cycle: regulation of cell growth, proliferation and cell death

As Figure 5.1 illustrates, and the hallmarks in Table 5.2 identified, cancer arises because cell division becomes unregulated (or uncontrolled) in a population of cells.

To understand the hallmarks of cancer we need to understand how cell division is normally regulated and how this becomes unregulated.

The growth and division of our cells and tissues must be strictly controlled to maintain a balance between cell division and cell death. Many tissues must be able to rapidly increase the number of cells by cell division to replace cells lost to injury and normal wear and tear. At the same time, cell division must be stopped when enough new cells have been made. In most tissues, there will also be some 'programmed cell death' or apoptosis. Cells that are damaged, or cells that, for example, 'over-grow' in the process of wound-healing need to be removed. In addition, 'old' cells that have undergone a set number of divisions, controlled by the length of the telomeres, also need to be removed. In such cases they undergo apoptosis – programmed cell death.

The cell cycle is the series of steps that a cell goes through as it divides into two daughter cells (Figure 5.2). It may be helpful to appreciate that the cell cycle has some similarities with the washing cycle on an automatic washing machine. In both, we can recognise a definite start and a finish, and a series of steps to go through until the cycle is complete. The steps of the cell cycle are summarised in Table 5.3.

Under normal circumstances, cells are signalled to 'enter' the cell cycle and start dividing by:

(a) a combination of hormones and growth factors which signal the cell to divide. These 'signalling molecules' attach to specific receptors on the cell (Chapter 1) and

(b) the cells responding to 'spatial signals' from neighbouring cells and the surrounding extracellular matrix that indicate how much room is available for new/replacement cells.

Under these conditions, which favour cell division, the cell proceeds through the phases of the cell cycle summarised in Table 5.3.

State	Description	Abbreviation	
Quiescent	Gap 0	G0	Resting phase where a cell has left the cell cycle and stopped dividing. Cells that are unable to divide, such as neurons, remain in G0 for their whole life. Many cells never rest (i.e. do not enter G0) and continue to divide throughout life. For example, epithelial cells.
Interphase	Gap 1	G1	In G1 cells grow in size, increase their supply of proteins, and increase their number of organelles such as mitochondria and ribosomes.
	Synthesis	S	DNA replication takes place during S phase. DNA replication means the exact copying of each strand of DNA.
	Gap 2	G2	During the gap between DNA synthesis (S phase) and mitosis the cell continues to grow.

(Continued)

Table 5.3 (Continued)

State	Description	Abbreviation	
Cell division	Mitosis	M	Mitosis (nuclear division) and cell division (cytokinesis).
			Each daughter cell receives an identical set of 46 chromosomes. Errors in mitosis can either result in cell death through apoptosis or cause mutations that may lead to cancer.

Table 5.3 Phases of the cell cycle

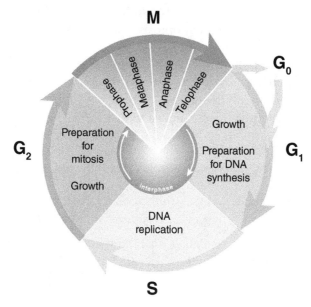

Figure 5.2 Cell cycle

Mitosis is the division of the nucleus that dividing body cells go through. This is shown in Figure 5.3. Almost all of the cells that make up the body contain a nucleus. The nucleus stores the genetic material. Figure 5.4 shows a typical body cell with the nucleus that contains the genetic material.

The genetic material is made of a long, thin molecule called deoxyribonucleic acid, or DNA. Each DNA molecule is 'wound-up' and 'packaged' into a structure called a chromosome. Human body cells have 46 chromosomes. Each chromosome is one of a pair – so each human body cell has 23 pairs of chromosomes. One of each pair originated from the egg cell, and the other of each pair from the sperm cell.

Figure 5.5 shows a single chromosome taken from the cell nucleus. It has been 'un-wound' to show how it is made from a single, long, thin molecule of DNA. A single gene is shown on the DNA molecule. A gene is a length of DNA that encodes the information to make a protein. In total, the human genome (which is all the DNA in a cell) encodes for around 30,000 proteins. When a cell divides it must copy the genetic material with no, or minimum copying errors.

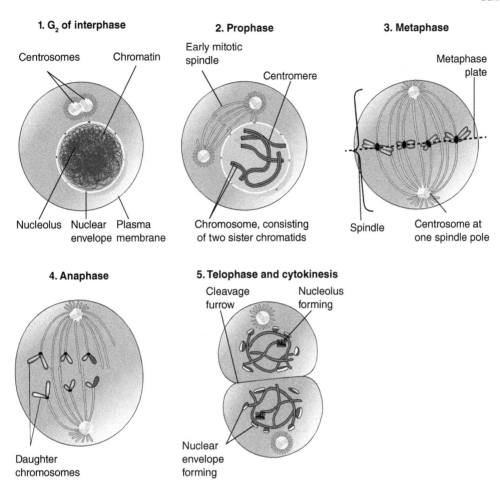

1. G₂ of interphase

Centrosomes Chromatin

Nucleolus Nuclear Plasma
envelope membrane

2. Prophase

Early mitotic spindle

Centromere

Chromosome, consisting of two sister chromatids

3. Metaphase

Metaphase plate

Spindle Centrosome at one spindle pole

4. Anaphase

Daughter chromosomes

5. Telophase and cytokinesis

Cleavage furrow Nucleolus forming

Nuclear envelope forming

Figure 5.3 Mitosis

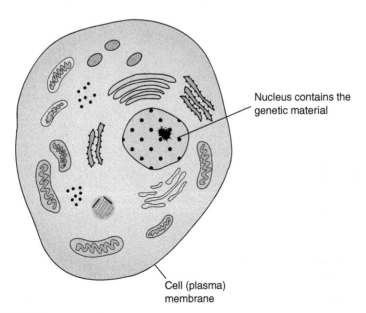

Nucleus contains the genetic material

Cell (plasma) membrane

Figure 5.4 Typical human cell

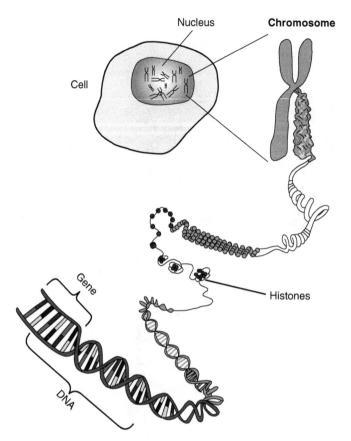

Figure 5.5   Single chromosome

Regulation of the cell cycle involves processes crucial to the survival of a cell. These include the detection and repair of genetic mutations and the prevention of uncontrolled cell division. Cell cycle 'checkpoints' are used to regulate progress of the cell cycle. There are several checkpoints, for example between G1 and S phase, and between G2 and M phase. There is also a mitotic checkpoint after M phase. The checkpoints ensure that damaged or incomplete DNA is not passed onto daughter cells. Errors in mitosis or DNA replication lead to the cell cycle being stopped for repair of damaged DNA or, if damage cannot be repaired, a cell is signalled to undergo apoptosis. Like the washing machine, these 'molecular' events that control the cell cycle are ordered and directional; that is, each process occurs in a step-like fashion and it is impossible to 'reverse' the cycle. Errors in mitosis or DNA replication are the source of mutations. If mutations occur in the genes that regulate the cell cycle, then this can lead to cancer.

A clearer understanding of the roles of numerous genes in regulating the cell cycle is emerging and is discussed in the next section.

Genes and cancer

There are many different types of cancers but all share one characteristic – uncontrolled growth that progresses towards limitless expansion of cells. As we have discussed, in normal tissues, cell replacement should equal cell death. Cells communicate with each other through signalling molecules (Chapter 1). In normal tissues, cells receive signals to stimulate cell division, to stop cell division and also to signal apoptosis (programmed cell death). Apoptosis, or 'cell suicide', is the mechanism by which old or damaged cells normally self-destruct. Apoptosis of 'old' cells is controlled by telomeres, the cellular 'counting device' on the end of chromosomes. The telomere shortens after every cycle of DNA replication (S phase of the cell cycle, Figure 5.2). Cell proliferation and apoptosis are regulated by proteins encoded by genes regulating the cell cycle, including proteins that control the cell cycle checkpoints. In cancer, the cancer cells are able to 'escape' these regulations on cell division and cell death by acquiring the capabilities, or hallmarks, summarised in Table 5.2 and discussed below.

Two families of genes normally control the events of the cell cycle. They are grouped according to whether a mutation of the gene leads to:

- Gain of function – mutation in genes called proto-oncogenes can make the cell independent of growth stimulating factors as identified by Hallmark 1, or
- Loss of function – mutations in tumour suppressor genes make the cell unable to conduct checks and signal for repairs during the cell cycle as identified by Hallmark 2. The cell can proceed through the cell cycle despite the accumulation of errors and, in addition, signalling apoptosis is avoided (Hallmark 3).

To acquire the hallmarks of cancer, a cell must generally develop mutations in a combination of these regulatory genes. These mutations are passed onto daughter cells when the cell divides. We will discuss these genes in more detail.

Proto-oncogenes are genes that normally code for proteins that form cell growth activating (signal transduction) pathways that promote cell proliferation (Chapter 1) (Figure 5.6).

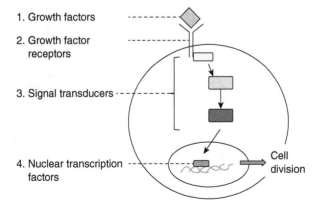

1. Growth factors

2. Growth factor receptors

3. Signal transducers

4. Nuclear transcription factors

Cell division

Figure 5.6   Proto-oncogenes and signal transduction

Proto-oncogenes that have acquired mutations are called oncogenes. Mutations in oncogenes result in proteins with a 'gain of function'. This means that the protein the gene encodes has a new or altered function. (The protein 'misbehaves' so to speak.)

Alternatively, the gene can be 'over-expressed'. This means that there is an over-production of the protein. This can also result in the function of the protein being altered. There are many proto-oncogenes and they can be grouped into four categories summarised in Table 5.4. Oncogenes relate to Hallmark 1, activating signal transduction pathways to stimulate the cell to enter the cell cycle.

Category of oncogene	
Growth factors	Growth factors are proteins that are manufactured and secreted into the extracellular space. They diffuse to nearby cells and attach to receptors on the target cell surface. The binding of growth factors to the cell surface receptor activates cell signalling (Chapter 1). This leads to activation of the cell cycle and cell division. Some growth factor genes acquire mutations in the process of carcinogenesis. These growth factor genes are called proto-oncogenes and, following mutation, they are referred to as oncogenes. For example, over-production of growth factors by proto-oncogenes that have acquired a mutation to become an oncogene can lead to excessive signalling (or stimulation) of cell division and growth of cells. By over-producing growth factors, the cancer cell may stimulate its own cell division (autocrine) as well as that of its neighbours.
	Examples of growth factors secreted by cancer cells include: epidermal growth factor (EGF) and vascular endothelial growth factor (VEGF). EGF is commonly over-secreted in some breast cancers.
Receptors	Growth factors cannot penetrate the cell membrane so their presence at the cell surface must be transmitted – transduced – into the cell by receptors on the cell surface (Figure 5.6). As discussed in Chapter 1, receptors are proteins on the outside of the cell and activate enzymes on the inside of the cell to promote signal transduction to the nucleus of the cell resulting in cell proliferation. The receptors are specific to particular growth factors.
	A mutation in a proto-oncogene which encodes for a cell surface receptor may lead the cell to produce cell surface receptors that should not be present, or to an over-production of cell surface receptors. The cell with 'new' growth factor receptors on its surface will then respond to growth factors present in its local environment. Cancer cells with an abnormally high number of growth factor receptors will be particularly sensitive to growth factors.
	An example of this is the 'over-expression' of human epidermal growth factor receptor type 2 (HER2) receptors in about 25% of breast cancers. These breast cancer cells have an abnormally high number of HER2 receptors on their surface. This means that they are very sensitive to the epidermal growth factor and readily stimulated by it. The drug trastuzumab (Herceptin) is a monoclonal antibody (MAB), a targeted therapy, which specifically attaches to the HER2 receptor on the surface of breast cancer cells preventing cell division.
Cytoplasmic signalling molecules	Another way in which mutation of a proto-oncogene may result in proliferation is through the manufacture of excessive or abnormal proteins that are needed for signal transduction pathways inside the cell (Chapter 1). These pathways involve proteins that transmit signals from activated cell surface receptors to the cell nucleus. Mutation of the gene that codes for a signal transduction protein results in activation of the pathway. This activation of the signal transduction pathway will occur even when there is no growth factor at the cell surface to signal the cell to divide.

	The best understood example of this mechanism is mutation of the *ras* gene family. *Ras* proto-oncogenes code for Ras proteins that transmit signals from receptors at the cell surface into the interior of the cell (signal transduction proteins). Normally, the Ras protein is activated then rapidly deactivated once the signal has been transmitted to the next part of the signal transduction pathway. A mutation in the *ras* gene can lead to the production of an altered Ras protein that is permanently active and continues to stimulate cell proliferation inappropriately. *Ras* gene mutations occur in about a third of all cancers and are a focus for new targeted cancer treatments.
Nuclear transcription factors	The pathway from growth factor stimulation of the cell surface receptor and the signal transduction pathway results in transcription of a set of genes in the nucleus that move the cell to enter S phase of the cell cycle. A number of proto-oncogenes have been identified that code for transcription factors (proteins) in the nucleus. These transcription factors promote cell division. *Myc, jun* and *fos* are examples of proto-oncogenes that code for nuclear transcription factors. Abnormalities of the *myc* genes have been found in breast and lung cancers, leukaemia and neuroblastoma.

Table 5.4 Proto-oncogenes

Whilst oncogenes stimulate cell proliferation, *tumour suppressor genes* inhibit cell division or induce apoptosis in cells. Proteins encoded by tumour suppressor genes normally stop the cell cycle in G1 phase at the checkpoint. To become a cancer cell, cells must not only 'short circuit' growth-promoting signals (Hallmark 1), but also 'evade' the normal mechanisms that stop cell division (Hallmark 2).

Cancers can arise when a tumour suppressor gene acquires mutations that result in loss of 'function' of the protein that the gene encodes. An example of a tumour suppressor gene is retinoblastoma gene (*Rb*). The *Rb* gene encodes for the Rb protein, or pRb, which is important in preventing a cell from proceeding through the cell cycle. pRb has been called the 'master brake' of the cell cycle blocking cell division (see Table 5.4). A mutation of the Rb gene can prevent the Rb protein from being made, or lead to the production of a faulty Rb protein that does not work. Without the Rb protein, the cell cycle will continue through G1 phase to S phase.

Each body cell has two copies of most genes, one from the mother's egg cell and one from the father's sperm cell. Tumour suppressor genes may acquire genetic mutations but, in order for cancer to develop, *both* copies of the tumour suppressor gene must be damaged. In familial cancers, which are quite rare, a person may inherit a mutated copy of a tumour suppressor gene from one parent. This increases their risk of cancer compared to someone who inherits two functional copies of the gene.

A non-functioning or 'defective' Rb protein is common to a number of cancers. Other tumour suppressor genes include *p53* and *BRCA1* and *BRCA2*. These are summarised in Table 5.5. With rare familial cancers, knowledge about the sequence of tumour suppressor genes provides the opportunity to screen individuals with a family history of cancer to determine whether they carry a defective gene.

Tumour suppressor gene	
p53 gene	*p53* is the most common tumour suppressor gene defect identified in cancer cells. More than half of all types of cancers lack functional *p53* gene. The p53 protein (TP53), like the Rb protein, inhibits the cell cycle. Normally p53 protein accumulates after DNA damage. TP53 protein binds to the damaged DNA and stalls cell division to enable DNA repair before DNA replication during S phase. Where DNA damage is too great and repair cannot take place, TP53 initiates apoptosis. *p53* is known as the 'guardian of the genome'.
	Mutation of *p53* gene and lack of TP53 function enables genetically damaged and unstable cells to survive and continue to replicate often acquiring further cancer-promoting mutations. *p53* gene is also important for cancer therapy. Chemotherapy and radiotherapy result in cellular damage that normally triggers TP53 protein to initiate cell suicide. Cancer cells which lack functional *p53* gene and TP53 protein may be resistant to some radiotherapy and chemotherapy.
BRCA1 and BRCA2	The breast cancer genes *BRCA1* and *BRCA2* are tumour suppressor genes identified through studies of inherited predisposition to particular cancers. Normally these genes produce tumour suppressor proteins that ensure the 'stability' of the cellular DNA. When either of these genes acquires a mutation, such that the protein is not made or does not function correctly, DNA damage may not be repaired. As a result, cells are more likely to develop additional genetic changes that can lead to cancer.
	A *BRCA1* or *BRCA2* mutation can be inherited from a person's mother or father. Each child of a parent who carries a mutation in one of these genes has a 50% chance of inheriting the mutation. Women with a family history of breast cancer and an inherited defect in these genes have between 45% and 90% lifetime risk of cancer. These genes also increase breast cancer risk in men. The onset of inherited breast cancer is earlier than non-inherited, sporadic forms of breast cancer and the occurrence of bilateral breast cancer is higher. The study of these genes is providing insight into breast cancer biology.
APC gene	The *APC* gene produces adenomatous polyposis coli (APC) protein that helps control how often a cell divides, how it attaches to other cells within a tissue, or whether a cell moves within or away from a tissue. This protein also helps ensure that the chromosome number in cells produced through cell division is correct. *APC* gene mutation can occur in colorectal cancer and is associated with certain forms of familial colorectal cancer (familial adenomatous polyposis (FAP)).

Table 5.5 Tumour suppressor genes

In summary, we have identified that proto-oncogenes and tumour suppressor genes normally regulate the cell cycle. In cancer, mutations in proto-oncogenes can lead to the formation of an oncogene that produces an onco-protein with a 'gain of function'. This can create 'gain of function' in growth factors, receptors, signalling pathways and transcription factors to promote unregulated cell division (Hallmark 1). Mutations in tumour suppressor genes lead to 'loss of function'. The tumour suppressor gene fails to produce a tumour suppressor protein or produces a faulty protein that does not function. This can result in the cancer cell evading normal growth inhibitory signals and apoptosis (Hallmarks 2, 3). Cancer cells may also acquire 'replicative immortality' as the regulation of telomeres is altered and enables the length of the telomeres to be maintained. 'Old' cells will continue dividing beyond their usual lifespan (Hallmark 4).

In addition to acquiring the capabilities of unregulated cell proliferation, evasion of apoptosis and immortality, cancer cells may also invade nearby tissues and metastasise to other parts of the body. We will now discuss these capabilities.

Like all cells, cancer cells require oxygen and nutrients to function (Hallmarks 5 and 9). Cancer cells continue to enter the cell cycle, undergo cell division and produce daughter cells to form a neoplasm (or tumour) (Hallmarks 6, 7). In order for neoplasms to grow in size, the cancer cells need to acquire a blood supply to provide oxygen and nutrients and remove waste products. Without a blood supply, cells at the centre of the neoplasm become short of oxygen (hypoxic) and die. Cancer cells can stimulate the formation of new blood vessels. This process is called angiogenesis (Hallmark 5). Many cancer cells start to produce vascular endothelial growth factor (VEGF). VEGF is an angiogenic growth factor, which means it stimulates the production of new blood vessels. It is thought that cancer cells produce VEGF in response to hypoxia. VEGF stimulates proliferation of vascular endothelial cells. These are the cells making up the wall of blood capillaries (the endothelium). This proliferation of endothelial cells leads to the development of new blood vessels.

Establishing a blood supply (Hallmark 5) enables the cancer cells that form the primary tumour to increase in number and for further mutations to occur, accumulate and confer advantage on cancer cells, enabling their growth and dominance in the tissue environment (Hallmark 7). The new blood supply also provides a pathway for metastases as cancer cells detach from the primary tumour and enter the bloodstream (Hallmark 6). The inhibition of angiogenesis, through the use of drugs such as bevacizumab, is an important targeted therapy developed to limit tumour growth and metastases. We will discuss targeted therapies in the treatment section.

Cancer cells can break away from the primary tumour in the tissue of origin and be carried in the blood or lymphatic system to other parts of the body where they can start to grow into new tumours. Tumours from cancer cells that have spread are called metastases. A cancer that has spread has 'metastasised'. Figure 5.7 illustrates a primary cancer of the colon with liver metastases. For cancer cells to access the blood and lymphatic circulation they must first pass through the basement membrane of the tissue of origin, move through the extracellular space and penetrate the basement membrane of the blood or lymphatic vessel. This complex process involves loss of adhesion between cells and the release of enzymes such as proteases that digest the basement membrane. The cancer cell squeezes through the basement membrane of its tissue of origin and also that of the blood or lymphatic vessel. The cell(s) then circulate through the blood or lymphatic vessels and, when the cell reaches the new tissue to be colonised, it must squeeze through the basement membranes by similar mechanisms. In the new tissue, the cancer cell must acquire nutrients and a blood supply (angiogenesis) adapting to an environment that differs from its tissue of origin.

The survival of cancer cells in the circulation, however, is not guaranteed. Cancer cells are exposed to immune cells and may be detected and destroyed (Hallmark 8, 10). They may also undergo apoptosis. Some cancer cells 'prefer' specific sites

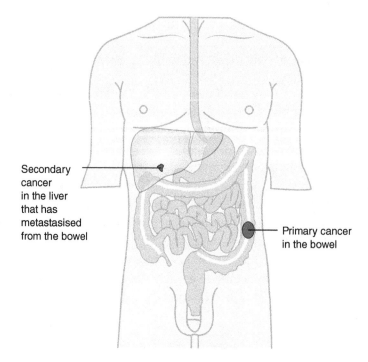

Figure 5.7   Diagram showing primary cancer and metastasis

to metastasise to. This may be related to circulatory flow. For example, cancer cells from the colon often metastasise to the liver because they travel in the portal vein. However, the patterns of spread for other cancers cannot be explained by blood flow patterns and is poorly understood. Lymphatic spread is more predictable. Generally, the lymph nodes that immediately drain the tissue of origin are colonised first and then the cancer cells spread from node to node.

Activity 5.3   Evidence-based practice and research

For the four common cancers and others you may be interested in, complete the table by identifying the sites of metastases.

Cancer	Sites of metastases
Breast	
Lung	
Colorectal	
Prostate	

There is no model answer for this activity.

Grading and staging

In clinical practice, in order to diagnose and determine the most appropriate treatment and care, a patient will undergo various investigations to establish the type of cancer and the extent of disease within their body. To establish the type of cancer, a detailed history, clinical examination and a biopsy will be taken. The biopsy may be from the primary tumour or from a metastatic lesion, including a lymph node. The cancer cells will be looked at in the laboratory to identify the type of cell. A process called grading of the cancer cells will also be undertaken.

Grading describes a neoplasm in terms of how abnormal the cancer cells look under a microscope compared to the normal cells from which they developed. There are different grading systems for cancers but, generally, there are three grades (Table 5.6). A low-grade cancer may grow more slowly and be less likely to metastasise than a high-grade one. Cancer cells, including those that have metastasised, can exhibit degrees of differentiation. Differentiation refers to how well-developed the cancer cells are and how they are organised in the tissue compared to the tissue of origin. If the cells and tissue structures are very similar to normal the neoplasm is called 'well-differentiated'. These cancers may grow and spread slowly. In 'poorly differentiated' or 'undifferentiated' neoplasms, the cancer cells look very abnormal and the cells are not arranged in the usual way – the normal structures and tissue patterns are missing. These cancers are generally considered more likely to invade surrounding tissues or to metastasise to other parts of the body.

Clinical examination, history, grading, blood and radiological investigations form part of the process of 'staging'. *Staging* describes the location and pattern of spread of cancer cells within the person. Staging is a way of describing factors such as grade, tumour size, extent of local invasion, lymph node and organ involvement and presence of distant metastases. A number of staging systems are used. The purposes of staging systems are to:

(a) provide a common language to describe the size and spread of cancer within the person;

(b) enable treatment results to be compared between research studies;

(c) develop standardised guidelines for treatment between hospitals and services.

In clinical practice, you may see the international TNM system commonly used. TNM stands for tumour, node, metastasis. Using numbers, the system describes the size of the primary tumour (T), whether the cancer has spread to the lymph nodes (N), and whether it has spread to a different part of the body (metastasised) (M). In practice, you may also see other number staging systems with Roman numerals (I–IV) being used. Grading and staging are summarised in Table 5.6.

Grading	Grading systems classify tumours into increasing degrees of malignancy:
Histology of cancer cells to determine the cell type the cancer arose from, the grade and degree of differentiation.	Grade 1: The cancer cells look very similar to normal cells and are growing slowly. Grade 2: The cells look unlike normal cells and are continually growing/dividing. Grade 3: The cancer cells look very abnormal and are continually dividing. Grade X: The grade cannot be assessed. An undetermined grade. Differentiation: May also be reported as undifferentiated, poorly differentiated, moderately or well differentiated.
Staging	**TNM staging system:**
Includes the results of radiography investigations, exploratory surgery or biopsy, and blood tests to identify tumour markers. CT, MRI and PET imaging techniques may be used for non-invasive imaging of the body.	T – the size of the neoplasm and how far it has spread into nearby tissue – it can be 1, 2, 3 or 4, with 1 being small and 4 large. N – whether the cancer has spread to the lymph nodes – it can be between 0 (no lymph nodes containing cancer cells) and 3 (many lymph nodes containing cancer cells). M – whether the cancer has spread to another part of the body – it can either be 0 (cancer has not spread) or 1 (cancer has spread). For example, a small cancer that has spread to the lymph nodes but not to anywhere else in the body may be summarised as T2 N1 M0. A more advanced cancer that has spread to lymph nodes and other body organs may be T4 N3 M1.

Table 5.6 Grading and staging

Scenario

You are caring for Frances. Frances is a 64-year-old woman who had cancer of the right breast diagnosed. A partial mastectomy was performed followed by radiotherapy. In addition, she was commenced on Tamoxifen 20 mg BD.

The pathology report included the following information:

Specimen: Wide local excision and axillary dissection.

Wide local excision specimen weighing 80 g. It consists of skin including nipple measures 50 × 10 mm and covers fatty tissue with maximum dimension of 80 mm. In tissue beneath nipple is pale irregular mass 25 × 20 × 20 mm irregular poorly defined margin. Closest excision margin is 5 mm from mass. Axillary dissection reveals 13 lymph nodes.

Sections show high-grade ductal carcinoma in situ with micro-calcification. Also invasive adenocarcinoma of ductal type. Grade II. Maximum tumour dimension is 22 mm. No evidence of vascular or lymphatic permeation. Both in situ and invasive carcinoma are completely excised by 5 mm margin. None of lymph nodes contains tumour.

Conclusion: Right breast in situ and invasive ductal carcinoma grade II. 22 mm complete excision.

Activity 5.4   Critical thinking

In the scenario with Frances, what cell type did her cancer develop from?

Using the TNM classification system below, what would be the TNM staging for Frances, assuming no evidence of metastases?

Stage	Description
Tis	Carcinoma in situ
T1	Tumour smaller than (<) 2 cm
T2	Tumour 2–5 cm
T3	Tumour larger than (>) 5 cm
T4	Tumour extends from breast into chest wall and/or skin and/or is inflammatory
N0	No spread to nearest lymph nodes
N1	Spread to lymph nodes on same side as breast cancer and is mobile
N2	Spread to lymph nodes on same side as breast cancer and is fixed
N3	Spread to internal mammary nodes on same side as breast cancer
M0	No spread to other parts of body
M1	Cancer spread to another part of body

A model answer is provided at the end of the chapter.

You might also look at histology reports for your patients who have been investigated for cancer.

As part of the staging process, patients may have blood tests that include identifying tumour markers. *Tumour markers* are substances (antigens) associated with tumour cells that may help to identify the tissue of origin (see Chapter 4). Some tumour markers are released into the circulation. Unfortunately, most tumour markers are not very specific for cancer as the normal cells in the tissue of origin may also produce them. Alpha-fetoprotein, for example, is measured in pregnant women as a screening test for developmental abnormalities. In cancer, it can also be used for a subset of tumours in non-pregnant women, men and children. Tumour markers are useful as indicators for further diagnostic investigations or to monitor tumour activity during and following treatment. An increase in a particular tumour marker may indicate progression and proliferation of the cancer cells. Table 5.7 provides examples of common tumour markers.

The results of grading and staging procedures, like those experienced by Frances, will inform clinical decisions about which cancer treatment may be used – singly or in combination – aimed at cure, control or palliation. Localised tumours may be managed with surgery and radiotherapy. Tumours that have metastasised are likely to require a systemic treatment. Chemotherapy, hormone therapy and targeted therapies are systemic treatments because they circulate in the bloodstream aiming to kill any cancer cells including those that have metastasised. We will now discuss cancer treatment in more detail.

Marker	Commonly associated tumour
Carcinoembryonic antigen (CEA)	Adenocarcinoma of colon, breast, ovary, lung, stomach
CA125	Ovarian, uterus, cervix
Alpha-fetoprotein (AFP)	Testicular, germ cell tumours
Prostatic-specific antigen (PSA)	Prostate

Table 5.7 Tumour markers

Treating cancer

Cancer treatment includes:

(a) Surgery

(b) Radiotherapy

(c) Chemotherapy

(d) Hormone therapy

(e) Biological therapies

This section will briefly discuss surgery and radiotherapy and focus on chemotherapy, hormone therapy and biological therapies.

Surgery

Most patients with 'solid' tumours, meaning sarcomas, carcinomas and lymphomas (National Cancer Institute, 2015), will have some surgical treatment. Surgery may be used to diagnose, treat or palliate cancer. A tumour or lymph nodes may be biopsied to diagnose the cancer type and grade. Surgery can be curative for localised tumours. The benefit of surgery can be removal of the tumour with minimal damage to other body cells. As reported in Frances's pathology report (Activity 5.4), the surgeon normally aims to remove a margin of normal tissue around the resected tumour to ensure complete removal. Lymph nodes may also be removed to assess for evidence of metastases.

Surgery for some tumours may be challenging if vital structures such as nerve or blood supply are involved. Surgery can also result in disfigurement and potential loss of function. Surgical resection may be used on its own or used in conjunction with radiotherapy and/or drug treatments.

Radiotherapy

Involves the use of high-energy radiation from X-rays, gamma rays, neutrons and protons to kill cancer cells. Ionising radiation may be used to:

1. kill cancer cells that are not accessible to surgery due to location;
2. kill cancer cells that remain undetected following surgery.

Radiotherapy can be used prior to, or following, surgery. Radiotherapy may also be used for palliation to reduce the tumour size and for symptom control, including the management of pain from bone metastases. Total body irradiation is used in preparation for bone marrow transplantation. Radiation kills cells by damaging their DNA. Cells that are dividing through the cell cycle are susceptible to radiotherapy – both normal and cancer cells. Radiation may not kill cells directly. Instead, radiation may trigger apoptosis.

External beam radiation is the most widely used. The radiation comes from a machine called a linear accelerator. The patient is only exposed to radiation whilst the machine is switched on. External beam radiation can be used to treat specific areas of the body. It can also treat more than one area such as the main tumour and nearby lymph nodes. The radiation is aimed at the cancer, but also affects the normal tissue in the treatment field. Ionising radiation does not distinguish between normal cells and cancer cells. As normal and cancer cells within the radiation field may be in different phases of the cell cycle and cycling at different rates, external beam radiation is usually given daily over several weeks to maximise cell kill and minimise side-effects. Cells in the mitosis (M) phase are more sensitive to radiation. The impact on normal cells in the treatment field results in side-effects experienced by patients.

Acute side-effects occur in cells that are rapidly dividing including skin, hair, mucosal lining of the GI tract, and epithelial linings such as the bladder and vagina. These effects may be experienced 10–14 days after radiotherapy starts and begin to improve 10–14 days after radiotherapy has finished. Late side-effects may occur in cells with a slower cell cycle, for example, bone, muscle and connective tissue. Due to the slow rate of division, these side-effects may take months or years to present and may persist.

Radiotherapy can also be delivered by implanting a radioactive source in (interstitial) or near (intracavity) the tumour to deliver a high radiation dose to the tumour while reducing the radiation exposure in the surrounding healthy tissues. This treatment is called brachytherapy. Interstitial brachytherapy involves directly inserting the source into the tumour or body tissue containing the tumour, for example, prostate implants.

Intracavity brachytherapy can be used to treat the cervix. The source is positioned in the vaginal vault/uterus. Systemic radiotherapy can also be delivered using radioactive substances that travel in the blood to the tissues. Radioactive iodine is an example used to treat an overactive thyroid and thyroid cancer. The patient takes a dose of radioactive iodine by mouth, as a liquid or in capsules, which kills thyroid cells. In this case the patient is radioactive for a period of time and precautions will be required to protect staff and families.

Chemotherapy

Surgery and radiotherapy are normally local or regional treatments. In contrast, chemotherapy drugs can affect cancer cells (and normal cells) located throughout the body. Your knowledge of the cell cycle is important to understanding chemotherapy as chemotherapy drugs interfere with some aspect of cell division (Figure 5.2). Chemotherapy agents may act by directly interfering with DNA, inhibit enzymes related to DNA/RNA synthesis or destroy cell proteins. Chemotherapy drugs may be used singly or, more usually, in combination. Each drug will act on cells in different phases of the cell cycle. This is because, at any one time, only a portion of cancer cells will be in a phase of the cell cycle susceptible to a particular chemotherapy drug.

Chemotherapy drugs may be classified as:

- cell cycle phase specific, acting on cells undergoing division within the cell cycle;
- cell cycle phase non-specific, active on cells in either dividing or resting phases including G0.

Cell cycle phase specific drugs, for example, include 'mitotic poisons' such as vincristine – a drug that prevents the formation of the spindle fibres necessary for nuclear division during mitosis (M) (Figure 5.3). Other mitotic poisons include taxanes, such as Paclitaxel. Taxanes interfere with microtubules – cell structures that move chromosomes during mitosis – to induce apoptosis (see Figure 5.3). S phase inhibitors, such as 5-Fluorouracil, block the synthesis of thymidine, one of the four nucleotides in DNA, required for DNA replication. Cell cycle phase non-specific drugs include 'alkylating agents' such as cyclophosphamide that bind to the DNA molecule disabling the mechanism for cell division.

Several cycles of chemotherapy are given to ensure that all cancer cells have been killed. Like radiotherapy, chemotherapy drugs are not selective, affecting dividing normal cells and cancer cells. Rapidly dividing normal cells, particularly those of the bone marrow, gastrointestinal epithelia, hair follicles, sperm and egg production are most affected resulting in the side-effects associated with chemotherapy. Bone marrow depression affects the number of red blood cells, white blood cells and platelets. It is the most serious side-effect predisposing the patient to anaemia, infection and bleeding. Neutropenia, a reduction in the number of neutrophils, occurs 7–10 days post-chemotherapy due to failure of production in the bone marrow or peripheral destruction. Neutropenia predisposes patients to bacterial and fungal infections and the development of neutropenic sepsis which is life-threatening. Other side-effects include anaemia, thrombocytopenia, stomatitis, mucositis, nausea, vomiting, fatigue and reduced fertility.

Hormone therapies

Hormone therapies are used to slow or stop the growth of 'hormone sensitive' tumours that require certain hormones to grow (endocrine stimulation). Hormone therapies can work by preventing the body from producing the hormone or by interfering with the action of hormones. Hormone therapies are used for both prostate and breast cancer.

Prostate cancer

Androgens are male sex hormones that control the development and maintenance of male characteristics. Testosterone and dihydrotestosterone (DHT) are the most common androgens. Testosterone is produced mainly in the testicles. Some prostate cancer cells may also be able to produce testosterone. Androgens are required for normal growth and function of the prostate gland. Androgens also stimulate the growth of both normal and prostate cancer cells by binding to, and activating, the androgen receptor expressed in prostate cells. Once activated, the signal transduction pathway is initiated stimulating cell division (Figure 5.6).

Prostate cancer cells are referred to as 'androgen dependent' or 'androgen sensitive' because, in the early stages, treatments that decrease androgen levels or block androgen activity can inhibit prostate cancer cell growth. To prevent cancer cell proliferation, androgen deprivation therapy may involve:

(a) *Reducing androgen production by the testicles* – includes the most commonly used hormone therapies. Drugs called luteinising hormone-releasing hormone (LHRH) agonists prevent the secretion of luteinising hormone from the pituitary gland and prevent testosterone being produced by the testicles. Men receiving an LHRH agonist for the first time may experience 'testosterone flare' due to a temporary increase in testosterone levels. LHRH agonists briefly cause the pituitary gland to secrete extra luteinising hormone before blocking its release. This 'flare' may temporarily worsen clinical symptoms.

(b) *Blocking the action of androgens in the body* – anti-androgen drugs compete with androgens for binding to the androgen receptor on prostate cells. Androgen antagonists promote apoptosis and stop prostate cancer growth.

(c) *Blocking the production of androgens throughout the body* – androgen synthesis inhibitors are drugs that prevent the production of androgens throughout the body, by the adrenal glands, the testicles and the prostate cancer cells themselves. Drugs, for example aminoglutethimide and abiraterone, block testosterone production by inhibiting an enzyme called CYP17.

Reducing the amount of androgens produced by the body can have wide ranging side-effects including: loss of libido, erectile dysfunction, loss of bone density, changes in blood lipids, growth of breast tissue (gynaecomastia) and hot flushes.

Breast cancer

The hormones oestrogen and progesterone act as growth factors (Table 5.4) that can promote the growth of some breast cancers. These are called 'hormone dependent' breast cancers. Oestrogen and progesterone are hormones produced by the ovaries in pre-menopausal women and by other tissues, such as fat and skin, in both pre-menopausal and post-menopausal women. Hormone dependent breast cancer cells contain hormone receptors that become activated when hormones bind to them (endocrine stimulation). The activated receptor causes the signal transduction pathway to become activated resulting in the stimulation of cell growth. Pathologists can determine whether breast cancer cells contain hormone receptors by testing samples of tumour tissue following biopsy. If cancer cells contain oestrogen receptors, the cancer is called oestrogen receptor positive (ER-positive). If the cancer cells contain progesterone receptors, the cancer is called progesterone receptor positive (PR-positive). Approximately 70% of breast cancers are ER-positive. Most are also PR-positive. Breast cancer cells can also be HER2-positive (see below). Breast cancers that lack oestrogen receptors are oestrogen receptor negative (ER-negative). These tumours do not require oestrogen to signal cell division. Breast cancers that lack progesterone receptors are called progesterone receptor negative (PR-negative).

For hormone-sensitive breast cancer, different types of hormone treatments are used:

(a) *Aromatase inhibitors* are used to block the activity of an enzyme called aromatase which the body uses to make oestrogen in the ovaries and other body tissues. Aromatase inhibitors are used for post-menopausal women because the ovaries in pre-menopausal women produce too much aromatase for the inhibitors to block production effectively. Drugs, for example anastrozole, are used to temporarily inactivate aromatase and prevent oestrogen being produced from body fat in post-menopausal women.

(b) *Tamoxifen* is an example of a drug that competes with oestrogen's ability to bind to oestrogen receptors and stimulate the growth of breast cancer cells. Tamoxifen acts as an antagonist blocking oestrogen activity in breast tissue. It can, however, behave as an oestrogen agonist in the uterus possibly increasing risk of endometrial cancers. Tamoxifen may be prescribed for pre- and post-menopausal women (like Frances) and men with ER-positive breast cancer.

(c) *Luteinising hormone (LH) blockers*: ovarian function can be suppressed temporarily with the use of luteinising hormone-releasing hormone (LHRH) agonist drugs. These drugs, for example goserelin acetate, are used for pre-menopausal women with oestrogen receptor positive breast cancer. They interfere with signals from the pituitary gland that normally stimulate the ovaries to produce oestrogen. This is called ovarian ablation.

Biological therapies

Biological therapies are the focus of attention in the development of new therapies for conditions including rheumatoid arthritis and inflammatory bowel disease (Chapter 10) as well as anti-cancer drugs. As you will see from the examples, understanding cell biology, carcinogenesis and the ability to identify different molecular and cellular parts in cancer cells have been key to the development of biological therapies.

Biological therapies interfere with specific molecules involved in the growth, progression and spread of cancer to block the growth and spread of cancer. The National Cancer Institute (2018) identify that biological therapies are different from chemotherapy in the following ways:

1. Biological therapies act on specific molecular targets associated with cancer whereas traditional forms of chemotherapy cannot distinguish between normal cells and cancer cells and can result in damage to normal cells/tissues.
2. Biological therapies are designed to interact with their target whilst chemotherapy drugs are used because they kill cells.
3. Biological therapies are cytostatic. This means that they block cancer cell proliferation whereas chemotherapy agents are cytotoxic killing cancer cells.

For people with cancer, biological therapies offer individualised or personalised medicines that use specific information about their tumour to help diagnose and plan treatment. Examples include HER2-positive breast cancer cells.

As we have discussed, proteins that are more abundant in cancer cells could be potential targets for cancer therapies especially if known to be involved in cell growth and survival. The human epidermal growth factor-2 protein (HER2) is an example as HER2 is expressed at high levels on the surface of some cancer cells. Several biological therapies are directed against HER2, including trastuzumab. This drug is approved to treat certain breast and stomach cancers that overexpress HER2. Trastuzumab is a monoclonal antibody (MAB) that targets the HER2 receptor preventing the receptor from sending the normal growth-promoting signals and slowing or stopping the cancer from growing. MABs may also be bonded to toxic substances such as radioactive particles or cytotoxic chemicals. By combining a radioactive particle with a MAB, for example, radiation therapy can be directly delivered to cancer cells without damaging surrounding normal cells. Similarly, combining chemotherapy drugs with a MAB enables cytotoxic therapy to be delivered directly to the cancer cells. Ado-trastuzumab emtansine (Kadcyla), for example, contains an antibody that binds to HER2 receptors on breast cancer cells. The cancer cells then ingest the antibody which releases molecules of chemotherapy.

Other MABs interfere with the action of proteins necessary for tumour growth. Bevacizumab, for example, inhibits angiogenesis by interfering with the action of vascular endothelial growth factor (VEGF). As discussed earlier, this protein is secreted by cancer cells to stimulate new blood vessel formation. When bound to bevacizumab, VEGF cannot attach to the cell receptor. This prevents the signalling that leads to new blood vessels.

Another approach to biological therapy is to identify whether cancer cells produce altered (mutated) proteins that promote cancer progression. For example, the cell growth signalling protein BRAF is present in an altered form in many melanomas resulting from mutation in the *BRAF* proto-oncogene. A drug called Vemurafenib targets the altered form of the BRAF protein for patients with melanoma whose cancer has a specific V600E BRAF mutation. Researchers also look for abnormalities in chromosomes that are present in cancer cells but not normal cells. Sometimes these chromosomal abnormalities result in the creation of a fusion gene (a gene that incorporates parts of two different genes) to produce a fusion protein that drives cancer development. These fusion proteins also offer potential targets for biological cancer therapies. For example, imatinib mesylate targets the BCR-ABL fusion protein. This is made from pieces of two genes that get joined together in some leukaemia cells and promotes the growth of leukaemic cells.

Whilst MABs are highly targeted drugs, adverse events do occur. Patients should be screened and, as a nurse, you should be aware of the risk of cytokine-release reactions. Patients may experience infusion-related or hypersensitivity reactions. Infusion-related reactions result from the release of cytokines. When a MAB binds to an antigen on the targeted cell, the immune response is triggered and numerous cytokines are released from activated white blood cells (Chapters 2 and 4). When cytokines are released into the circulation, patients may experience systemic symptoms including fever, nausea, hypotension, tachycardia, headache, rash and sore throat.

Hypersensitivity reactions may arise caused by an interaction between factors released by immunoglobulin E and mast cells causing an antigen–antibody reaction. Symptoms may be mild, moderate, severe and life-threatening. Pre-infusion hydrocortisone and/ or antihistamines may be prescribed to prevent life-threatening complications.

MAB-associated systemic and cutaneous adverse events can also lead to cardiac events. Trastuzumab is associated with cardiac dysfunction including cardiomyopathy, ventricular dysfunction, arrhythmias and acute coronary syndromes such as myocardial infarction. Regular cardiac screening is commonly undertaken.

Scenario

Frances asks you about why she was not offered Herceptin as treatment for her breast cancer. You are aware that trastuzumab is a MAB and check Frances's pathology report for the HER2 status of her breast cancer cells.

The report states:

Oestrogen and progesterone receptor status is positive and HER2 staining is negative.

Activity 5.5   Critical thinking

Drawing on the information about biological therapies and your understanding of HER2 receptor status, how might you respond to Frances's question in the scenario above?

A suggested answer is given at the end of the chapter.

Conclusion

As there are more than 200 different types of cancer, cancer can affect people in many different ways. Understanding the process of carcinogenesis can help you understand how a normal cell becomes a cancer cell and acquires the capabilities known as the hallmarks of cancer. We can also understand why people develop the signs and symptoms that they experience, and how drugs such as hormones, chemotherapy, biological therapies and other interventions are used to treat, manage or palliate cancer and its effects. We have identified the risk factors for cancer and the strategies for prevention and early detection of the four most common cancers in the UK. The discussion demonstrates the significance of understanding cancer biology and the development of personalised treatment through the use of biological therapies to enhance the survival and limit the side-effects of drugs experienced by people affected by cancer.

It is now time to review what you have learned within this chapter by undertaking some multiple choice questions.

Activity 5.6   Multiple choice questions

1. Cancer is a group of diseases characterised by:

   a) Unregulated cell growth
   b) Invasion into surrounding tissues
   c) Spread to distant organs/sites
   d) All of the above

2. The four most common cancers in the UK are:

   a) Lung, colorectal, prostate, breast
   b) Skin, lung, colorectal, prostate

(Continued)

(Continued)

   c) Lung, stomach, prostate, breast

   d) Breast, colorectal, prostate, lymphoma

3. The cell cycle:

   a) Regulates cell growth and proliferation

   b) Is reversible

   c) Has 7 phases

   d) Does not include gaps

4. Mutations in proto-oncogenes lead to:

   a) Over-activity of the gene

   b) Formation of an oncogene

   c) Promotion of cell proliferation

   d) All of the above

5. Mutations of tumour suppressor genes:

   a) Leads to gain of function

   b) Needs to occur in both copies of the gene in cancer

   c) Leads to the formation of an oncogene

   d) Cannot be inherited

6. *p53* gene:

   a) Is a tumour suppressor gene

   b) Produces p53 protein

   c) Is called the 'guardian of the genome'

   d) Is all of the above

7. *BRCA1* and *BRCA2* genes:

   a) Are proto-oncogenes

   b) Are tumour suppressor genes

   c) Are implicated in familial colorectal cancer

   d) Produce growth factors

8. Angiogenesis:

   a) Stops blood vessel development

   b) Stops metastases

   c) Is a tumour marker

   d) Requires vascular endothelial growth factor (VEGF)

9. Radiotherapy:

   a) Only targets cancer cells

   b) Is a localised treatment

   c) Uses ionising radiation

   d) Is a palliative treatment

10. Trastazumab:

    a) Is a biological therapy

    b) Acts on the HER2 receptor

    c) Is associated with cardiac dysfunction

    d) Is all of the above

Chapter summary

In this chapter we have:

- Described what cancer is, the process of carcinogenesis and how cancer cells differ from normal cells.
- Explained the role of proto-oncogenes and tumour suppressor genes in cell growth and how mutations in these genes can lead to unregulated cell growth.
- Described the hallmarks of cancer cells.
- Described how cancer cells are graded and how cancers are staged to inform the selection of cancer treatment.
- Explained the pharmacological treatment options available for cancer including chemotherapy and biological therapies.

Activities: Brief outline answers

Activity 5.4 Critical thinking (p135)

The TNM staging for Frances is T2N0M0.

The report states that the maximum tumour dimension is 22 mm (T2). No evidence of vascular or lymphatic permeation. Both in situ and invasive carcinoma are completely excised by a 5 mm margin. None of the lymph nodes contains tumour (N0). Assuming no metastases are identified (M0).

Activity 5.5 Critical thinking (p143)

Frances's report identifies that HER2 staining is negative. As a targeted therapy, Frances's cancer would not respond to trastazumab, but should respond to the prescribed Tamoxifen as her tumour is oestrogen receptor positive.

Activity 5.6 Multiple choice questions (pp143–5)

1. Cancer is a group of diseases characterised by:

    a) Unregulated cell growth

2. The four most common cancers in the UK are:

    a) Lung, colorectal, prostate, breast

3. The cell cycle

    a) Regulates cell growth and proliferation

4. Mutations in proto-oncogenes lead to:

    d) All of the above

5. Mutations of tumour suppressor genes:

    b) Needs to occur in both copies of the gene in cancer

6. *p53* gene:

    d) Is all of the above

7. *BRCA1* and *BRCA2* genes:

    b) Are tumour suppressor genes

8. Angiogenesis:

    d) Requires vascular endothelial growth factor (VEGF)

9. Radiotherapy:

    c) Uses ionising radiation

10. Trastazumab:

    d) Is all of the above

Further reading and useful websites

http://learn.genetics.utah.edu/content/basics/

This 'tour the basics' website provides an excellent, interactive introduction to genetics. It is from the Genetic Science Learning Site from the University of Utah. We strongly recommend this for understanding genes, DNA and chromosomes from the beginning.

www.cancerresearchuk.org/cancer-info/cancerstats/

CRUK website provides a wealth of information about cancer – including the latest statistics for different cancers and information for professionals.

www.cancerresearchuk.org/sites/default/files/state_of_the_nation_apr_2018_v2_0.pdf/

CRUK 2018 Cancer in the UK.

www.cancerresearchuk.org/health-professional/cancer-statistics-for-the-uk/

CRUK 2018 Cancer statistics for the UK.

www.cancerresearchuk.org/health-professional/cancer-statistics/childrens-cancers/

CRUK 2018 Children's cancer statistics.

Section 2 Protective mechanisms

Chapter 6　Pain

Chapter aims

After reading this chapter, you will be able to:

- explain the protective function of pain;
- describe the sensory and emotional aspects of pain;
- explain how nerve impulses arise from 'noxious' stimuli and how these impulses are conveyed to the brain;
- describe how pain can be modulated;
- apply a knowledge of pain physiology to pain assessment;
- describe the different drugs used for treating pain, their mechanisms of actions and the common adverse effects.

Introduction

Almost 10 million Britons suffer pain daily resulting in a major impact on their quality of life and more days off work.

(British Pain Society, 2014)

The International Association for the Study of Pain (IASP, 2014) recognises that nurses play a critical role in effective pain management because they have frequent contact with patients in a variety of settings (including home, hospital, outpatient clinic and community). This frequent contact will place you as the nurse in a unique position to identify patients who have pain and to perform a comprehensive pain assessment. This assessment should include the impact of pain on the patient and the patient's family members. You will then be able to initiate actions to manage the pain and evaluate the effectiveness of the pain management.

An understanding of the physiology of pain and its pharmacological treatments have been recognised as pivotal for nurses to make an appropriate assessment of the patient and to manage pain effectively. With this in mind, this chapter introduces you to the physiology of pain and its pharmacological treatments. We start the chapter by examining the nature of pain as a sensory and emotional experience. The nature of pain is developed further by examining the physiology of pain and the body's own **endogenous** pain inhibiting systems. We will examine pain assessment and the pharmacological treatment of pain using the World Health Organization Analgesic Ladder (WHO, 2010). You will then be in a position to understand the correct use of analgesics, their sites and mechanisms of action.

What is pain?

On a physiological level, pain is an unpleasant sensation that alerts us to injury or to the presence of a potentially injurious stimulus. For example, pain may prevent someone putting weight on a twisted ankle. Accidently touching a hot saucepan causes an immediate reflex withdrawal of the arm, preventing damage to the hand. Interestingly, this reflex occurs a fraction of a second before we have consciously experienced the pain.

Pain as a sensation is protective, providing important information about our environment (the presence of a hot saucepan) or about tissue injury (such as a twisted ankle). Pain also affects us emotionally. For example, an undiagnosed pain can be very worrying; it may make us irritable or anxious. Our emotional experience of pain can affect our behaviour. We may avoid particular activities including work or socialising.

It is important to appreciate that the sensory and emotional aspects of pain can arise without any apparent cause. By 'apparent cause', it is usually meant 'without any apparent tissue injury'. People with clinical depression often describe themselves as in pain. This is a clear example of the emotional aspect of pain and of pain experienced in the absence of tissue damage.

These features of pain are captured in the International Association for the Study of Pain's influential definition of pain:

> *Pain is an unpleasant sensory and emotional experience associated with actual or potential tissue damage, or described in terms of such damage.*

> (IASP, 2012)

This definition is particularly powerful because it captures not only the physiological nature of pain (as an unpleasant sensation) but also the emotional aspect of pain. The emotional experiences that accompany pain remind us that pain is a cause of suffering. This is especially so when the pain is chronic. The IASP definition also reminds us that pain can be experienced even in the absence of tissue injury.

Scenario

You are a nurse in the accident and emergency department when Lola, a 15-year-old girl, presents with a painful and swollen wrist. Whilst making an assessment of Lola, you discover the cause of her injury. Lola explains that she was on her skateboard going downhill at speed. Suddenly, the front wheels of the skateboard became stuck in a gap between paving flagstones and came to an abrupt stop. Lola explains that she fell onto her outstretched right arm and heard a sharp 'crack'. She felt an immediate, acute, severe pain in her right forearm.

You examine Lola's arm. There is no broken skin but there is tenderness, swelling and some bruising. Lola's injury is consistent with her account of the accident.

You ask Lola to rate her pain on a scale of one to ten, with ten being the worst possible pain. Lola rates her pain as 'eight'. She is given paracetamol and opioid analgesia. After 30 minutes you reassess Lola's pain which she reports as now 'two'. An X-ray shows an incomplete fracture of the radius with little displacement of the bone. Lola's arm was immobilised in a cast for five weeks.

We will use the scenario described above to illustrate the physiology of **nociceptive pain** in the subsequent sections of this chapter. Lola's pain is a typical example of nociceptive pain. Nociceptive pain refers to pain brought about by the activation of **pain fibres**. Pain fibres are the ends of specialised **nerve fibres** and are located around the body. Pain fibres are given the name **nociceptors**, to distinguish them from other sensory fibres such as those for touch. Nociceptors are so-called because they detect 'noxious' or tissue-damaging stimuli.

Nociceptive pain occurs as a protective, physiological response to tissue injury or to stimuli that could cause tissue damage. As such, nociceptive pain is a normal protective response. There is a second type of pain called **neuropathic pain** which is due to damage to the nerve fibres themselves. Neuropathic pain can occur as a long-term complication of diabetes (Chapter 12), or following damage to the **spinal cord** or brain such as in a stroke. In the sections below, we describe the physiology of nociceptive pain.

The physiology of nociceptive pain

We will divide the following account of nociceptive pain into four parts:

1. *Nociception*: the conversion of noxious stimuli into nerve impulses by nociceptors.
2. *Transmission*: the movement of nerve impulses along defined pathways to reach the brain.

3. *Perception*: the conscious experience of pain which arises through stimulation of higher brain centres.

4. *Modulation*: an increase or decrease in our perception of pain. We will introduce the gate control theory to explain this.

1. Nociception

Pain, like other sensations (such as touch, taste, smell), arises from activity in the nervous system. Pain is experienced when specific areas of the brain are activated by incoming 'pain messages'. Pain-causing stimuli, such as high temperature or intense pressure, are detected by the ends of nociceptors. Nociceptors are located in most tissues of the body (but not in the central nervous system). The best understood nociceptors are those in the skin and form the basis of the description below.

There is a relatively high number of nociceptors in the skin compared to other areas of the body. This may be expected as the skin is the barrier between the body and the outside world, which is where most damaging assaults to the body originate. Each pain fibre is a single nerve cell, or neurone (Figure 6.1). One end of the nociceptor is located in the skin where it detects pain stimuli. The axon of the pain fibre travels within a **spinal nerve** to reach the spinal cord. The **cell body** of the pain fibre is located in the **dorsal root ganglion**. The dorsal root ganglion is a swelling in the spinal nerve close to where it meets the spinal cord. Pain fibres end in the **dorsal horn** of the spinal cord where they connect with other neurones (Figure 6.2).

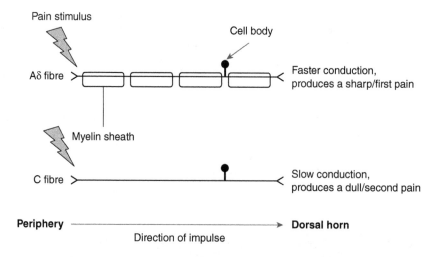

There are two types of pain fibre: Aδ and C. Aδ fibres are wider than C fibres and have a myelin sheath. They conduct nerve impulses faster than C fibres. Aδ fibres respond to intense pressure and produce a 'first', sharp pain. C fibres are thinner and are not myelinated. They conduct impulses more slowly. They respond to inflammatory chemicals and produce a 'second', dull aching pain.

Figure 6.1 Nociceptors (pain fibres)

It is important to note that each spinal nerve carries thousands of nerve fibres. Only some of these fibres carry pain information. Others carry information about touch, pressure and temperature. Yet other fibres carry nerve impulses in the opposite direction to the skeletal muscles for movement.

The endings of nociceptors in the skin can be activated by three types of stimuli:

(i) *Temperature:* a very hot (> 45°C) or a very cold (< 5°C) stimulus can activate nociceptors. Examples include touching a hot pan or putting your hand in a bucket of ice.

(ii) *Intense pressure:* this might include treading on a drawing pin or slicing your finger in a blender (as happened to Ruby in Chapter 2).

(iii) *Certain chemicals:* you will have experienced pain from a chemical source if you have accidently rubbed chilli powder in your eye. The skin itself is a fairly good protection against chemicals. The most important chemicals stimulating nociceptors come from within the body and are those released from damaged tissues. These are termed inflammatory mediators (Chapter 2; Table 2.2). Of these two types, bradykinins and prostaglandins stimulate nociceptors and cause pain.

Within the skin some pain fibres only detect intense pressure; some only detect very hot or very cold stimuli. Others can detect extremes of temperature and inflammatory chemicals. Each pain fibre contains receptors in their cell membrane. These receptors are **ion channels** which open when stimulated by one of the three types of pain stimuli. Once open the ion channels allow sodium (Na^+) and calcium (Ca^{2+}) ions to flow through the membrane into the cell. The movement of these ions into the cell can generate a nerve impulse (or **action potential**). This process of converting a stimulus into an electrical nerve impulse is called signal transduction (Chapter 1). In respect of pain stimuli which activate nociceptors, the process is called **nociception.**

You may have noticed that a few minutes after experiencing a painful injury the pain increases in intensity. The area around the injury may also feel tender. This increase in pain and tenderness is known as hyperalgesia. It is due to the action of inflammatory chemicals released from damaged cells and the nerve endings themselves. The inflammatory chemicals 'sensitise' the nerve endings of pain fibres making them more responsive to pain stimuli. An important family of inflammatory mediators that sensitise pain fibres are the prostaglandins.

We met prostaglandins in Chapter 2, where we noted that prostaglandins are released from damaged cells, macrophages and neutrophils during an inflammatory response. Prostaglandins are formed from arachidonic acid which is a component of the phospholipid molecules which make up the cell membrane. Some of the phospholipids in the cell membrane in response to inflammatory stimuli are be converted to arachidonic acid by the enzyme phospholipase. Arachidonic acid is then converted to prostaglandins by cyclooxygenase enzymes (COXs). We will see shortly, under 'Non-steroidal anti-inflammatory drugs (NSAIDs)', that NSAIDs act by inhibiting the COX enzyme and so reduce prostaglandin synthesis.

$$\text{Phospholipid} \xrightarrow{\textit{phospholipase}} \text{arachidonic acid} \xrightarrow{\textit{cyclooxygenases (COXs)}} \text{prostaglandins}$$

Prostaglandins bind to receptors on the nerve endings of pain fibres and lower the threshold for activation. This means the pain fibres 'fire' at greater frequency (send out more nerve impulses) causing more pain messages to reach the brain.

Injury to skin, muscle or bone causes an immediate fast, sharp pain, followed seconds later by a dull, aching sensation. This is accounted for by the presence of two types of pain fibre in the skin and somatic tissues: A-delta (Aδ) and C which have a different structure (Figure 6.1). Aδ fibres conduct nerve impulses at a relatively fast speed. These produce an immediate or 'first pain' sensation which is sharp and well-localised. C fibres conduct the nerve impulse at a relatively slow speed; these produce a 'second' dull, aching pain.

Scenario

Whilst assessing Lola's fractured wrist as a nurse in accident and emergency, you make a mental picture of what has caused Lola's pain.

You are aware that bones, including Lola's radius, are covered with a fibrous sheath, the periosteum. The periosteum is supplied with a large number of Aδ pain fibres. The intense pressure causing Lola's radius to fracture will have activated many of these Aδ fibres. This will have caused Lola to have felt an immediate (or first) sharp pain, which will be well localised to the site of the fracture. Moments later Lola may have experienced a second dull pain from C fibres stimulated by inflammatory chemicals released from the damaged bone.

You are aware that the current tenderness Lola is experiencing in the affected area is due to an inflammatory response and she is likely to be experiencing hyperalgesia. You take great care not to touch the damaged area unnecessarily.

Following this scenario we look at how pain messages are transmitted to the brain.

2. Transmission

Nerve impulses generated through nociception reach the brain in a matter of milliseconds. Figure 6.2 shows the pathway by which Aδ and C fibres enter the spinal cord through the dorsal root of the spinal nerve and synapse in the dorsal horn of the spinal cord.

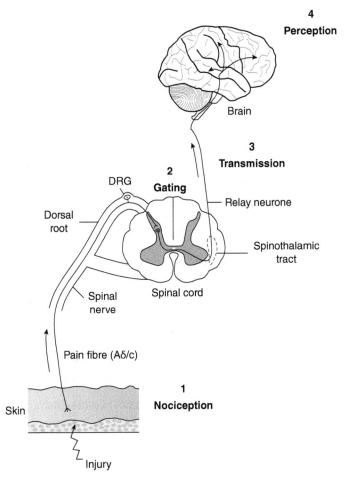

The figure shows the pathway of pain impulses from the skin to the brain. A pain fibre and a relay neurone are shown. DRG = Dorsal root ganglion

Figure 6.2 The pain pathway

Synaptic transmission

To fully understand pain transmission and **pain modulation** you will need to know about synaptic transmission (Figure 6.3). This is the process by which a nerve signal is passed on from one neurone to another across a microscopic gap called the synapse. We introduced the synapse and the role of neurotransmitters in Chapter 1.

The result of synaptic transmission is to increase or decrease the probability that the post-synaptic neurone will fire a nerve impulse, or action potential. If binding of the neurotransmitter makes the post-synaptic neurone more likely to fire, the neurotransmitter is described as excitatory. By contrast, if binding of the neurotransmitter makes the post-synaptic neurone less likely to fire, the neurotransmitter is described

(Continued)

(Continued)

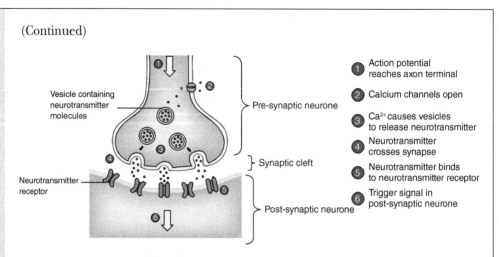

Vesicle containing neurotransmitter molecules

Neurotransmitter receptor

Pre-synaptic neurone

Synaptic cleft

Post-synaptic neurone

1 Action potential reaches axon terminal

2 Calcium channels open

3 Ca^{2+} causes vesicles to release neurotransmitter

4 Neurotransmitter crosses synapse

5 Neurotransmitter binds to neurotransmitter receptor

6 Trigger signal in post-synaptic neurone

Figure 6.3 Synaptic transmission

as inhibitory. Whether a neurotransmitter is excitatory or inhibitory depends upon the nature of the receptor. Many neurotransmitter receptors are ion channels. Binding of an excitatory neurotransmitter, such as glutamate, to its receptor will open the ion channel and ions (usually Na^+) will flow into the cell. This makes the post-synaptic neurone more likely to produce an action potential.

Endorphins are inhibitory neurotransmitters important in reducing pain transmission. Endorphins work by binding to the pre-synaptic neurone near the axon terminal. This has the effect of decreasing the amount of neurotransmitter (e.g. glutamate) released by the pre-synaptic neurone (Rang et al., 2015).

In the dorsal horn, the nerve endings of Aδ and C fibres release two main neurotransmitters: glutamate and substance P, which are excitatory. Release of these neurotransmitters excite **relay neurones** within the dorsal horn. The relay neurones cross over to the opposite side of the spinal cord. They then travel in specific **white matter tracts** of the spinal cord to eventually reach sites in the brainstem and midbrain (the thalamus).

The junction or synapse between Aδ or C fibres and the relay neurones in the dorsal horn has been identified as a possible 'pain gate' – where pain messages may be blocked. This pain gate forms an important part of the gate control theory. We will come back to this under 'Modulation', below.

The white matter tract carrying most pain messages is called the spinothalamic tract. This carries nerve fibres to the thalamus. Before reaching the thalamus, some of the relay neurones send branches to various centres in the brainstem. These include the periaqueductal grey – a centre associated with descending pain modulation pathways and activation of the **sympathetic nervous system** and a '**fight or flight**' response is triggered (Cortelli et al., 2013).

3. Perception

Perception refers to the conscious experience of pain. From the thalamus pain signals are sent out to higher brain centres including the anterior cingulate cortex and the somatosensory cortex. It is through the activation of these higher centres that the perception of pain occurs. Figure 6.4 shows some of the brain areas activated by pain signals, including the higher brains areas associated with pain perception.

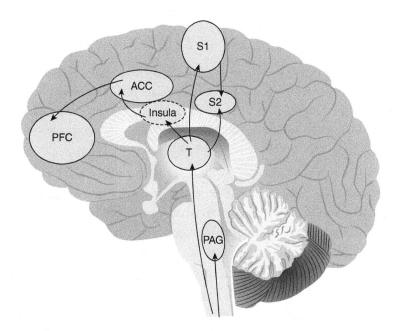

Our understanding of the brain areas activated in the experience of pain come largely from neuroimaging studies. There is no single 'pain area' which processes pain messages. Instead there is a highly complex network of areas involved. Pain messages ascend the spinal cord to the brain. En route, a subset of messages activate an area of the brainstem called the periaqueductal grey (PAG). The PAG is associated with descending modulation of pain (see text under 'Descending modulation' for details). The thalamus (T) in the midbrain receives pain messages and relays these to higher areas of the brain, namely: the primary and secondary somatosensory cortex (S1, S2); the anterior cingulate cortex (ACC) and the insula. Activation of S1 and S2 are associated with the ability to localise the pain and describe the nature of the pain (for example, as stabbing, aching or shooting). Messages are also relayed to the anterior cingulate cortex (ACC) and insula. The ACC is associated with the emotional or 'aversive' aspects of pain (Xiao and Zhang, 2018); whereas activity in the insula reflects 'How much the pain hurts' (Segerdahl et al., 2014). The prefrontal cortex (PFC) has a role in attentional processing of pain and may in addition be associated with pain modulating pathways (Lorenz, 2007).

Figure 6.4 Brain areas activated during the experience of pain

We can see from Figure 6.4 that many areas of the brain are activated in response to pain. There is no single brain area responsible for pain. This accords well with the multi-dimensional nature of the experience of pain. For example, and simplifying from very complex functional neuroimaging studies, activation of a region of the cortex called the anterior cingulate cortex (ACC) and the insula are associated with the 'emotional and motivational' aspects of pain (Vogt, 2005; Segerdahl et al.,

2015) including the 'unpleasantness' or 'suffering' aspects of persistent pain. These regions of the brain form part of the 'emotional brain', or limbic system (MacLean, 1990) and are associated with other emotions, such as fear, happiness and sadness. The somatosensory cortex is associated with the 'sensory-discriminative' aspects of pain. These aspects of pain include the intensity of the pain, how the pain feels (for example, stabbing, shooting or aching) and its location (site from which the pain is arising). The scenario below describes Lola's experience of pain.

Scenario

Whilst assessing Lola in A&E you note that her heart rate and blood pressure are slightly raised and her skin feels damp. You appreciate that pain messages will have stimulated a 'fight or flight' response in Lola. Sympathetic fibres to her heart and blood vessels will have increased her heart rate and caused her blood pressure to rise. Fibres to the skin will have caused Lola to perspire.

You are aware that Lola will have perceived pain when her somatosensory cortex and anterior cingulate cortex were activated by pain signals. Activation of her somatosensory cortex caused the sensation of a sharp stabbing pain, followed by a dull, aching pain. This sensation was easy to localise – it was clearly coming from her fractured right wrist.

Activation of Lola's anterior cingulate cortex produced an emotional response: Lola's arm hurt a lot and she was initially very upset and frightened. However, once Lola's pain subsided with the analgesia she became less upset. You were able to reassure her that her wrist would heal within a matter of months and that she would still be able to access social media using her left hand. Feeling reassured and feeling the effects of the analgesia, Lola no longer felt upset. Addressing the emotional impact of pain is a very important part of pain management.

In the scenario above, you can see how Lola's experience of pain changed – not only through the analgesia but through being reassured about her injury. This change in pain perception is called modulation. In the section below we discuss modulation of pain using the gate control theory.

4. Modulation

Our perception of pain is influenced by many factors. At one extreme, some people experience stress-induced analgesia. Here, a person does not feel pain despite the presence of an injury. Even in less extreme cases, the pain experienced is always a result of a complex interaction of sensory and emotional factors.

Activity 6.1   Reflection

Think of the worst pain you have ever experienced, and the circumstances surrounding it. What made this experience so painful? Can you think of an example where something should have been very painful, but it wasn't particularly?

This is a personal reflection but we have made some possible suggestions at the end of the chapter.

Activity 6.1 will enable you to appreciate the factors and circumstances that influence our experience of pain. These factors are said to 'modulate' pain. Understanding how pain is modulated is a very important part of pain management.

To account for how the many different factors alter our experience of pain, Ronald Melzack and Patrick Wall published 'the gate control theory of pain' (Melzack and Wall, 1965). They argued that the transmission of pain impulses could be decreased at the dorsal horn of the spinal cord. Specifically, they proposed the existence of a 'gate' in the dorsal horn that 'opens' or 'closes' to increase or decrease the number of pain messages reaching the brain (Figure 6.4). This gate would be 'opened' by tissue injury but 'closed' by other factors including the psychological state of the patient, massaging the painful area or analgesia.

The gate control theory significantly altered the way we think about pain. Pain is no longer seen as the result of a straightforward pain pathway taking pain impulses from the site of injury to the brain. Perception of pain is viewed as heavily modified by activity in the dorsal horn. Nursing care can influence this through administration of analgesia as well as emotional, informational and physical support of the person in pain.

The gate control theory proposes two main ways that pain can be modulated at the dorsal horn:

(i) Segmental or counter-stimulation. The gate is 'closed' through massage or transcutaneous electrical nerve stimulation (TENS).

(ii) Descending modulation. The gate is 'closed' through nerve impulses coming from the brain.

Segmental or counter-stimulation

Massaging the skin over the injured area can help reduce pain. Massage stimulates 'touch fibres' (Aβ fibres). Nerve impulses from Aβ fibres travel to the dorsal horn at the same 'segmental' level of the spinal cord as the incoming pain messages. The spinal cord is divided into segments (C1-S5) with each segment receiving a spinal nerve from each side of the body. The incoming Aβ fibres reduce the transmission of impulses from C fibres to the relay neurones (Figure 6.5).

This is also the basis of the TENS machine used to help relieve pain (see Activity 6.2).

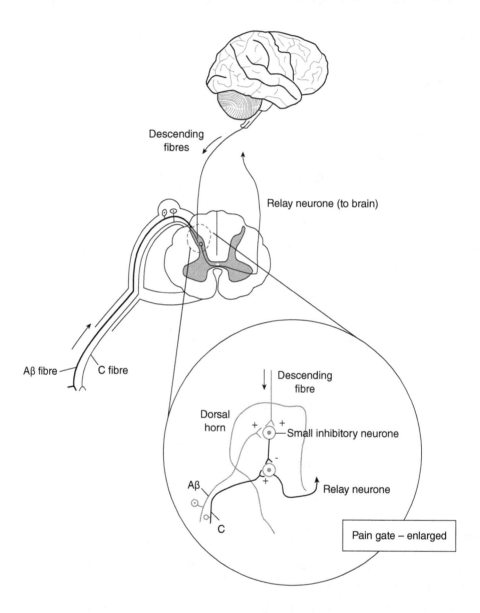

The figure shows how Aβ touch fibres from the skin travel into the dorsal horn with C pain fibres. Descending fibres from the brain end at the same point in the dorsal horn. This is the location of the pain gate.

The smaller diagram shows the detail of the pain gate. Aβ and descending fibres both activate a small inhibitory neurone. This inhibitory neurone reduces activity of the relay neurone. By contrast the C pain fibres activate the relay neurone. The balance of these opposing effects determines the number of pain messages reaching the brain.

Figure 6.5 The pain gate

Activity 6.2   Critical thinking

Transcutaneous electrical nerve stimulation (TENS) for pain relief was a direct development of the gate control theory of pain. TENS is hypothesised to work according to the segmental or counter-stimulation modulation of pain. Electrodes placed on the skin deliver an electric current to stimulate nerve fibres in the skin that synapse in the spinal cord at the same segmental level as the active pain fibres. Using your understanding of the gate control theory (in relation to segmental or counter-stimulation modulation), explain a possible mechanism by which TENS might help reduce pain.

An answer is provided at the end of the chapter.

Activity 6.2 enabled you to apply your understanding of pain modulation by segmental or counter-stimulation. We now look at **descending modulation**.

Descending modulation

The gate control theory predicts that our psychological state can affect how we experience pain. Our psychological state includes our mood, our level of attention to the pain and our anxieties over the pain. It is believed that these psychological factors help reduce pain by activating nerve pathways from the brain to the dorsal horn (Figure 6.5).

These nerve pathways have their nerve endings in the dorsal horn where they release a number of neurotransmitters that inhibit synaptic transmission between the C fibres and the relay neurones. These neurotransmitters include: **endorphins**, serotonin and **noradrenaline**. Opioid analgesics and tramadol act to mimic the effect of these neurotransmitters and so block transmission in the dorsal horn. We will return to these under 'Management of pain: pharmacological interventions'.

Pain assessment

To be able to manage pain effectively it is essential to undertake a comprehensive, holistic assessment. This will enable the multi-professional team to identify the cause(s) of pain, the factors that are influencing the pain, the impact of pain for the patient and the most appropriate treatment and care.

The physiology of pain offers a multi-dimensional explanation for the individual experience of pain. Pain assessment should include the sensory dimension of pain; the emotional response of the patient to the pain, and how it impacts on a person's ability to function and participate in society. Whilst it is beyond the scope of this chapter to review all aspects of pain assessment and the use of pain assessment tools, Activity 6.3 will help you consider the importance of multi-dimensional pain assessment.

Activity 6.3   Critical thinking

Pain assessment

In clinical practice, you are asked to assess your patient's pain. Frank is a 66-year-old with a 1-year history of prostate cancer. The prostate cancer is being treated with hormone therapy. He has been admitted to the medical ward complaining of severe back pain. Consider what questions you might ask, observations you might make and information you might need to find out about Frank to assess each dimension of his pain. Use the table below to help you.

Pain assessment: Frank		
Past history		
Previous treatment		
Observations		
Dimension of pain:	**Components to be assessed:**	**What questions might you ask:**
Sensory	Pain intensity Location Character ('what the pain feels like')	
Emotional	Relations with others Enjoyment of life Mood	
Impact on daily activities	Sleep Walking General activity Working	

In order to help with this, you might find the questions on the following pain assessment tool useful: **www.npcrc.org/files/news/briefpain_short.pdf/**

Suggested answers are given at the end of the chapter.

Types of pain

Patients' descriptions of 'what their pain feels like' – its character – alongside your understanding of their past and current medical history and treatment are important for identifying the type of pain the patient is experiencing. Earlier in the chapter we identified pain as nociceptive and neuropathic. There are different pain types within the broad groups of nociceptive and neuropathic based on where in the body the pain is felt. Nociceptive pain can include: **visceral** and somatic. These are summarised in Table 6.1. All types of pain can be either acute or chronic. The pain types can be felt at the same time or singly and at different times.

Type of pain	Key features	Description	Response to opioids
Nociceptive pain – somatic (soft tissue)	Somatic pain is caused by the activation of pain receptors in either the body surface or musculoskeletal tissues. Somatic pain is caused by a combination of factors, such as inflammation, repetitive trauma, excessive activity, vigorous stretching, and contractions due to paralysis, spasticity, disuse and misuse.	Localised ache, throbbing, gnawing. Can be aggravated by activity and relieved by rest.	Good: > 80% pain control easily achievable by non-opioid/opioid.
Nociceptive pain – somatic (bone pain)		Well-localised, aching pain, local tenderness. Worse on movement. Somatic tissues are supplied by a high density of Aδ fibres and C fibres making it easy to localise.	Variable response to opioids. NSAIDs + non-opioid/opioid often more effective. In cancer – radiotherapy may be important treatment option.
Nociceptive pain – visceral	Visceral pain arises from damage or distension of internal organs (or viscera). It is the most common form of pain. Visceral pain includes pain from the stomach, kidneys, gallbladder, urinary bladder and intestines. Visceral pain is often 'referred' to the surface of the body. For example, pain from myocardial infarction is often felt as radiating to the neck, jaw and down the left arm.	Visceral pain is vague, not well localised. It is usually described as pressure-like, deep squeezing, dull or diffuse. The viscera are supplied by C fibres. These are at low density making visceral pain hard to localise.	Good: > 80% pain control easily achievable by non-opioid/opioid.
Neuropathic	Neuropathic pain is caused by injury to the brain, spinal cord or peripheral nerves. This type of pain usually occurs within days, weeks or months of the injury and tends to occur in waves of frequency and intensity.	Neuropathic pain is typically a burning, tingling, shooting, stinging or 'pins and needles' sensation. Some people also complain of a stabbing, piercing, cutting and drilling pain.	Often poor response to non-opioids/opioids: management of poor opioid-responsive pain may include a variety of treatments involving adjuvant analgesic drugs and non-drug measures including steroids, NSAIDs, anticonvulsants, antidepressants, TENS.

Table 6.1 Pain types

Table 6.1 also highlights that the different types of pain respond differently to the various analgesics. If the type of pain and its causes are not identified accurately it will not be possible for the appropriate medication to be prescribed. We know from clinical practice that particular types of pain can be responsive, partially responsive or are poorly response to opioid-type drugs. For some pain types a combination of drugs is required to manage the pain effectively. Identifying the pain type will, therefore, help you to select which analgesia, or combination of drugs, the pain is most likely to respond to and help the patient to have reduced pain or be pain-free as quickly as possible. Table 6.1 identifies the different types of pain, their key features and response to non-opioids and opioids. We discuss the pharmacological interventions in more detail in the next section.

Management of pain: pharmacological interventions

This section provides you with an introduction to the pharmacological interventions for pain management. You have seen from Table 6.1 that the type of pain has a significant impact on the choice of analgesics. To assist clinical decision-making and a logical approach to treatment decisions, analgesics are broadly classified into three groups:

1. Non-opioid analgesics – this includes paracetamol, aspirin and non-steroidal anti-inflammatory drugs (NSAIDs).

2. Opioids – in clinical practice, this group may be further divided into 'weak opioids' (for mild to moderate pain) and 'strong opioids' (for moderate to severe pain). This distinction is, however, based on the international implementation of the World Health Organization Analgesic Ladder rather than pharmacological considerations.

3. Adjuvant analgesics – a group of drugs whose primary purpose or design was not as an analgesic but they do have analgesic effects in particular clinical circumstances. These include steroids, anxiolytics, antidepressants and anticonvulsants.

Effective pain management should be guided by the World Health Organization Analgesic Ladder. This is explained below.

World Health Organization Analgesic Ladder

In 1986, the WHO published a set of guidelines regarding the use of analgesics in treating cancer pain. It described a three-step approach of sequential use of drugs commensurate with the level of pain as reported by the patient. This is known as the WHO Analgesic Ladder and is shown in Figure 6.6.

This stepwise concept with practical recommendations has been widely adopted as a standard for pain management. Moving up from no treatment, the original model starts with non-opioids (for example aspirin, paracetamol or non-steroidal anti-inflammatory drugs (NSAIDs) for mild pain), then increasing to weak opioids like codeine as the second step for intermediate level pain. Finally, strong opioids like morphine, fentanyl and methadone are the third step for severe pain. Activity 6.4 aims to show you how the stepwise approach can work in practice.

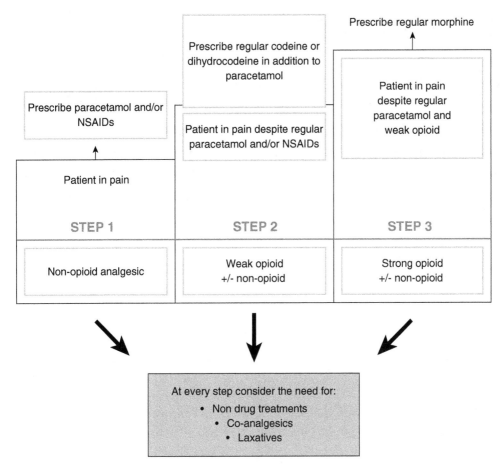

Figure 6.6   The WHO Analgesic Ladder

Activity 6.4   Decision-making

You work in a nursing home. One of the residents is an elderly man called Kenneth who suffers from lower back pain. You regularly administer paracetamol 1 g four times a day to manage the pain. Until recently this had kept the pain well managed. However recently Kenneth has told you he is in pain. Considering the WHO Analgesic Ladder, which pharmacological treatments might be an option for Kenneth?

A suggested answer is given at the end of the chapter.

It is not possible to provide a fully comprehensive account of every analgesic available here. You are reminded to consult formularies for more specific detail about doses, adverse effects and interactions as well as regional, national and international clinical guidelines to aid your clinical decision-making.

Non-opioid analgesics

Paracetamol

Paracetamol is a well-known analgesic and antipyretic (fever reducing) drug with little anti-inflammatory activity. It is a very useful drug when used regularly (that is, four times a day).

The mechanism by which paracetamol produces its effects is undefined. It relieves pain but does not significantly reduce inflammation. Side-effects from paracetamol are uncommon with usual doses although some nausea might occur. In overdose, paraceta-mol is very toxic to the liver. This is because the usual metabolic pathways, which convert paracetamol into more water soluble metabolites, become overloaded by excess amounts of paracetamol. As a result toxic metabolites are formed which damage the liver.

In general, paracetamol causes few clinically relevant drug interactions. These can be found in Appendix 1 of the British National Formulary.

Non-steroidal anti-inflammatory drugs (NSAIDs)

As their name suggests this group of analgesics have anti-inflammatory properties as well as pain relieving properties. The name sets them apart from another group of drugs with powerful anti-inflammatory properties: the steroids (Chapter 2), hence the non-steroidal part. The group includes drugs such as ibuprofen, diclofenac, aspirin and naproxen. These drugs have very different chemical structures but all act in the same way and all have similar side-effects.

As we saw earlier in the chapter, prostaglandins help to sensitise nerve endings to pain. The NSAIDs work by blocking the synthesis of prostaglandins in the body by inhibiting enzymes called cyclooxygenases.

Side-effects and considerations for practice

Prostaglandins have many functions in the body in addition to their role in pain. Reducing the level of prostaglandins leads to some well-known side-effects and con-traindications to the use of NSAIDs. These are as follows:

- *Gastrointestinal ulcers:* NSAIDs can cause ulcers and should not be used in people with an active ulcer. Prostaglandins reduce acid secretion in the stomach therefore reducing prostaglandins with NSAIDs increases acid production. Prostaglandins are also important in producing the mucus which helps to protect the gastric mucosa. Therefore reducing prostaglandins increases the risk of gastric mucosa ulceration.

Taking the drugs with food only partially helps as the effect is systemic, that is, it is caused by the drug in the bloodstream. People at risk might be prescribed a 'proton pump inhibitor', such as lansoprazole, to counter this effect. The proton pump inhibitor works by reducing stomach acid production (Chapter 10).

- *Worsening of asthma*: Prostaglandins help to keep the airways in the lungs open. Blocking prostaglandins in an asthmatic patient can lead to worsening asthma attacks in some, but not all, patients.
- *Impaired renal function*: Prostaglandins help maintain renal blood flow. In patients with impaired renal function, for example the elderly, blocking prostaglandins with an NSAID can lead to further renal impairment and even renal failure.

Although NSAID drugs are similar, with a common mechanism of action and similar side-effects, there are some differences. The risk of gastrointestinal effects such as ulcers varies, with ibuprofen believed to be 'kinder' on the gastrointestinal tract than others. Also people might get more pain relief from one NSAID than with another and a process of trial and error might be needed to find the right one.

NSAIDs can cause many drug interactions and these should always be checked in the British National Formulary as consequences may be severe. One important example is the interaction between methotrexate and NSAIDs. This does not occur in everyone, but in some individuals methotrexate toxicity is increased, possibly due to decreased renal excretion. Many other interactions can be explained by considering the adverse effects of NSAIDs. For example increased kidney toxicity occurs with other drugs that can also cause kidney toxicity such as ACE inhibitors and diuretics. Increased gastrointestinal bleeding and ulceration occurs with other drugs also causing ulcers or increased bleeding such as corticosteroids, selective serotonin reuptake inhibitor (SSRI) antidepressants (for example fluoxetine) and antiplatelet agents such as clopidogrel and warfarin.

Opioid analgesics

Morphine is the archetypal opioid analgesic. It comes from the opium poppy which has been used for medicinal purposes for thousands of years. Since the isolation of morphine from the opium poppy, many synthetic compounds with pain relieving properties have been developed. The collective term for these and any substance that produces morphine-like effects is opioid analgesics. Opioids are useful for many kinds of acute and chronic pain but they are less useful for neuropathic pain.

Opioids act as agonists at opioid receptors (Chapter 1) and there are three main types of receptor: *mu, delta* and *kappa*. Different opioids have differing affinities for each receptor which may help to explain their slightly different effects. Opioid receptors are widely distributed in the brain and spinal cord but also exist in the periphery. Stimulating these receptors reduces pain signals. As explained previously opioids act at the synapse of the dorsal horn and inhibit the transmission of impulses here. They also increase the firing of neurones in the inhibitory descending pathways which leads to a reduction in the transmission of pain signals to the brain. They affect higher brain centres and alter the conscious experience of pain. This might lead to a patient describing still feeling pain but caring much less about it.

There are many different opioids and they differ from each other in terms of potency, half-life and some side-effects. Different pain types have a variable response to non-opioids and opioids. In some patients even large doses of morphine may not control pain. In these cases a switch to another opioid, known as opioid rotation, might be of benefit. However not all pain is opioid sensitive. It would also be important to reassess the pain and consider the addition of a different type of analgesia.

Activity 6.5   Research

The pharmacokinetics and potencies of opioids vary and great care must be taken when switching routes of administration or switching opioid (Chapter 1).

a) Look at the 'Prescribing in palliative care' section in the front of the BNF. If a patient was prescribed Morphine MST Continus tablets 60 mg twice a day plus morphine oral solution 10 mg four times a day, what dose of subcutaneous diamorphine would this equate to?

b) 5 mg s/c morphine is equivalent to 3 mg of diamorphine. Is morphine more or less potent than diamorphine?

c) How does understanding the pharmacokinetics of morphine help to explain the difference in oral and parenteral doses?

A suggested answer is given at the end of the chapter.

Examples of different opioids

Morphine has a relatively short half-life which helps to explain why it needs to be given every 4 hours to maintain analgesia. Long-acting (slow release) formulations of morphine can be given less often; examples include MST Continus and Morphne XL. These medicines have been made in a special way (i.e. formulated) so that the morphine is absorbed more slowly from the GI tract into the blood stream and the effects last longer. You must check that you have selected the correct formulation before administering it to a patient.

Diamorphine. The actions and uses are similar to morphine. It is more soluble and so is especially useful for syringe drivers.

Methadone. This has a long half-life of 15–60 hours and is therefore much longer acting than morphine (which has a half-life of 2 hours). It is useful as opioid replacement therapy in addiction as supervised once daily dosing is possible. Euphoric effects are less than with morphine.

Fentanyl. Many formulations are available, for example, buccal tablets and patches, but nothing that can be swallowed. It undergoes extensive first pass metabolism which means that very little would reach the general circulation after an oral dose. Patches have been formulated to have a long duration of action and are applied every 72 hours.

Buprenorphine. Again first pass metabolism means it is often given sub-lingually where it is absorbed straight into the bloodstream from the blood vessels under the tongue. It can also be given as a patch. It is a partial agonist which means it has both agonist and antagonist (i.e. opioid blocking) properties. This can mean that giving it to a patient who is used to taking a pure agonist such as morphine may cause some withdrawal symptoms as it might block some of the effect.

Codeine. This is often described as a weak opioid and is more suitable for mild to moderate pain (step 2 in the WHO Analgesic Ladder). Constipation can be a major problem. In 2013 the MHRA advised that it should not be used in children under 12 due to increased toxicity in some children after surgery (Chapter 1). Codeine is really a pro-drug and is metabolised by the liver to the active metabolite morphine. Some people are ultra-rapid metabolisers and it is thought the children who had problems fell into this group. Conversely some people are poor metabolisers and do not get much analgesic effect from codeine.

Activity 6.6   Critical thinking

You are caring for a frail elderly patient with swallowing difficulties who is in acute pain. A colleague suggests you ask the doctor to prescribe a fentanyl patch. What problems might there be in choosing this as the first opioid the patient has had?

A suggested answer is given at the end of the chapter.

Side-effects and considerations for practice

Opioids are very powerful analgesics, but unfortunately they also have some problematic effects that can limit their use:

Constipation. Opioid receptors are present in the bowel. When opioids act on these receptors, gastrointestinal motility is reduced.

Nausea and vomiting. Opioids activate the chemoreceptors trigger zone in the brain inducing vomiting (Chapter 7). An anti-emetic drug may need to be given to prevent this. For example metoclopramide may be given when morphine or diamorphine is used for the pain associated with a myocardial infarction.

Respiratory depression. Too much opioid can stop a person breathing, which is usually the cause of death by opioid overdose. When breathing slows, carbon dioxide levels in the blood increase. This increased carbon dioxide is usually a signal to increase respiration. Opioids reduce the sensitivity of the brain's respiratory centre to carbon dioxide levels and therefore breathing is not stimulated as expected.

Euphoria or dysphoria: Euphoria describes an intense pleasurable feeling and is mediated mainly by mu receptors. Dysphoria is the opposite and mediated mainly by kappa receptors. This may explain why some opioids produce more euphoria and some more dysphoria.

Tolerance: During opioid consumption the body compensates by reducing the number of opioid receptors available. The amount of opioid needed for the same effect may therefore need to be increased over time. This tends to be most problematic when opioids are being abused. When they are used for pain, once the pain is stable, dose adjustment is not usually required. Increases might be needed if the pain changes or increases.

Physical dependence: Even after using opioids for pain, stopping them suddenly may cause withdrawal symptoms such as restlessness, runny nose, shivering and diarrhoea. The use of opioids results in changes to the central nervous system and these symptoms are the result of the body trying to rebalance itself once the opioid is stopped.

Addiction: In this case psychological dependence is more dominant. This tends to be less of a problem if opioids are used for cancer pain or acute pain. Fear of this can lead to underdosing patients or delaying the use of opioids when they are needed.

Opioids are known to be central nervous system depressants and as such may interact with other central nervous system depressants such as alcohol, antidepressants, benzodiazepines and antipsychotics. Severe drowsiness and reduced alertness may result. For a full list of interactions the British National Formulary should be consulted.

Research summary: Opioid use in chronic pain

Concerns have been expressed that prescribing opioids for chronic pain is on the rise and that this has been accompanied by an increase in deaths (Dhalla et al., 2011). Although there is clear evidence that opioids help with acute pain and cancer pain, much less is known about their effectiveness in chronic non-cancer pain (CNCP). Systematic reviews show few well designed long-term clinical trials, limited benefits and problematic side-effects (Freynhagen et al., 2013). In chronic pain, as well as a reduction in pain intensity, other factors are increasingly important such as sleep, mood, physical, vocational, social and emotional wellbeing. Opioids have not been proved to help with these.

As well as the side-effects previously listed, there are further problems that need consideration when opioids are prescribed long term. They can cause hormonal problems leading to adrenal insufficiency and infertility. Opioids also suppress the immune system, however, the clinical relevance of this is unclear (BPS, 2010). Surprisingly, opioids may also increase pain (hyperalgesia). This pain might feel different to the original pain, for example being more spread out around the body (BPS, 2010).

Tramadol

Tramadol is sometimes grouped together with opioid analgesics but there are some important differences. It was thought to be less addictive. However due to concerns that abuse of this drug was on the increase it is also classified as a controlled drug.

Tramadol is an agonist at opioid receptors but it also increases the neurotransmitters noradrenaline and serotonin. Some of the fibres that form part of the inhibitory descending pathways (mentioned previously under 'Modulation') release noradrenaline and serotonin at the 'gate' in the dorsal horn. This reduces pain transmission.

Side-effects and considerations for practice

Side-effects are similar to those caused by opioids. Common side-effects include dizziness, nausea, fatigue and headache.

Many interactions that occur with opioids also occur with Tramadol. In addition, as it also increases serotonin and noradrenaline, it can interact with other medicines that also increase these neurotransmitters. Examples include triptans used to treat migraine and antidepressants. A full list of interactions can be found in the British National Formulary. The next activity explores this interaction in more depth.

Activity 6.7   Research: Drug interactions

Look up the interaction between Tramadol and SSRI antidepressants in the most recent British National Formulary (BNF). What might happen if both are given together? Why does this interaction occur?

A suggested answer is given at the end of the chapter.

It is now time to review what you have learned within this chapter by undertaking some multiple choice questions.

Activity 6.8   Multiple choice questions

1. The physiology of nociceptive pain includes four stages: nociception, transmission, perception and modulation. Which of these is the conversion of a noxious stimulus into a nerve impulse?
   a) Nociception
   b) Transmission

(Continued)

(Continued)

    c) Perception

    d) Modulation

2. Which type of nerve fibre is associated with a slow, dull 'second' pain?

    a) α

    b) Aβ

    c) Aδ

    d) C

3. During an inflammatory response, which inflammatory mediators 'sensitise' nociceptors?

    a) Bradykinins

    b) Histamine

    c) Serotonin

    d) Prostaglandins

4. Pain arising from a 'pulled' muscle would be classified as:

    a) Nociceptive – somatic

    b) Nociceptive – visceral

    c) Neuropathic – somatic

    d) Neuropathic – visceral

5. Which type of pain tends to be well-localised?

    a) Somatic

    b) Visceral

    c) Neuropathic

    d) Referred

6. Which of the following is an example of a non-steroidal anti-inflammatory drug (NSAID)?

    a) Paracetamol

    b) Fentanyl

    c) Amitriptyline

    d) Diclofenac

7. NSAIDs must be used with caution in patients with renal disease because:

    a) They can irritate the kidneys and further reduce renal function.

    b) They inhibit the synthesis of prostaglandins which are needed to maintain renal blood flow.

    c) They are excreted by the kidney and plasma levels will increase in patients with renal disease.

    d) They can acidify urine and affect the removal of waste products.

8. An adult patient with asthma is being treated for lower back pain with regular paracetamol. Despite this prescription they are still in pain. What would be a suitable choice of additional analgesia?

   a) Ibuprofen
   b) Morphine
   c) Codeine
   d) Tramadol

9. Patients using fentanyl patches are advised to avoid baths when wearing a patch because:

   a) Hot water causes vasodilation and can increase absorption of fentanyl leading to an overdose.
   b) Hot water causes the adhesive on the patch to dissolve resulting in a detached patch and increased pain.
   c) Lying down in a bath can reduce your blood pressure; this exacerbates the side-effect of postural hypotension caused by fentanyl.
   d) Fentanyl is an analgesic. If the bath were too hot pain stimuli would be reduced and severe scolding could result.

10. Which one of the following statements is TRUE?

   a) Opioids can cause the side-effect respiratory depression due to stimulation of the chemoreceptor trigger zone.
   b) Opioids can cause nausea and vomiting due to irritation of the stomach lining.
   c) Opioids can precipitate asthma attacks due to reduction of prostaglandin synthesis.
   d) Opioids can cause constipation due to their action on opioid receptors in the gastrointestinal tract.

Chapter summary

Pain is a protective mechanism that helps to alert us to injury. Nociceptive pain is brought about by activation of pain fibres called nociceptors. Extremes of temperature and intense pressure can activate nociceptors. Chemicals can also activate nociceptors, including chemicals such as prostaglandins which are released by the body in response to tissue injury. These act to sensitise nerve endings and are part of inflammation. Pain fibres enter the dorsal horn in the spinal cord where they synapse with other nerves

(Continued)

(Continued)

which relay the message to the brain. The gate control theory describes how these pain signals can be modified to increase or decrease the intensity of pain signals. This helps to explain the role that emotions have in pain and how it is experienced, a key consideration for nursing care. Holistic pain assessment is vital and aims to consider causes, the impact of pain for the patient and the most appropriate treatment and care. Effective pain management can be guided by the WHO Analgesic Ladder. Step 1 involves non-opioid analgesics such as paracetamol and non-steroidal anti-inflammatory drugs (NSAIDs). These drugs act by reducing prostaglandin synthesis. Step 2 involves the addition of opioids; these are analgesics with a similar structure to morphine. These drugs work as agonists at opioid receptors in the central nervous system which reduce pain signals and affect how we experience pain.

Activities: Brief outline answers

Activity 6.1 Reflection (p159)

There are very many factors you could have identified. These may include: the nature and degree of the injury, your anxieties over the cause of the pain, your previous experience of pain, anxieties over the consequences of the pain.

People often report cutting their finger, for example during food preparation, but not feeling any pain until moments later, after which, the pain may be very intense.

Activity 6.2 Critical thinking (p161)

According to the gate control theory, TENS works by stimulating Ab fibres entering the spinal cord at the same segmental level as the activated pain fibres. This will reduce the synaptic transmission from C fibres to the relay neurones. This will reduce the number of pain signals reaching the brain.

Activity 6.3 Critical thinking (p162)

Pain assessment: Frank		
Past history	1-year history prostate cancer	
Previous treatment	Hormone therapy	
Observations	Pale, tense, avoids eye-contact	
Dimension of pain:	**Components to be assessed:**	**What questions might you ask:**
Sensory	Pain intensity – how severe is your pain? Location – where is your pain? Where does it hurt? Character – 'what the pain feels like' – how often does the pain occur?	You might use a visual analogue scale or ask the patient to rate their pain on a scale of 0–10. You might use a body diagram to record the location of your patient's pain. Your patient may have more than one site of pain and/or their pain may radiate.

		Descriptive words may include: sharp, stabbing, shooting, pins and needles, deep, dull, aching. Patients may also describe if the pain is intermittent or continuous.
Emotional	Relations with others – how is your pain affecting how you get on with people? Enjoyment of life – how is the pain affecting your ability to enjoy things? Mood – How is your pain affecting your mood? How are you feeling?	It may also be important to ask Frank what he thinks is causing his pain. What helps the pain and what makes it worse?
Impact on daily activities	Sleep – how is your sleep? Walking – is your ability to walk affected? Is it painful when you walk? General activity Working	It may be important to explore if the patient is experiencing other symptoms. You should also be aware of the patient's medical history, his current medication and the extent of his cancer. You should ask about social and home circumstances in case additional support and/ or referral to other members of the multi-professional team is required in hospital or following discharge from hospital.

Activity 6.4 Decision-making (p165)

Looking at the Analgesic Ladder, Kenneth might be ready to move to step 2. A weak opioid such as codeine or a non-steroidal anti-inflammatory drug could be added. The choice would depend on other medicines Kenneth is taking and his general physical health. NSAIDs for example can be toxic to the kidney, especially in older people. The constipating effects of codeine and possible adverse effects on falls and cognition would also need to be considered in an elderly patient. It is also important to remember that non-pharmacological interventions need to be considered.

Activity 6.5 Research (p168)

Total dose of morphine in 24 hours should be calculated which is 160 mg. From the table in the BNF 3 mg subcutaneous diamorphine is equivalent to 10 mg oral morphine. This equates to 48 mg diamorphine.

The BNF states it is only an approximate guide and in reality the new dose given might also reflect how well the pain is currently controlled. To compare potencies we need to look at equivalents for the same route. Potency refers to the amount of drug needed for the same effect. In this case less diamorphine is needed and it is therefore more potent. If we compare the oral and IV doses of morphine we can see that 5 mg IV morphine is approximately equivalent to 10 mg oral morphine. This demonstrates that not all of the oral morphine reaches the systemic circulation. Some may not be absorbed from the GI tract but most of the losses are due to first pass metabolism (Chapter 1).

Activity 6.6 Critical thinking (p169)

Even the lowest strength patch of fentanyl patch is 12 micrograms which is equivalent to 30 mg of morphine. This might be too much for a frail elderly patient. Side-effects would need monitoring closely. There have been cases of significant respiratory depression and fatalities in opioid naïve patients, i.e. those not already on opioids (Janssen-Cilag Ltd, SPC). Also the dose from a patch will take time to build up so will not provide immediate pain relief. The maximum analgesic effects and side-effects cannot be properly evaluated until 24 hours have elapsed.

Activity 6.7 Research (p171)

The interaction between an SSRI antidepressant and Tramadol may cause increased serotonergic effects and an increased risk of CNS toxicity. This is because both drugs increase serotonin. This can lead to serotonin syndrome which is characterised by tachycardia, shivering, twitching, over-responsive reflexes, agitation and can lead to seizures.

Activity 6.8 Multiple choice questions (pp171–3)

1. The physiology of nociceptive pain includes four stages: nociception, transmission, perception and modulation. Which of these is the conversion of a noxious stimulus into a nerve impulse?

    a) Nociception

2. Which type of nerve fibre is associated with a slow, dull 'second' pain?

    d) C

3. During an inflammatory response, which inflammatory mediators 'sensitise' nociceptors?

    d) Prostaglandins

4. Pain arising from a 'pulled' muscle would be classified as:

    a) Nociceptive-somatic

5. Which type of pain tends to be well-localised?

    a) Somatic

6. Which of the following is an example of a non-steroidal anti-inflammatory drug (NSAID)?

    d) Diclofenac

7. NSAIDs must be used with caution in patients with renal disease because:

    b) They inhibit the synthesis of prostaglandins which are needed to maintain renal blood flow.

8. An adult patient with asthma is being treated for lower back pain with regular paracetamol. Despite this prescription they are still in pain. What would be a suitable choice of additional analgesia?

    c) Codeine

9. Patients using fentanyl patches are advised to avoid baths when wearing a patch because:

    a) Hot water causes vasodilation and can increase absorption of fentanyl leading to an overdose.

10. Which of the following statements is TRUE?

    d) Opioids can cause constipation due to their action on opioid receptors in the gastrointestinal tract.

Further reading

Macintyre, P and Schug, S (2015) *Acute Pain Management: A Practical Guide* (4th edition). London: CRC Press/Taylor and Francis.

This book provides a very comprehensive and up-to-date guide to all aspects of the management of acute pain.

Simonsen, T, Aarbakkee, J, Kay, I, Coleman, I, Sinnott, P and Lysaa, R (2006) *Illustrated Pharmacology for Nurses.* London: Hodder Arnold.

A comprehensive pharmacology textbook for nurses. Chapter 14 covers analgesics.

Swift, A (2018) Understanding pain and the human body's response to it. *Nursing Times* [online]; 114: 3, 22–6.

A recent and comprehensive review of pain physiology related to nursing practice.

Useful websites

www.who.int/cancer/palliative/painladder/en/

WHO Pain Relief Ladder for cancer pain relief.

www.who.int/medicines/areas/quality_safety/guide_perspainchild/en/

WHO guidelines for persisting pain in children.

www.britishpainsociety.org/people-with-pain/frequently-asked-questions/

British Pain Society (2014) FAQs. This site provides a source of information from the British Pain Society on information on frequently asked questions on pain.

Chapter 7 Nausea and vomiting

Chapter aims

After reading this chapter you will be able to:

- define what is meant by nausea, vomiting and retching;
- explain the purpose of nausea and vomiting and the physiology of vomiting;
- describe the different pathways which can stimulate vomiting;
- identify the different neurotransmitters which stimulate the vomiting response;
- explain the range of drugs which can be used to manage nausea and vomiting and their sites of action.

Introduction

Nausea and vomiting are important as biological systems for drug side-effects, disease co-morbidities, and defenses against food poisoning.

(Horn, 2008)

Nausea and vomiting are distressing and debilitating. They are frequently reported by patients with a range of conditions including infection, pain, following surgery, drug side-effects and advanced cancer. However, as the quote by Horn identifies, nausea and vomiting are important protective mechanisms against the ingestion and effects of toxins. Vomiting can remove a noxious substance from the stomach. Nausea, as an unpleasant sensation of unease and discomfort associated with the urge to be sick, may help us to avoid further ingestion of substances that the body has recognised as harmful.

Nausea and vomiting are complex and multifactorial in nature. This means that they may occur due to a number of psychological and physical causes. This can make assessment and management of nausea and vomiting challenging. Drug treatments are commonly used for managing nausea and vomiting with a range of options available. Current recommendations to manage nausea and vomiting are based on the presumed cause(s) and our knowledge of the vomiting, or emetogenic (nerve), pathways which stimulate and activate the vomiting response. Drugs are chosen to match the most likely emetogenic stimulus. The drugs act to block the neurotransmitter(s) that stimulate the vomiting response (NHS Scotland, 2014). In clinical practice, however, this is often complicated by the challenges of identifying the cause(s) and the fact that many anti-emetic drugs work on multiple receptors.

In this chapter, we will explore why we experience nausea and vomiting. The common causes (aetiology) will be identified and we will relate these to the physiology of vomiting and the emetogenic pathways. With this knowledge, we can identify the neurotransmitters that are involved in stimulating the vomiting response. This is important for your clinical decision-making when considering which anti-emetic drug(s) may be effective. We will discuss the clinical assessment required and the drug options. Non-drug interventions for nausea and vomiting are also an important aspect for effective management but are beyond the scope of this chapter. You may wish to research nursing care and non-pharmacological management as part of your learning about nausea and vomiting.

Why do we experience nausea and vomiting?

As humans, we have developed responses that enable our survival. For survival, it is important that we can identify foods that are safe to ingest. Our sensory systems help us to identify spoiled foods using olfactory (odour) cues. Taste can also be an effective deterrent to eating when food is sour or bitter. Smell and taste could be described as the 'gatekeepers' of the gastrointestinal (GI) tract preventing us from ingesting potentially harmful substances. These are, however, not always effective in detecting the quality of food. Nausea and vomiting are behavioural mechanisms to protect against ingested toxins. Nausea enables us to avoid the ingestion of toxins, and vomiting expels toxins from the stomach. Together nausea, vomiting and diarrhoea (which we introduce in Chapter 10) are important for helping to prevent the ingestion and absorption of toxins from the GI tract.

Today, in the UK and other high-income countries, we are surrounded by food that is relatively safe, nutritious and abundant. But, in terms of evolution, our physiological capabilities developed when we hunted for our next meal instead of going to the supermarket (Horn, 2008). Despite this evolution, we still deal with the danger of food poisoning if food contains harmful pathogens and toxins (Chapter 3). Nausea and vomiting can also arise in those with food allergies or food intolerance. Pregnant women, during the first trimester of pregnancy, are particularly susceptible to nausea and vomiting. These are believed to play an adaptive role in survival of the foetus. The first trimester is a period of rapid foetal growth. During this period, the developing foetal central nervous system (CNS) is highly susceptible to the effects of toxins. Pregnant women can appear to be 'picky' eaters and may avoid meat and fish products. This enables pregnant women to avoid foods that are more likely to contain pathogens that might harm the foetus. Many of the drugs that we discuss in this book have side-effects of nausea and vomiting. These include antibiotics, cancer chemotherapy and some analgesic drugs. Nausea and vomiting, therefore, serve important roles in survival. By their nature, as protective responses, they have a low threshold for being activated.

Activity 7.1   Evidence-based practice and research

Nausea and vomiting are common and distressing symptoms.

Before reading further, consider:

- What is meant by the term 'nausea' and what is its purpose?
- What happens physically before, during and after vomiting?
- What is the purpose of vomiting?
- What is meant by the term 'anticipatory nausea and vomiting' and when might this occur?
- What is retching and why does this happen?
- How is regurgitation different from vomiting?
- What causes of nausea, regurgitation, retching and vomiting can you identify?

There is no model answer for this activity. However, you can compare your answer to the section 'Explaining terms'.

Explaining terms

In Activity 7.1 you were asked to define several terms. Compare your answers with the descriptions below.

Nausea is an 'aversive' experience that often accompanies vomiting. 'Aversive' means that the person feels a strong dislike for something, perhaps the taste or smell from the food they are eating. This aversive experience is likely to stop them eating any more. This can prevent the further ingestion of potentially harmful toxins into the GI tract and absorption into the circulation. Nausea is, however, a non-specific symptom. This means it can be triggered for a number of reasons. For example, nausea often occurs with motion (as 'motion sickness'), pregnancy, dizziness, migraine, fainting, pain or food poisoning. Nausea may occur as a side-effect of drugs. Nausea can also be experienced in anxiety and depression.

Patients may describe nausea as an unpleasant 'wave-like' sensation at the back of the throat and epigastrium (this is the central region of the abdomen below the sternum). Symptoms associated with **autonomic nervous system** stimulation may occur such as pallor, cold sweats, excess salivation, tachycardia and diarrhoea. Nausea is generally associated with some degree of anorexia or loss of appetite. A person can suffer nausea without vomiting. Vomiting can also occur without nausea. In clinical practice, nausea can be more difficult to manage than vomiting using anti-emetic drugs. For example, the severity of drug-induced vomiting from cancer chemotherapy can be controlled with anti-emetic medications, but nausea can persist. This suggests that nausea and vomiting are separate physiological processes and require separate assessment and management.

Vomiting or emesis is the involuntary, forceful expulsion of the contents of a person's stomach through the mouth. Vomiting can be caused by a wide variety of stimuli. It may present as a specific response to gastritis (inflammation of the stomach), or as a non-specific symptom of disorders including brain tumours and elevated intracranial pressure. Vomiting may be preceded by nausea, but not always. The process of vomiting results from a complex interaction between the relaxation of the GI tract, contraction of the diaphragm and abdominal muscles, and 'reverse peristalsis' in the small intestine. This is discussed more fully in the next section. Vomiting is different from 'regurgitation', although the two terms are often used interchangeably.

Regurgitation is the return of undigested food to the oesophagus and the mouth without the force associated with vomiting.

Anticipatory nausea and vomiting (ANV) are commonly referred to when discussing patients receiving chemotherapy. For this patient group, anticipatory nausea appears to occur in about one in three patients; anticipatory vomiting occurs in about one in ten patients. A number of mechanisms have been proposed to explain ANV. For example, ANV can be explained by classical conditioning (also known as Pavlovian conditioning). In classical conditioning, a previously neutral stimulus (for example, a smell or sight associated with the chemotherapy environment) elicits a conditioned response after a number of treatments called 'learning trials'. In cancer chemotherapy, the first few chemotherapy treatments are the learning trials. The chemotherapy drugs are the 'unconditioned stimuli' that result in post-chemotherapy nausea and vomiting in some patients. The drugs become associated with neutral, environmental stimuli (for example, the smell of the setting, the sight of the oncology nurse or the chemotherapy room). These previously neutral stimuli then become 'conditioned' stimuli. The conditioned stimuli (for example, the smell of the setting) then trigger ANV. ANV is a learned response that, in other life situations such as an experience of food poisoning, would result in an adaptive avoidance of the stimulus (spoiled food). However, for the person receiving chemotherapy, avoidance of the stimuli (the setting, the nurse or the smells associated with the chemotherapy) may not be possible as they undergo several cycles of treatment. It is, therefore, important to manage chemotherapy related nausea and vomiting effectively from the beginning of the course of treatment in order to reduce the possibility of ANV developing. ANV is not only experienced by people receiving chemotherapy. ANV can develop as a conditioned response in any situation where a neutral stimulus (sights, smells, sounds, a person, a food) becomes associated with experiencing nausea and vomiting. An example of this is provided in the case study below: Judy.

Retching, also known as 'heaving', is the attempt to vomit. It involves reverse peristalsis into the stomach and oesophagus without vomiting. The function is thought to enable mixing of gastric contents, which are acidic, with intestinal refluxate in order to buffer the gastric contents and give it momentum in preparation of vomiting. This can be as distressing as vomiting itself.

Case study: Judy

On a school trip to Germany, Judy (15 years old) and her classmates travelled on the overnight ferry from the north-east of England to Holland – a 12-hour crossing. The crossing was particularly 'rocky' with strong gusty wind, heavy rain and high waves. To try to distract themselves, the classmates went to the on-board café where there was music playing. Everyone began to feel nauseous due to the rolling boat, the smell of food and the sound of people being sick in the public toilets nearby.

Judy had previously been on a couple of boat trips and experienced nausea. On those occasions (which might be described as learning trials), she had used acupressure bands on her wrists to try to alleviate the nausea. Unfortunately, however, this latest experience reminded her of previous trips and she started to feel anxious about being sick. Judy also recognised and associated the perfume her friend was wearing with the previous boat trips and her feelings of nausea. The combination of the rolling ship, the smell of the perfume, the smell of food, the sounds of people vomiting and the odour of vomit from the toilets nearby resulted in Judy vomiting. It took Judy several days to recover once the group arrived at their destination.

On the return journey, Judy started to feel anxious when she saw the gangplank to the boat. She noticed the slight rocking movement of the boat in dock, the smell of her friend's perfume and immediately felt sick and vomited. Judy developed anticipatory nausea and vomiting related to these 'neutral stimuli' becoming conditioned stimuli. She now avoids sailing and prefers to fly. Her friend also tries to avoid wearing the particular perfume when they meet.

Activity 7.2   Critical thinking

Use Judy's experience and your own from clinical practice to identify common stimuli for nausea and vomiting.

A suggested answer is given at the end of the chapter.

Through Activity 7.2 you will have identified many stimuli that can trigger nausea and vomiting. In the next section we look more closely at how nausea and vomiting arise through the co-ordinated actions of both the central and peripheral nervous systems.

The neurophysiology of vomiting (emetogenesis)

Vomiting is controlled by the medulla oblongata of the brainstem. Within the medulla oblongata are neurones making up the 'vomiting centre'. The vomiting centre is not a discrete structure but a diffuse network of interconnecting neurones. The network of interconnected neurones which form the vomiting centre 'integrate' incoming (afferent) signals from several parts of the body. If stimulated above a certain threshold, the vomiting centre sends out efferent signals to cause vomiting.

'Input' or afferent signals to the vomiting centre come from:

- Higher cortical centres of the brain (the cerebral cortex and limbic system).
- The chemoreceptor trigger zone (CTZ).
- The labyrinth/vestibular system of the inner ear through the vestibulocochlear nerve (cranial nerve VIII).
- The GI system and the pharynx (throat) through the vagus nerve (cranial nerve X) and spinal sympathetic nerves.

The afferent signals to the vomiting centre are shown in Figure 7.1 and are summarised in Table 7.1.

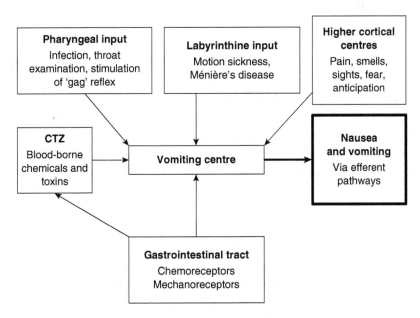

Figure 7.1   Afferent pathways to the 'vomiting centre'

When stimulated above a threshold level by one or more of these afferent inputs, the vomiting centre triggers the vomiting response through its efferent pathways.

First, we will look at the afferent input in more detail. This level of detail is important for developing your understanding of the assessment of nausea and vomiting, and to inform your decision-making when administering anti-emetic drugs.

Afferent input to the vomiting centre

- *Chemoreceptor trigger zone (CTZ)*: the CTZ is made up of interconnecting nerve networks located in the area postrema of the brain. The CTZ is outside the blood–brain barrier and receives input about blood-borne drugs, hormones, electrolytes and toxins. This means that the chemicals and toxins in the blood and the cerebrospinal fluid can diffuse through to the CTZ and interact with receptors in the CTZ.

  Neurones in the CTZ and area postrema are thought to have two types of receptors: receptors at the surface of the neurone and receptors that are found deeper on the dendrites. The surface receptors are called chemoreceptors. These chemoreceptors are activated from contact with emetic substances (such as toxins and chemicals) circulating in the blood. The activation of these chemoreceptors triggers action potentials relaying information about the level of emetic substances in the blood to the vomiting centre. The chemoreceptors continually send this information about how much emetic substances are in the blood even if the threshold level to stimulate vomiting is not reached.

  The CTZ and area postrema have a number of receptors thought to be involved in stimulating nausea and vomiting such as serotonin (5-HT_3) receptor, dopamine (D_2) receptor, histamine (H1 and H2) receptor, acetylcholine (Ach) receptor, substance P (NK1) receptor and opioid (Mu2) receptor. As identified earlier in the chapter, the vomiting response has a low threshold for being activated. Vomiting can be stimulated when a certain amount (threshold) of blood-borne toxin binds to a certain amount of chemoreceptors in the CTZ to trigger action potentials to activate the vomiting centre. For example, opioid receptors in the CTZ monitor levels of opioids in the blood and, when a threshold amount of opioids bind to a certain number of opioid receptors in the CTZ, the opioid receptors increase firing of action potentials which signals the vomiting centre to initiate the vomiting response.
- *Pharyngeal input*: the vagus nerve (cranial nerve X) supplies sensory nerve fibres to the pharynx or throat. These sensory fibres are activated when the pharynx is irritated by the presence of infection such as *Candida albicans*, an instrument to examine the mouth or by a person causing a 'gag' reflex to stimulate vomiting. Signals from these sensory fibres are transmitted to the vomiting centre.

- *Labyrinth stimulation/vestibular system*: the labyrinth is part of the inner ear that is responsible for the sensations of balance and movement. The vestibular system reacts to position change and sends information to the brain via the vestibulocochlear nerve (cranial nerve VIII). It plays a role in motion sickness. These position changes stimulate histamine (H1) receptors in the inner ear, and nerve impulses are sent to the 'vomiting centre' via the chemoreceptor trigger zone (CTZ). Drugs such as opioids can also directly stimulate the vestibular apparatus and may result in nausea and vomiting via the same pathway.

- *Cerebral cortex and limbic system*: these are thought to cause nausea and vomiting when stimulated via the senses (particularly smell), anxiety, learned associations (ANV), pain, meningeal irritation or increased intracranial pressure. Activation of these higher centres in the brain is relayed to the CTZ and vomiting centre. Relevant neurotransmitters are thought to include histamine and acetylcholine that attach to H1 and acetylcholine (Ach) receptors respectively.

- *Peripheral pathways*: the main emetogenic input from the periphery is from the GI tract, serosa and viscera (Chapter 10). Sensory signals are transmitted from the GI tract by the vagal and spinal sympathetic nerves. Enterochromaffin cells in the GI mucosa release serotonin (5-HT) in response to toxins in the blood or GI tract. Serotonin binds to 5-HT_3 receptors on the vagus nerve and, as a receptor agonist, promotes signals to the 'vomiting centre' that may initiate the vomiting pathway. Mechanoreceptors in the intestinal wall are also activated by abnormal contractions (diarrhoea due to infection/inflammation), distortion (for example, tumour) and distension (for example, overeating, constipation).

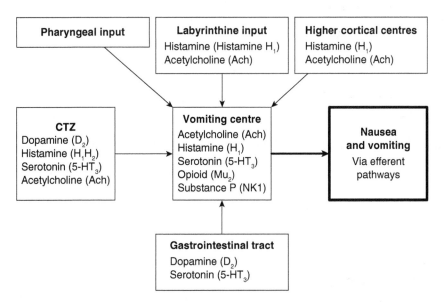

Figure 7.2 Neurotransmitters involved in signalling to the vomiting centre. This figure identifies the neurotransmitters that promote signalling to the vomiting centre. The neurotransmitters are receptor agonists. The receptors are shown in brackets.

Input and mechanism leading to nausea and vomiting	Stimuli
Higher centres – cerebral cortex is stimulated by a number of stimuli. These higher cortical centres stimulate the 'vomiting centre'	Sensory input including pain, foul smells, horrific sights. Memory, fear, anxiety, anticipation
Increased intracranial pressure within the cerebral cortex activates histamine receptors. This may stimulate meningeal mechanoreceptors which stimulate the 'vomiting centre'	Haemorrhage Meningitis Primary tumour or metastases
Labyrinth stimulation – movement related or opioids cause sensitivity of vestibular nerves	Motion sickness Ménière's disease Opioids
Blood-borne chemicals and toxins stimulate vomiting through their action on the chemoreceptor trigger zone (CTZ)	Chemical causes – electrolyte imbalance (uraemia and hypercalcaemia), hormones (pregnancy and hyperglycaemia) Toxins – infection and food poisoning Drugs – digoxin, chemotherapy, opioids, anaesthetic agents, antibiotics, alcohol excess
Gastrointestinal tract – mechanoreceptors respond to stretch, compression and distortion within the GI tract stimulating the vagus nerve which signals to the vomiting centre	Obstruction, constipation, squashed stomach syndrome, enlarged liver, stretching/ movement of organs during surgical procedures
Gastrointestinal tract – serotonin is released in response to toxins or irritants and attaches to 5HT3 chemoreceptors stimulating the vagus nerve which signals to the vomiting centre	NSAIDs, chemotherapy, inflammation, allergies, infection
Pharyngeal stimulation	*Candida albicans* (thrush), throat examination

Table 7.1 Common stimuli of nausea and vomiting (adapted from Mannix, 2010)

Efferent pathways: what is the process of vomiting?

The act of vomiting involves three types of efferent pathways initiated by the 'vomiting centre':

1. *Motor*: the neural pathways involved in the motor act of vomiting involve the phrenic nerve to the diaphragm, the spinal nerves to the abdominal and intercostal muscles, efferent visceral autonomic fibres to the GI tract, and the viscera efferent fibres to the voluntary muscles of the pharynx and larynx.

2. *Parasympathetic*: increase in salivation. This protects the oesophagus, oral cavity and tooth enamel from stomach acid as the stomach contents are expelled through the mouth.

3. *Sympathetic nervous system*: sweating and increased heart rate occur due to sympathetic nervous system activity.

Prodromal phase (pre-ejection): Involves relaxation of gastric muscles followed by 'retroperistalsis' of contents from the small intestine into the stomach through a relaxed pyloric sphincter. The pressure within the thorax (intrathoracic) is lowered by inspiration together with an increase in abdominal pressure as abdominal muscles contract to propel stomach contents into the oesophagus. The oesophageal sphincter relaxes to enable this. The stomach does not contract during vomiting. The stomach, oesophagus and their sphincters are relaxed during vomiting. The force that expels the contents comes from contraction of the diaphragm and the abdominal muscles.

Ejection phase: Retching occurs and involves contraction of the abdominal muscles, diaphragm and muscles used for inspiration. This is followed by vomiting requiring more vigorous contractions of the abdominal muscles and relaxation of the upper oesophageal sphincter.

Consequences of vomiting

Severe and prolonged nausea and vomiting can have harmful consequences.

*   Dehydration, particularly in children.
*   Reluctance to continue with potentially beneficial treatments.
*   Electrolyte disturbances.
*   Malnutrition which may result in starvation and vitamin deficiency.
*   Mallory–Weiss tear (gastro-oesophageal laceration syndrome): involves bleeding from laceration in the mucosa at the junction of the stomach and oesophagus resulting in haematemesis (vomiting up blood) after violent retching.
*   Metabolic alkalosis: vomiting results in the loss of acidic gastric juices from the gastrointestinal tract so that there is an abnormal loss of hydrogen ions (H^+) from the body. This leads to an acid–base disturbance associated with an increase in bicarbonate (HCO_3^-) and a reduction in plasma concentrations of hydrogen ions (H^+). Alkalosis may lead to tetany (muscle spasms due to low calcium levels), seizures and decreased mental status. Metabolic alkalosis also decreases coronary blood flow and predisposes people to arrhythmias. Hypoventilation may occur which causes hypoxemia.

Scenario: Adam

Imagine you are the nurse caring for Adam. Adam is a 70-year-old man who had a tumour removed from his descending colon about 18 months ago. At that time there was no evidence of residual cancer. He is admitted to the ward with abdominal pain

(Continued)

(Continued)

and vomiting of 3 days duration. The symptoms have worsened during that time and he is now in constant pain and nauseated, vomiting intermittently. He is dehydrated and unable to keep anything down. His medical assessment suggests an obstruction that is confirmed on abdominal X-ray at the site of the previous surgery. He also has an enlarged liver on examination. The doctors suspect recurrence of the bowel cancer with liver metastases.

Surgery is not appropriate, palliative treatment is proposed.

Activity 7.3   Decision-making

Refer to the scenario with Adam.

- Make an assessment – what do you need to know about Adam's nausea and vomiting?
- List the possible causes of his nausea and vomiting.
- Which afferent pathways are involved?
- How might you manage his symptoms? Consider:
    o   What drugs might be prescribed?
    o   What drugs should be avoided? Why?
    o   What routes of administration might be used?
    o   What non-pharmacological interventions and nursing care might you implement?

Compare your answers with the clinical assessment and pharmacological management sections and answers at the end of the chapter.

Clinical assessment and management

Nausea and vomiting are distressing and debilitating symptoms resulting from disease processes as well as infection, and the side-effects of treatment and medication. As we have discussed, a number of neurotransmitters and receptors have been identified as being associated with the emetogenic pathway. The 'vomiting centre' integrates information received from the CTZ, chemoreceptors and mechanoreceptors in the GI tract, the vestibular system and higher order centres in the cortex. It is thought that the effect of anti-emetic drugs is directly related to their ability to bind to and antagonise (block) specific receptors. However, there also appears to be overlap between the neurotransmitters with some neurotransmitters acting in more than one emetic pathway. This helps to explain why different anti-emetic drugs can be effective for treating multiple causes of nausea and vomiting. Some anti-emetic drugs, which act on single receptor groups, may be required in combination to effectively treat nausea and vomiting that have multiple causes. Your clinical assessment and choice of anti-emetic must therefore take into consideration which emetogenic pathway is, or are, being triggered and the most likely cause(s) of these symptoms.

Although nausea and vomiting are often associated, they should be assessed separately. Their management relies on your, and the multi-professional team's, ability to identify the aetiology and mechanisms of nausea and/or vomiting in an individual patient and then match this with the appropriate drug(s). Much of this is dependent on taking a careful history, carrying out a focused physical examination, arranging appropriate investigations, and then combining the results with evidence-based knowledge of the emetogenic pathways and the available anti-emetics.

It is important to remember that some patients, like Adam, may have multiple stimuli contributing to his nausea and vomiting.

NICE (2016a) suggests that assessment should include asking about:

- Nausea: onset, frequency, intensity, relieving and exacerbating factors, relationship to vomiting.
- Vomiting: onset, frequency, quantity, force, colour, timing and pattern.

  o   The pattern of nausea and vomiting can provide clues to the causes of the symptoms. Nausea that is relieved by vomiting, for example, suggests a GI cause, whilst nausea and vomiting accompanied by pain or colic suggests gastric stasis. Headaches, especially early morning headaches, accompanied by nausea and vomiting may indicate increased intracranial pressure. Movement-related nausea suggests vestibular dysfunction. Polyuria accompanied by confusion and nausea may suggest electrolyte imbalances such as hypercalcaemia or hyponatraemia.

  o   Observation of the vomit itself – colour, odour, volume – will help to guide the diagnosis and management decisions. Large volume vomit with oesophageal reflux may indicate gastric stasis, whilst intermittent nausea with faeculent vomiting may indicate bowel obstruction.

- Other associated or concurrent symptoms (for example constipation, heartburn, diarrhoea, flatus, cough, headache or confusion).
- Treatment history including current medication (for example opioids, antibiotics, chemotherapy, digoxin, anti-emetics).
- Medical history.
- Effect on nutrition including food and fluid intake.
- Impact on activities of daily living and quality of life.

You should also be aware of any laboratory tests for metabolic or blood-borne factors which will detect abnormalities related to nausea and vomiting (for example hypercalcaemia, hyponatraemia) and also assess for complications of these symptoms such as dehydration and metabolic alkalosis. Some patients, like Adam, may require radiological investigations to assess for constipation or bowel obstruction.

NICE (2016a) also recommends physical examination of your patient for identifying other reasons for nausea and vomiting. The medical and nursing examination might include:

- Checking the mouth and oropharynx for signs of infection (thrush), ulceration or tenacious sputum which may be causing pharyngeal stimulation.
- Chest percussion for signs of infection, observing or asking about presence of a cough.
- Checking the abdomen for signs of ascites, constipation, hepatomegaly or distension suggesting impaired gastric emptying resulting in stimulation of mechanoreceptors.
- Checking for signs of papilloedema – papilloedema is optic disc swelling that is caused by increased intracranial pressure or cerebral metastases.
- Assessment of anxiety – there may be a psychological element to the symptoms that produces distress and affects quality of life which needs to be explored during the assessment process.

Once a thorough history has been taken, and a physical examination undertaken, the most likely cause(s) can be developed. Any drug management will focus on prescribing the appropriate antagonist to block the receptor(s) and action of the neurotransmitter(s) that may be stimulating the vomiting response.

Pharmacological management

In practice, there are often a number of causes and a full assessment of these symptoms should be made. When deciding which anti-emetic, or combination of drugs, might be appropriate to manage your patient's nausea and vomiting:

- Consider the pathway by which the cause(s) may be triggering the vomiting reflex.
- Consider the chemical/neurotransmitter(s) involved in the emetogenic pathway.
- Select the drug that is able to block (antagonise) this pathway.
- Select the appropriate route of drug delivery (tablet, injection, subcutaneous, rectal, patch).
- Optimise the dose of the medication.

Below is a list of commonly used anti-emetic drugs selected for their effectiveness as antagonists to specific receptors. As you will see:

- Some drugs which are used as anti-emetics in clinical practice may also be prescribed as treatments for other conditions but have been found to have anti-emetic properties when used at particular doses.

- Some drugs act on specific receptors whilst others may antagonise (block) a range of receptors that normally respond to different neurotransmitters.

Local guidelines and formularies should be checked or pharmacist advice sought with regard to recommended prescribing doses or drug combinations prior to treating.

We will now consider the drugs in more detail.

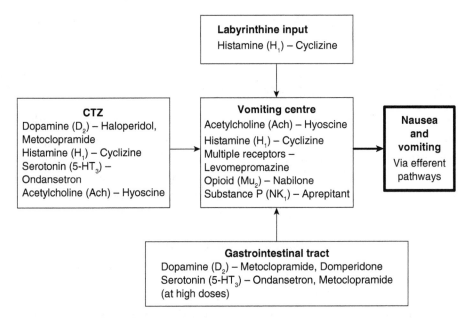

Figure 7.3 Pharmacological management. This figure identifies the neurotransmitters that promote signalling to the vomiting centre. The neurotransmitters are receptor agonists at the receptors (shown in brackets). Examples of anti-emetic drugs are provided. Anti-emetics are antagonists at these receptors blocking the action of the neurotransmitter.

Dopamine antagonists

Dopamine receptors are present in the CTZ. These drugs are potent dopamine D_2 receptor antagonists and blocking these receptors can result in reduced nausea and vomiting. Examples of dopamine antagonists are haloperidol, metoclopramide and domperidone, but there are important differences between them.

Haloperidol acts as an anti-emetic mainly by blocking D_2 receptors in the CTZ. It can also be used as an antipsychotic as it antagonises other dopamine receptors in the brain which are thought to be involved in psychosis. When used as an anti-emetic, it is commonly used in the context of chemical or metabolic causes of nausea and vomiting including hypercalcaemia and morphine toxicity (NICE, 2016a).

As well as antagonising D_2 receptors in the CTZ, metoclopramide also blocks D_2 receptors in the GI tract. Metoclopramide relaxes the pyloric sphincter and increases the strength of gastric contractions. This adds to the anti-emetic effect.

191

Metoclopramide is known as a prokinetic drug because of this action. Prokinetic drugs are useful for nausea and vomiting induced by gastric stasis, for example due to hepatomegaly, opioids or functional/partial obstruction. Metoclopramide is also used for gastroparesis – a condition that leads to poor emptying of the stomach. At higher doses, metoclopramide may also act as a 5-HT$_3$ antagonist. This contributes to the anti-emetic effect as it prevents stimulation of 5-HT$_3$ receptors on the vagus nerve and in the CTZ.

Domperidone is very similar in its action to metoclopramide. However, it does not readily cross the blood–brain barrier so has fewer effects on the brain.

Side-effects and implications for practice

Metoclopramide and haloperidol can cause movement disorders such as parkinsonism and dyskinesia. Because these drugs are relatively non-specific they also antagonise other dopamine receptors in the brain. As we see in Chapter 12 blocking dopamine can cause symptoms resembling Parkinson's disease. However, at the low doses used for anti-emetic purposes, these effects are uncommon (NICE, 2016a). Domperidone rarely has this effect as it works on peripheral dopamine receptors rather than those in the brain.

As domperidone and metoclopramide stimulate gastrointestinal motility they should not be used when nausea and vomiting is caused by bowel obstruction (for example, in patients like Adam, with bowel obstruction).

Prokinetics (metoclopramide and domperidone) should not be given concurrently with drugs with antimuscarinic activity (hyoscine) because antimuscarinic drugs competitively block the action of prokinetics (NICE, 2016a).

Histamine antagonists

Histamine antagonists, also known as antihistamines, work by blocking H$_1$ receptors in the vomiting centre, reducing the excitability of the inner ear labyrinth, and blocking conduction in the vestibular–cerebellar pathway. They may also have an effect on the H$_1$ receptors in the CTZ. Examples of histamine antagonists include cyclizine and promethazine. Cyclizine is used to treat nausea, vomiting and dizziness associated with vagus nerve-mediated motion sickness, vertigo and mechanical bowel obstruction (NICE, 2016a). It can also be used post-operatively following administration of general anaesthesia and opioids.

Side-effects and implications for practice

These drugs cross the blood–brain barrier and, blocking histamine receptors in the brain, can cause drowsiness (Chapter 1). They also have slight anti-muscarinic activity that can lead to side-effects such as dry mouth and urinary retention.

Activity 7.4   Evidence-based practice and research

Why are non-sedative antihistamines such as loratadine and cetirizine not useful for nausea and vomiting?

Compare your answer with that at the end of the chapter.

Anticholinergic/antimuscarinic anti-emetics

Anticholinergics are a class of drugs that block the binding of the neurotransmitter acetylcholine (Ach) to acetylcholine receptors present in nerve fibres in the central and peripheral nervous system. Acetylcholine receptors are classified into two groups – muscarinic or nicotinic. Acetylcholine is a muscarinic receptor agonist. Antimuscarinic antagonists block the muscarinic receptor and are used as anti-emetics. Examples include hyoscine hydrobromide (scopolamine). Hyoscine hydrobromide inhibits para-sympathetic nerve impulses, part of the autonomic nervous system that are responsible for involuntary movement of smooth muscles. This makes it a useful anti-emetic as it can reduce GI motility, lessen spasms and reduce secretions. Hyoscine hydrobromide also has an effect on the central nervous system due to its ability to cross the blood–brain barrier. This group of anti-emetics is useful for motion-related nausea and post-operative nausea and vomiting. They can, however, cause urinary retention and diminished bowel movement (ileus).

Serotonin (5-HT) antagonists

Examples of 5-HT$_3$ receptor antagonists include ondansetron and granisetron. They achieve their anti-emetic effect by blocking specific serotonin (5-HT) receptors both peripherally and in the central nervous system. These drugs are selective and have little affinity for other receptors involved in nausea and vomiting. 5-HT$_3$ antagonists were initially developed for reducing acute vomiting post-chemotherapy. Cancer treatments, such as chemotherapy and radiotherapy, are thought to cause the formation of 'free radicals' that cause serotonin to be released by enterochromaffin cells in the small intestine. Serotonin stimulates 5-HT$_3$ receptors on vagal afferent nerve fibres within the GI tract. As you can see in Figure 7.2, these nerve fibres project to the vomiting centre to initiate the vomiting response. In addition, serotonin circulating in the blood may bind to 5-HT$_3$ receptors in the CTZ. In current practice, 5-HT$_3$ antagonists are most commonly used for acute emesis following chemotherapy and for post-operative nausea and vomiting.

Levomepromazine

Levomepromazine is thought to act predominantly by blocking dopamine type 2 (D$_2$) receptors in the brain (NICE, 2016a). It may also antagonise a variety of receptors including histamine, muscarinic and serotonin receptors. The multi-modal action of levomepromazine is useful for example within palliative care for the treatment of intractable nausea and vomiting, and for delirium in the last days of life.

Neurokinin 1 (NK1) receptor antagonist

NK1 antagonists have antidepressant, anxiolytic and anti-emetic properties. An example of this type of drug is aprepitant. Aprepitant is used for vomiting associated with the treatment of cancer. Chemotherapy induced vomiting may occur in acute and delayed phases. Whilst the acute phase of vomiting responds to 5-HT$_3$ antagonists, until the development of NK1 receptor antagonists, the delayed vomiting phase has been difficult to manage. NK1 receptor antagonists work by blocking brain NK1 receptors from the peptide substance P neurotransmitter.

Having discussed the action for a range of anti-emetics, we will now consider your decision-making when selecting an appropriate anti-emetic drug in clinical practice.

Selecting an appropriate anti-emetic drug

Case study

James has Parkinson's disease. He has been prescribed apomorphine, a dopamine agonist, for his symptoms. He is suffering with the side-effect of nausea.

Activity 7.5   Decision-making

Discuss the suitability of the following in treating James's nausea:

Metoclopramide, cyclizine, haloperidol, domperidone.

Compare your answer with that at the end of the chapter.

The choice of anti-emetic drug is often dependent not only on the patient's health status and severity of nausea and/or vomiting but also on a drug's potential adverse effects and the available routes of administration. Often oral administration of drugs is not possible, and should not be considered when absorption via the GI tract may be impaired. Alternative routes, including rectal suppositories, subcutaneous infusions or transdermal patches, may be required. Due to the range of factors that may contribute to nausea and vomiting, a combination of drugs (and non-pharmacological care interventions) may be needed. It should also be remembered that, for some causes of nausea and vomiting, anti-emetic drugs may not be required. For example, nausea and vomiting due to constipation might be more appropriately treated by addressing the cause of the constipation.

Other drugs

Steroids

The anti-emetic properties of corticosteroids such as dexamethasone are not fully understood. They may act by inhibiting prostaglandin synthesis and also reduce the permeability of the area that houses the CTZ, reducing the effect of emetic toxins. Corticosteroids are widely used both prophylactically and as anti-emetics in chemotherapy. They have been shown to improve the effects of other anti-emetics (for example, metoclopramide and 5-HT$_3$ receptor antagonists). In addition, they are useful for reducing nausea and vomiting associated with raised intracranial pressure, bowel obstruction and hepatomegaly (enlarged liver).

Benzodiazepines

Although benzodiazepines are not indicated for use as single-agent anti-emetics, they can be useful in nausea and vomiting related to anxiety. When benzodiazepines, such as lorazepam, are used in conjunction with other anti-emetics, patients may benefit from their sedative, anxiolytic and amnesic properties in anticipatory nausea and vomiting (Rhodes and McDaniel, 2001). Benzodiazepines enhance the effect of the neurotransmitter gamma-aminobutyric acid (GABA) at the GABA$_A$ receptor resulting in sedation and anxiolytic (anti-anxiety) properties.

Non-pharmacological management of nausea and vomiting

Non-drug interventions can be helpful in managing nausea and vomiting, used alone or in combination with anti-emetic therapy, including:

- Ensuring the patient has easy access to a bowl, tissues and water.
- Creating an environment which eliminates sights, smells or sounds that can initiate nausea.
- Small meals served at room temperature.
- Offering cool, carbonated fluids.
- Other non-pharmacological methods such as acupuncture/acupressure bands show variable results in the treatment of nausea and vomiting.
- Relaxation therapy including music therapy, muscle relaxation and guided imagery are other non-pharmacological interventions associated with the reduction of nausea and vomiting.

It is now time to review what you have learned within this chapter by undertaking some multiple choice questions.

Activity 7.6   Multiple choice questions

1. Name the neurotransmitter molecule that is released in response to toxins or irritants in the GI tract:
   a) Serotonin (5-HT)
   b) Histamine
   c) Acetylcholine
   d) Neurokinin

2. Name the region in the brain that is directly stimulated by factors in the circulation that trigger emesis:
   a) Vomiting
   b) CTZ
   c) Higher cortical
   d) Pharyngeal

3. Factors in the circulation can affect this region of the brain because it has an incomplete . . .

4. The drug aprepitant is an antagonist for which neurotransmitter?
   a) Histamine
   b) Dopamine
   c) Acetylcholine
   d) Substance P

5. Which of the following is used to prevent nausea and vomiting?
   a) Dopamine antagonist
   b) Muscarinic antagonist
   c) Histamine antagonist
   d) All of the above

6. Vomiting:
   a) Is the same as regurgitation
   b) Involves contraction of the stomach
   c) Is involuntary
   d) Always preceded by nausea

7. Anticipatory nausea and vomiting (ANV):
   a) Only affects people receiving chemotherapy
   b) Does not require any treatment
   c) Is a conditioned response
   d) Cannot be prevented

8. Nausea is:

   a) An aversive experience
   b) An unpleasant wave-like sensation at the back of the throat
   c) Associated with excessive salivation
   d) All of the above

9. The vomiting centre is a neural network in the:

   a) Medulla oblongata
   b) CTZ
   c) Gastrointestinal tract
   d) Cortical centres

10. Levomepromazine is an anti-emetic which antagonises which receptors?

    a) Histamine
    b) Dopamine
    c) Muscarinic
    d) All of the above

Chapter summary

Nausea and vomiting cause distress, anxiety and reduced quality of life as well as other complications such as dehydration, malnutrition and electrolyte imbalance. As we have discussed, several organs and systems, and multiple neurotransmitters and receptors are responsible for the afferent messages that are relayed to the 'vomiting centre', which processes the information and co-ordinates vomiting. Current drug treatments are aimed at blocking these receptors. Adequate management or palliation of nausea and vomiting requires you to have knowledge of the emetic pathways, the neurotransmitters and receptors involved, to inform your assessment of each symptom. A targeted approach to drug treatment using established guidelines is recommended. Treatment may combine drug and non-pharmacological interventions. As a nurse, you can have a significant impact on your patients' experiences of nausea and vomiting through your understanding of the underlying physiological mechanisms. This knowledge will help you to select the appropriate use of drug and non-pharmacological strategies that are most likely to result in controlling or limiting these symptoms.

Activities: Brief outline answers

Activity 7.2 Critical thinking (p182)

You may have identified some of the following as stimulating nausea and vomiting: sights, smells or taste; distension of the gastrointestinal tract (from over-eating, constipation or disease); motion sickness experienced in, for example, a car or boat; blood-borne toxins, drugs or electrolyte imbalances; raised intracranial pressure from perhaps a brain tumour, haemorrhage or meningitis.

Activity 7.3 Decision-making (p188)

It is important that a comprehensive assessment of Adam's nausea and vomiting is undertaken drawing on the guidance from NICE (2016a). Adam has a bowel obstruction and evidence of liver metastases confirmed by radiological examination. His vomit is likely to be faecalent (contain faeces) and he is experiencing abdominal pain, distension and colic.

Potential afferent pathways stimulating the vomiting response for Adam include:

- Via mechanoreceptors in the gastrointestinal tract in response to distortion from the tumour site, gastric stasis and compression due to enlarged liver.
- Via chemoreceptors in the gastrointestinal tract and CTZ in response to electrolyte imbalance and dehydration, opioids administered for pain.
- Via the vagus nerve from his enlarged liver.
- Via higher cortical centres due to his anxiety and pain.

You will need to consider the route of administration of any anti-emetic and/or analgesia for Adam as he is unable to absorb any anti-emetics or medication via the oral route. A subcutaneous infusion of medication may be required. Depending on local policy for symptom management, initially he may be prescribed subcutaneous cyclizine for nausea and vomiting and diamorphine for pain. As domperidone and metoclopramide stimulate gastrointestinal motility they should not be used when nausea and vomiting is caused by bowel obstruction. Adam may also be prescribed steroids such as dexamethasone to reduce his hepatomegaly. Regular evaluation and reassessment of Adam will be required and adjustments made to the drugs used. For example, levomepromazine may be prescribed. You might look up your organisation's policies for symptom management in palliative care.

To help manage Adam's anxiety, he (and his family) will require informational and emotional support about his condition. Oral assessment and oral care will be important as will easy access to receptacles for vomiting and privacy during episodes of vomiting. Fluid replacement may also need to be considered.

Activity 7.4 Evidence-based practice and research (p193)

Loratadine and cetirizine are non-sedative because they do not cross the blood–brain barrier. As a result they would not reach the histamine receptors that need to be blocked in the vomiting centre to reduce nausea and vomiting.

Activity 7.5 Decision-making (p194)

The cause of the nausea is likely to be stimulation of dopamine receptors. You might have considered that blocking the receptors with a drug such as metoclopramide or haloperidol would improve the nausea. This is true but unfortunately would also make the motor symptoms of Parkinson's disease worse. Choosing a drug such as domperidone would be better as this has fewer effects on the central nervous system but would still block dopamine receptors in the CTZ and periphery to counteract nausea. Cyclizine is an antihistamine. This might be useful but, as we know the problem is likely to be caused by dopamine stimulation, counteracting this is a more logical choice.

Activity 7.6 Multiple choice questions (pp196–7)

1. Name the neurotransmitter molecule that is released in response to toxins or irritants in the GI tract:

    a) Serotonin (5-HT)

2. Name the region in the brain that is directly stimulated by factors in the circulation that trigger emesis:

    b) CTZ

3. Factors in the circulation can affect this region of the brain because it has an incomplete . . .

    Blood–brain barrier

4. The drug aprepitant is an antagonist for which neurotransmitter?

    d) Substance P

5. Which of the following is used to prevent nausea and vomiting?

    d) All of the above

6. Vomiting:

    c) Is involuntary

7. Anticipatory nausea and vomiting (ANV):

    c) Is a conditioned response

8. Nausea is:

    d) All of the above

9. The vomiting centre is a neural network in the:

    a) Medulla oblongata

10. Levomepromazine is an anti-emetic which antagonises which receptors?

    d) All of the above

Further reading and useful websites

The following NICE websites are recommended for further reading. The NICE websites provide guidance for the assessment and management of nausea and vomiting for different patient groups and also offer additional case scenarios to enhance your clinical decision-making through the implementation of evidence-based guidelines.

https://cks.nice.org.uk/nauseavomiting-in-pregnancy#!topicsummary/

NICE (2018a) *Nausea/Vomiting in Pregnancy.*

www.nice.org.uk/advice/esuom34/chapter/Key-points-from-the-evidence/

NICE (2014d) *Management of Vomiting in Children and Young People with Gastroenteritis: Ondansetron.*

https://cks.nice.org.uk/palliative-care-nausea-and-vomiting#!topicsummary/

NICE (2016a) *Palliative Care: Nausea and Vomiting.*

Section 3

Systems diseases and conditions

Chapter 8 Cardiovascular disease and hypertension

Chapter aims

After reading this chapter you will be able to:

- recognise cardiovascular disease as the leading cause of death in the United Kingdom;
- describe the risk factors, pathophysiology and clinical features for cardiovascular diseases including atherosclerosis, ischaemic heart disease and heart failure;
- describe the risk factors, pathophysiology and clinical features of hypertension;
- relate the signs and symptoms of these diseases to the underlying pathophysiology;
- explain how medications for atherosclerosis, hypertension, ischaemic heart disease and heart failure act;
- describe drug interactions, cautions and contraindications of medications used for cardiovascular diseases.

Introduction

Cardiovascular disease causes more than a quarter of all deaths in the United Kingdom (UK), or around 160,000 deaths each year (British Heart Foundation, 2016). Cardiovascular disease is also the major cause of death in other high income countries. The most common complications of cardiovascular disease are coronary heart disease and stroke.

NICE (2014a) defines cardiovascular disease as 'disease of the heart and blood vessels caused by the process of atherosclerosis'. Atherosclerosis is the build-up of fatty plaques in the wall of the arteries causing damage and restriction to blood flow. The damage to arteries takes many years to develop and, as such, cardiovascular disease usually affects people older than 50 years. It is also more common in men than women.

However, people much younger than 50 can be at risk of cardiovascular disease. Those with a family history of severe **hyperlipidaemia** may be at risk of cardiovascular disease in childhood. People with severe and enduring mental illnesses are at increased risk for a range of physical illnesses and conditions, including cardiovascular disease. Depression is associated with a significantly increased mortality from cardiovascular disease. It is estimated that those with schizophrenia and bipolar disorder die an average 25 years earlier than the general population, largely because of physical health problems (Mental Health Foundation, 2016).

In this chapter we begin by examining the risk factors and pathogenesis of atherosclerosis. We outline the main consequences of atherosclerosis which include: ischaemic heart disease, stroke and peripheral vascular disease. We then look at hypertension (high blood pressure). Hypertension is itself a risk factor for atherosclerosis. In addition, if left untreated, hypertension can cause other problems such as long-term kidney damage, cerebral haemorrhage (a type of stroke) and aortic **aneurysm**.

We then examine in more detail how atherosclerosis can affect blood supply to the heart muscle. Atherosclerosis is the main cause of ischaemic heart disease. This is where the blood supply to the heart muscle is reduced. The main consequences of ischaemic heart disease are stable angina and acute coronary syndromes.

Finally, we examine heart failure which is when the heart is unable to pump out enough blood to meet the demands of the body. Heart failure can be the end result of any chronic impairment of heart function, including myocardial infarction and chronic hypertension.

In this chapter, we have integrated the pharmacological treatments for the various conditions described. After each section on a particular cardiovascular disease, we give the main pharmacological treatments. This format will help you to understand how the pharmacological treatments relate to the different cardiovascular conditions covered.

Activity 8.1   Reflection

Complete this activity before continuing with this chapter. The aim is to identify your current knowledge on the risk factors for cardiovascular disease.

Tim is a practice nurse specialising in cardiovascular health. He works in a local medical centre. Part of Tim's role is to assess cardiovascular risk of patients aged 40 years and over. From your current knowledge of cardiovascular disease, what do you think the main risk factors are for cardiovascular disease in those aged over 40 years?

An outline answer is given at the end of the chapter.

Through completing Activity 8.1, you will begin to recognise the risk factors for cardiovascular disease. Many of these are potentially modifiable. This means that with effective screening, comprehensive advice on diet, weight management, levels of activity and pharmacological treatment, a person's risk of cardiovascular disease can be reduced. To provide the most effective health promotion information, it is important to understand these risk factors and how they contribute to cardiovascular disease. This is what we will look at next.

Risk factors for cardiovascular disease

Table 8.1 lists the risk factors for cardiovascular disease. These are classified as potentially modifiable and non-modifiable.

Potentially modifiable[1]	Non-modifiable
Smoking/tobacco use	Age
Poor diet	Male gender
High blood cholesterol	Family history of cardiovascular disease
High blood pressure	Ethnic origin
Insufficient physical activity	
Overweight/obesity	
Diabetes	
Psychological stress (linked to people's ability to influence the potentially stressful environments in which they live)	
Excess alcohol consumption	

Table 8.1 Risk factors for cardiovascular disease

[1] Yusuf, 2004 quoted in NICE Public Health Guidance 24: Prevention of Cardiovascular Disease (2010).

Age is an important non-modifiable risk factor for atherosclerosis and reflects the time needed for an atherosclerotic plaque to become advanced and trigger disease. Cardiovascular disease usually occurs in middle or later life. This is significant because in the UK and other high income countries, the population is ageing. As such, cardiovascular disease is likely to become an increasing problem. Males are more likely to experience cardiovascular disease than females. The incidence of cardiovascular disease in women increases once they have entered menopause. This suggests that female sex hormones may contribute to a lower risk. However, a large number of randomised control trials have shown that hormone replacement therapy does not reduce risk of cardiovascular disease in postmenopausal women (Ramrakha and Hill, 2012).

Family history of cardiovascular disease is another non-modifiable risk factor. Cardiovascular disease is multifactorial with genes, lifestyle and other environmental factors combining to produce increased risk. The genetic influence is considered significant if cardiovascular disease is present in a first-degree male relative before the age of 55 years and in a first-degree female relative before the age of 65 years.

Cardiovascular disease is up to 50% higher in those individuals living in the UK whose ethnic origin is South Asian. This reflects genetic factors and also an increased prevalence of risk factors including: type 2 diabetes, reduced physical activity and increased levels of triglycerides.

There are a significant number of potentially modifiable risk factors for atherosclerosis (Table 8.1). Smoking is estimated to increase the risk of cardiovascular disease by around 60%. This is the equivalent of 30,000 deaths per year from cardiovascular disease in the UK. Importantly, stopping smoking carries an immediate beneficial effect on cardiovascular disease. The development of effective local smoking cessation services by the NHS has been a key policy of the National Service Framework for Coronary Heart Disease (DH, 2000).

High blood cholesterol is also an important potentially modifiable risk factor for cardiovascular disease. Blood cholesterol levels can be reduced through careful attention to diet and increasing physical activity. Effective pharmacological intervention, through the use of cholesterol-lowering drugs called statins, may be advised. We discuss statins in the section 'Drugs used to reduce cardiovascular risk'.

Cholesterol is a type of lipid (fat molecule). It is found in a number of dietary sources and is manufactured within the body by the liver. Cholesterol is a vital component of cell membranes; it is also an important component of bile needed for fat digestion (Chapter 10). Cholesterol is also used to make steroid hormones (Chapter 2).

Lipids are insoluble in water. As such, cholesterol and triglycerides do not dissolve in the plasma, which is a watery fluid. Free cholesterol or triglyceride would in effect 'clog up' any blood vessel (like pouring fat down the drain). Cholesterol and triglycerides are carried in the blood as **lipoprotein particles**. These are microscopic 'spheres' made from lipid and protein molecules, which allow transport of cholesterol in the bloodstream. There are a number of different types of lipoprotein particle. Two in particular are associated with risk for cardiovascular disease:

- Low density lipoprotein particles (LDL particles) which are a risk factor for cardiovascular disease.
- High density lipoprotein particles (HDL particles) which help to lower the risk associated with LDL cholesterol.

LDL particles are made in the liver and transport cholesterol from the liver to sites in the body where it is needed. HDL particles transport cholesterol from tissues back to the liver.

Our plasma cholesterol levels depend upon our dietary intake and the amount made by the liver. The amount of cholesterol made by our liver will significantly depend upon our genetic make-up. In relation to this, there are a number of important genetic conditions which lead to very high blood cholesterol levels.

The most common of these is familial hypercholesterolaemia (FH) which is estimated to affect 110,000 people in the UK, or 1 in 500 people. FH is caused by a mutation in the gene encoding the LDL receptor. LDL receptors are located in the cell membrane of liver cells. As blood flows through the liver, LDL particles in the plasma attach to the LDL receptors and are taken up by the liver cells. This reduces plasma levels of LDL particles.

We have two copies of the LDL receptor gene; one copy of the gene is inherited from each of our parents. Those with FH will have inherited a mutated, non-functional copy of the LDL receptor gene. Their liver cells make only around half the number of LDL receptors. This reduces the clearance of LDL particles from the plasma. Those with FH have total plasma cholesterol levels of 7.5 mmol/L or above (5 mmol/L is considered healthy). Rarely, a person may have inherited two faulty copies of the LDL receptor gene. Their liver cells will have no functional LDL receptors. As such, total plasma cholesterol levels can be very high (over 13 mmol/L).

Raised levels of cholesterol of 7.5 mmol/L found in patients with FH are associated with accelerated atherosclerosis and coronary heart disease. Men with cholesterol levels of 7.5 mmol/L have by the age of 50 years a greater than 50% risk of coronary heart disease, and women have a greater than 30% risk by age 60 years. Those with cholesterol levels 13 mmol/L or over have symptoms of coronary heart disease in childhood and which is likely to cause early death from coronary heart disease (NICE, 2008). You can find out more about FH using the recommended reading at the end of this chapter.

Atherosclerosis

Atherosclerosis is a progressive disease of large- and medium-sized arteries. It is characterised by the build-up of fatty plaques, called an **atheroma**, within the wall of the artery. The atheroma causes a gradual narrowing of the lumen of the blood vessel called **stenosis**. Stenosis will reduce the blood flow through the artery and can cause ischaemia (impaired blood flow).

'Atheroma' comes from the Greek word for 'porridge'. At post-mortem, an atheroma looks and feels like hardened porridge in the artery wall. The atheroma develops over many years. This is estimated at over 40 years. Atheroma is believed to evolve from minor lesions called **fatty streaks** which are collections of lipid-filled foam cells (see below). Fatty streaks are thought to be a normal feature of arteries. However, for those living in high income countries, the fatty streaks can show harmful progression to more significant lesions as they enlarge.

Atherosclerosis develops through a chronic inflammatory response (Chapter 2). The current 'response to injury theory' proposes that a damaging inflammatory response develops in response to injury of the inner lining, or endothelium, of the artery.

Damage to the endothelium can occur from exposure to a variety of sources:

- Toxins from tobacco.
- Exposure to high levels of low density lipoprotein particles (LDL).
- Hyperglycaemia in diabetes mellitus.
- Microorganisms, possibly *Chlamydia pneumoniae* which has been isolated from atheromatous plaques.
- 'Shear stress' from blood flow – especially at artery branch points. Shear stress is increased in hypertension.

The damage to the endothelium makes it more 'permeable' to plasma LDL particles. Significant amounts of LDL particles begin to collect in the inner wall (or **intima**) of the blood vessel through the damaged endothelium. The damaged endothelial cells and the accumulation of LDL particles activate the inflammatory response (Chapter 2). Circulating white blood cells called monocytes attach to the endothelium and migrate into the intima where they become macrophages. Here they act as 'scavenger cells' and engulf LDL particles (through phagocytosis; Chapter 2). Macrophages containing engulfed LDL-cholesterol are called foam cells. Foam cells are unable to break down the cholesterol and soon die. This leads to a build-up below the endothelium of dead foam cells with their engulfed cholesterol. This produces a raised area referred to above as a fatty streak.

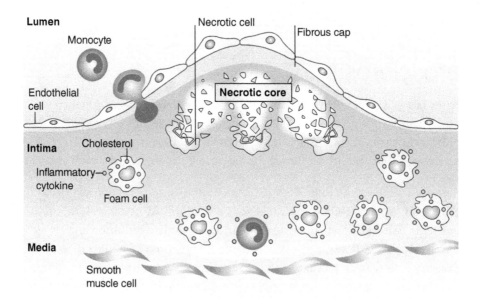

The figure shows the structure of an advanced atheromatous plaque in the wall of an artery. The fibrous cap comprises smooth muscle cells and collagen. The necrotic core of the plaque consists of cholesterol and necrotic cell debris. Smooth muscle cells migrate from the media into the intima. Monocytes are shown adhering to the endothelial cells in the lumen. These enter the intima to become cholesterol engulfing foam cells.

Figure 8.1 Advanced atheromatous plaque. (Reprinted by permission from Macmillan Publishers Ltd: *Nature Reviews Molecular Cell Biology* (vol. 11, no. 2), copyright, 2010)

A fatty streak may progress into a more advanced fibrous plaque. The damaged endothelial cells and macrophages release growth factors. These growth factors stimulate the growth and movement of smooth muscle cells from the **media** (middle layer of the artery) to the intima. The smooth muscle cells produce fibrous material, such as collagen, which forms a fibrous cap on the plaque. An advanced atheromatous plaque has the structure shown in Figure 8.1. It has a necrotic (or 'dead') core of foam cells, cholesterol and cell debris. The necrotic core is covered with a fibrous cap composed of smooth muscle cells and collagen.

The presence of an advanced plaque reduces the diameter of the lumen. The plaque can also cause a weakening of the arterial wall and this can lead to an aneurysm and possible rupture of the vessel.

Atheromatous plaques can be stable or non-stable: a stable plaque can cause vessel stenosis and weakening; an unstable plaque is potentially more serious because the surface of the plaque can become eroded, or ulcerate, or rupture. This can cause a **thrombus** to form on the plaque which may completely block the artery (occlusion). Debris from a ruptured plaque may generate emboli causing blood vessel blockage away from the original site of the plaque. This can be one cause of a stroke.

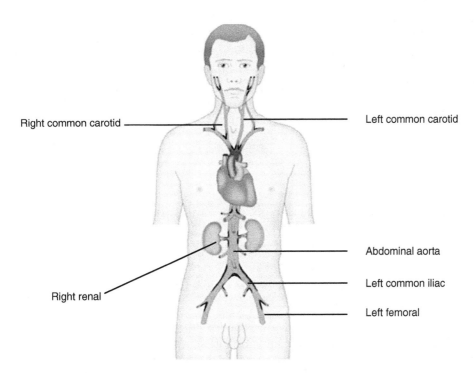

The figure shows the main sites of atherosclerosis (shaded dark grey). These are branch sites in arteries exposed to high blood pressure. The coronary arteries are not shown in this diagram but see Figure 8.4.

Figure 8.2 Main sites of atherosclerosis

The most common sites for atherosclerosis are large arteries exposed to high blood pressure (Figure 8.2). These include: the coronary arteries, the abdominal aorta, the iliac and femoral arteries (supplying the legs), and at the branch point in the carotid arteries which supply the head, and the renal arteries which supply the kidneys.

The potential consequences of atherosclerosis depend upon which artery or arteries are involved. Table 8.2 shows some of the main cardiovascular conditions caused by atherosclerosis. These are grouped by the artery involved.

Artery	Conditions/manifestation
Coronary arteries	Ischaemic heart disease (coronary artery disease): angina, acute coronary syndrome, sudden death, heart failure
Carotid artery	Cerebral infarction (stroke)
Aorta	Aortic aneurysm – localised dilation of the aorta due to weakening of the wall. Can tear and cause aortic dissection
Femoral and iliac arteries	Peripheral vascular disease

Table 8.2 Examples of important cardiovascular conditions

Drugs used to reduce cardiovascular risk

Drugs can be used to reduce some of the risk factors for atherosclerosis identified in Table 8.1. These include drugs used to lower cholesterol and drugs used to reduce blood pressure. We often talk about drugs being used for primary or secondary prevention. Primary prevention refers to the prevention of cardiovascular disease in those at risk; secondary prevention refers to slowing progression of disease in those who show signs of cardiovascular disease.

Case study

Muhammed is a 58-year-old man who comes to your clinic for a blood pressure check. He used to smoke but gave up when he was diagnosed with hypertension. Today, his blood pressure is controlled at 135/85 mmHg. His urea and electrolytes were also checked recently which showed that his kidney function was normal. He does not have symptoms of cardiovascular disease but his father had a 'heart attack' when he was 52. He is overweight with a BMI of 27. He is prescribed atorvastatin (a statin) 20 mg daily, amlodipine (a calcium channel blocker) 10 mg daily and lisinopril (an angiotensin converting enzyme inhibitor) 10 mg daily. The medication prescribed is all used to reduce the risk to Muhammed of cardiovascular disease.

Muhammed in the case study was prescribed a statin (atorvastatin), and amlodipine and lisinopril to reduce his blood pressure. In the section below, we examine statins which are used to lower cholesterol. Drugs used to treat high blood pressure are considered under 'Hypertension' below.

Statins

Examples of statins include atorvastatin, simvastatin and pravastatin. Statins are used to lower cholesterol which can slow the progression of atherosclerosis. This can prevent cardiovascular disease in those at risk (primary prevention). NICE (2014a) recommends that everyone who has a greater than 10% risk of developing cardiovascular disease in the next ten years should be prescribed a statin. Statins are also prescribed for people who have evidence of cardiovascular disease to prevent the condition worsening (secondary prevention). It is important to remember that lifestyle factors, such as diet, exercise and smoking, also need addressing.

Statins work by reducing cholesterol synthesis in the liver. Most cholesterol is made in the liver. The pathway of cholesterol synthesis in the liver requires an enzyme called 3-hydroxy-3-methylglutaryl-coenzyme A (HMG-CoA) reductase. Statins inhibit this enzyme thereby reducing cholesterol synthesis. This leads to a reduction of cholesterol in the blood.

Statins are metabolised by cytochrome P450 enzymes in the liver (Chapter 1). When other drugs or grapefruit juice are given which inhibit these liver enzymes drug interactions can occur. This can have serious consequences for patients.

Side-effects of statins

Statins can cause muscle pain in up to 5% of patients. In most cases this is mild but, in rare cases, statins can cause a condition called rhabdomyolysis. Muscle is broken down and myoglobin from the muscle is released into the bloodstream. This can damage the kidneys and deaths have been reported. The risk of muscle toxicity is increased when high doses are used or if statins are given with other medications which reduce the metabolism of statins. Patients starting on statins should be warned to report muscle pain. Statins can also increase plasma glucose and reduce insulin sensitivity. This effect is dose-related – the higher the dose the bigger the effect. This leads to a small increase in the risk of developing type 2 diabetes. Statins should also be used with caution in patients with liver disease as there have been reports of liver toxicity. Statins can increase the levels of liver enzymes when treatment is started, but levels often return to normal with continuing treatment. NICE (2008) suggests monitoring liver enzymes as a precaution.

Activity 8.2   Critical thinking

Esther is a 72-year-old woman who attends your nurse-led clinic.
She is attending for a cholesterol check and is prescribed simvastatin

(Continued)

(Continued)

40 mg once a day. You question her about her general health and she complains of muscle cramps in her legs which are worse at night. On further questioning she also explains that 5 days ago she was prescribed erythromycin 500 mg twice a day by the accident and emergency department for an infected wound on her finger. You recognise this as a possible case of rhabdomyolysis.

Can you explain the drug interaction between simvastatin and erythromycin that is causing the muscle pain? What would you do next?

An outline answer is available at the end of the chapter.

This activity illustrates the importance of monitoring side-effects. In this case, the side-effects were caused by a drug interaction.

Hypertension

Blood pressure varies from person-to-person with no clear cut-off point between normal blood pressure and hypertension. In light of this, definitions of hypertension vary. However, a commonly used definition of hypertension is 'persistently elevated blood pressure at a level where the benefit of treatment is clear cut for that individual' (Carton, 2012). Currently, in the UK, all patients with blood pressure over 160/100 mmHg should be treated. Decision to treat levels greater than 140/90 mmHg depends upon other risk factors.

It is estimated that as many as 7 million people in the UK are living with undiagnosed high blood pressure, without knowing they are at risk (British Heart Foundation, 2016). If left untreated hypertension is a risk factor for cardiovascular disease because it accelerates the progression of atherosclerosis. In addition, long-standing hypertension is associated with heart failure through increasing the work of the left ventricle. Hypertension increases the 'afterload' on the heart. This can cause the eventual weakening of the left ventricle (see under Heart failure, below). Hypertension may also lead to chronic kidney disease through damaging effects on small arteries and arterioles supplying the kidney. Other vascular disorders associated with hypertension include retinopathy, cerebral haemorrhage, dissecting aneurysm of the aorta and subarachnoid haemorrhage.

Ninety-five per cent of cases of hypertension have no known cause. These are referred to as essential hypertension. Five per cent are caused by an underlying disease such as chronic kidney disease. These cases are called secondary hypertension.

Normal blood pressure regulation

In this section we briefly review normal blood pressure regulation. Hypertension refers to high systemic blood pressure and results from a failure in normal regulation of blood pressure. Systemic blood pressure refers to the pressure of blood exerted on the walls of the arteries of the systemic circulation. The systemic circulation supplies oxygenated blood to all organs of the body. Systemic blood pressure is generated by contraction of the left ventricle with each heartbeat and 'drives' blood through the systemic circulation. Systemic blood pressure depends upon the volume of blood pumped out of the left ventricle (the **cardiac output**) and the resistance to this blood flow from the systemic blood vessels (the **systemic vascular resistance**).

Arterial blood pressure = cardiac output × systemic vascular resistance

Blood pressure is maintained in the short-term through adjusting cardiac output and systemic vascular resistance. For example, a momentary drop in blood pressure, occurring on standing up from a sitting position, causes a reflex increase in output from the sympathetic nervous system to the heart muscle and arterioles. In response, the heart contracts faster and with greater force, increasing the cardiac output. The arterioles vasoconstrict – or narrow increasing systemic vascular resistance. Together increasing cardiac output and increasing systemic vascular resistance produces an increase in blood pressure.

Longer-term adjustments to blood pressure involve adjustments to blood volume. Blood volume is regulated through the kidneys which are able to excrete more, or less, water (Chapter 14). An increased blood volume from, perhaps, increased salt and water intake, increases blood pressure through its effect on cardiac output. Increased blood volume results in an increased volume of blood returning to the right side of the heart. This is termed an increased 'preload'. When more blood returns to the heart, the ventricles fill with more blood and become stretched. The more the walls of the ventricles are stretched, the more forcefully they contract. The more forcefully the ventricles contract, the more blood is pumped out with each heartbeat. The volume of blood pumped out of the heart with each heartbeat is referred to as the stroke volume. Increases in stroke volume directly increase the cardiac output. The effect of an increased cardiac output is an increase in systemic blood pressure.

Following an increase in systemic blood pressure the kidneys excrete more sodium and water. The loss of sodium and water decreases the blood volume and blood pressure returns to normal. This regulatory process takes a number of days to come into full effect.

In the section 'Drugs used to treat hypertension', we will look in more detail at how these regulatory mechanisms can be altered by drugs used to reduce blood pressure.

Essential hypertension

There are a number of identifiable risk factors for essential hypertension. These are:

- family history of hypertension
- age
- ethnicity
- socioeconomic status
- stress.

These risk factors indicate hypertension is due to a combination of genetic and lifestyle factors, as well as age. There is no unifying account of the pathogenesis of essential hypertension. Patients often show both an increase in cardiac output and systemic vascular resistance. In a person who does not have hypertension, an increase in systemic blood pressure will be compensated for by a decrease in blood volume through the kidney, as described above. One mechanism for essential hypertension affects this compensatory process and is the inability of the kidneys to excrete sodium and water. Increased sodium and water retention will lead to increased blood volumes. In addition, many patients with hypertension show increases in systemic vascular resistance. In older adults, this may be due to hardening of the arteriole wall (arteriosclerosis) which increases resistance to blood flow. Arteriosclerosis is linked to the gradual increase in blood pressure with age. Other forms of hypertension may be mediated by enhanced sympathetic activity or increased levels of angiotensin II. Angiotensin II is a naturally occurring hormone that causes **vasoconstriction** and salt retention by the kidney.

Secondary hypertension is much less common than essential hypertension. It refers to hypertension due to a definable cause. The causes are various and can include endocrine disease, kidney disease and certain tumours. It may be a side-effect of medication.

Drugs used to treat hypertension

There are four main groups of drugs used to treat hypertension. These are angiotensin converting enzyme (ACE) inhibitors, calcium channel blockers, beta-blockers and thiazide diuretics. Muhammed, in the case study above, is on the calcium channel blocker, amlodipine, and the ACE inhibitor, lisinopril. Drug choice for a patient is determined by considering patient factors and applying guidelines such as those shown in Figure 8.3. The aim of treatment is to reduce blood pressure to 140/90 mmHg for people under 80 and 150/90 for those above 80 (NICE, 2011a).

Angiotensin converting enzyme (ACE) inhibitors

The renin angiotensin aldosterone system is an important way in which the body regulates blood pressure. Angiotensinogen is a peptide produced by the liver which enters

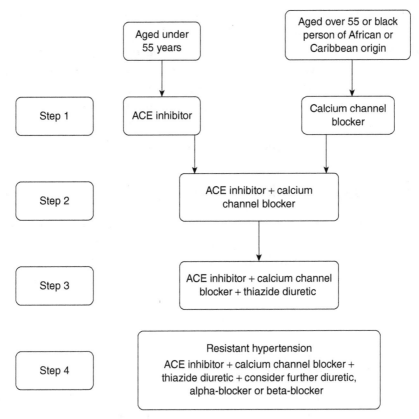

Figure 8.3 Adapted from NICE (2011a) Cg127. *The Clinical Management of Primary Hypertension in Adults*

the bloodstream. Renin, an enzyme produced by the kidney, diffuses into the bloodstream and converts angiotensinogen to angiotensin I. Angiotensin converting enzyme (ACE) is an enzyme that converts angiotensin I to angiotensin II. Angiotensin II is a potent vasoconstrictor which increases blood pressure. Blocking this enzyme with an ACE inhibitor will therefore lower blood pressure. Angiotensin II also stimulates aldosterone release from the adrenal cortex. This increases sodium and water reabsorption in the kidney. Reducing angiotensin II will therefore reduce sodium and water retention which again lowers blood pressure as fluid volume is reduced. Examples of ACE inhibitors include ramipril, lisinopril and enalapril.

As well as to reducing hypertension, ACE inhibitors are also used long term for people who have had a myocardial infarction or those who have heart failure or diabetes. They prevent further deterioration of organs, such as the heart and kidney, because they reduce the stress on these organs by reducing blood pressure.

Side-effects of ACE inhibitors

ACE inhibitors can cause hypotension which can make a patient feel dizzy. This is especially a problem when the first dose is given to people who have heart failure or who are on a diuretic. In some patients ACE inhibitors can cause renal injury as they reduce blood flow to the kidney. For this reason, patients need to have their kidney function checked before and during drug treatment. A persistent dry cough is a common problem with ACE inhibitors. The enzyme ACE is involved in the breakdown of bradykinin. When ACE is blocked, bradykinin builds up which causes the cough. Changing a patient to an angiotensin II receptor blocker (ARB) can be helpful in this case. ACE inhibitors can also cause angioedema. This leads to swelling of the lips, tongue and face. Again, this is caused by a build-up of bradykinin. This can be life-threatening if swelling also occurs in the airways. The ACE inhibitor would need to be discontinued and supportive therapies given.

Angiotensin receptor blockers (ARBs)

These drugs are related to ACE inhibitors. ARBs prevent angiotensin II binding to receptors on arterioles, preventing vasoconstriction. Their overall effect is similar to the ACE inhibitors as they dilate blood vessels and lower blood pressure. Importantly, ARBs do not cause a cough because they do not cause a build-up of bradykinin. They are usually used for people who cannot tolerate ACE inhibitors because of the cough. Examples of ARBs are losartan, candesartan and valsartan.

Calcium channel blockers

Calcium channels exist in smooth muscle in the walls of blood vessels and the heart. Calcium enters smooth muscle cells of blood vessels via the calcium channels to cause vasoconstriction. This would result in an increase in blood pressure. When these channels are blocked, calcium cannot enter the cells and vasodilation occurs which reduces blood pressure. When calcium channels in the heart are blocked this leads to a reduction in heart rate and a reduction in the force of contractions. Some calcium channel blockers work more on the heart and others work more on the blood vessels. In hypertension, calcium channel blockers which work more on the blood vessels are the most useful. Examples of calcium channel blockers used to treat hypertension include amlodipine and nifedipine.

Calcium channel blockers are also used to prevent angina. This will be described in the section on angina.

Side-effects of calcium channel blockers

Side-effects of calcium channel blockers result from the general vasodilation they cause. This includes headache, dizziness and flushing. Gastrointestinal disturbances and ankle oedema are also common.

Thiazide diuretics

Thiazide diuretics inhibit the reabsorption of sodium in the kidney. Excretion of sodium, potassium and water is increased as a result. Thiazides are moderately potent diuretics and only low doses are needed in hypertension. They are usually given in the morning so that diuresis does not interfere with sleep. Bendroflumethiazide is an example of a thiazide diuretic but current guidance suggests the use of chlorthalidone and indapamide for hypertension (NICE, 2011a).

Side-effects of thiazide diuretics

Electrolyte imbalances such as low potassium (hypokalaemia) and low sodium (hyponatraemia) may occur. Glucose levels can be elevated which makes them less suitable for diabetic patients. Postural hypotension and cramp are also common problems. They can also cause gout.

Beta-blockers

Beta-blockers are **beta adrenergic receptor** antagonists. This means that they block the binding of noradrenaline to beta adrenergic receptors on the heart and arterioles. As a result they reduce heart rate and decrease the force of heart contractions. They also relax smooth muscle in arteries, reducing blood pressure by reducing peripheral resistance. Examples of beta-blockers used to treat hypertension include propranolol, atenolol and bisoprolol.

Side-effects of beta-blockers

In patients with asthma, life-threatening **bronchoconstriction** may occur. This is the result of blocking beta receptors in the smooth muscle of the bronchioles in the lung (Chapter 9). Cold extremities can occur as beta-blockers cause peripheral vasoconstriction. Reduced cardiac output can make patients feel tired. Sometimes beta-blockers slow the heart too much causing heart block or signs of heart failure. In diabetic patients they can mask symptoms of hypoglycaemia and should be used with caution. Fat-soluble beta-blockers, such as propranolol, can enter the brain and cause sleep disturbances and nightmares.

Activity 8.3   Evidence-based practice and research

Use Figure 8.3 to determine whether Muhammed in the case study is on an appropriate treatment for hypertension. What stage of treatment is he at?

If you were a nurse prescriber, what type of medication would you start for an Afro-Caribbean woman aged 52 with hypertension? Assume the patient is on no other medication.

An outline answer is available at the end of the chapter.

This activity will have helped you understand how antihypertensive drugs are chosen for people. In the section below, we consider ischaemic heart disease. Ischaemic heart disease (IHD) is one of the most important consequences of atherosclerosis.

Ischaemic heart disease (IHD)

Scenario

You are a community nurse visiting Angus, aged 75 years, at home. He suffers from angina. You notice that he keeps a glyceryl trinitrate (GTN) spray on his kitchen table. You ask him how he uses the spray. He tells you that when he is out walking, especially if he is going up a hill, he sometimes experiences a tight and painful sensation in his chest. If this happens he stops walking and sprays two puffs of his GTN spray under his tongue and the pain usually goes away. If it does not he waits five minutes and sprays another two puffs under his tongue. He has been told that if that does not work after five minutes he should call an ambulance as he might be having a heart attack, but that luckily has not happened.

Angus in the above scenario suffers from stable angina. Angina is one way IHD can be experienced. As described, stable angina is a temporary chest pain which tends to occur on exertion and may be relieved by rest or taking a medication called GTN. In the next section, we consider the different types of IHD and the drugs used to treat these.

IHD results in over 117,000 deaths a year in the UK. The UK has one of the highest incidences of IHD in the world. The most common cause of IHD is obstruction in one or more coronary arteries due to atherosclerosis. IHD caused by atherosclerosis is referred to as coronary artery disease or coronary heart disease.

IHD occurs when the coronary blood supply is insufficient to meet the demands for oxygenated blood of the heart muscle (myocardium).

IHD can be experienced as:

- angina pectoris
- myocardial infarction
- sudden cardiac death
- heart failure.

Angina pectoris

Angina pectoralis is defined as chest pain or discomfort due to myocardial ischaemia (inadequate blood flow to the heart muscle). Ischaemia is usually due to coronary stenosis caused by atheroma. There are other possible causes including: tachycardia, anaemia, aortic stenosis, enlargement of the left ventricle and artery spasm.

Angina is termed 'stable' if symptoms have been present for at least two months without changes in severity or triggering factors. With stable angina, there is a fixed narrowing (stenosis) of the coronary arteries. Angina typically occurs on exertion and disappears on resting. Angina may also be triggered by emotional stress.

Angina arises with ischaemia, when the oxygen supply to the heart muscle becomes inadequate for its metabolic needs. The severity of angina is not always related to the level of ischaemia and ischaemia may be present without angina. The degree of pain may be related to the production of a molecule called adenosine which is released during myocardial ischaemia. Adenosine is thought to directly stimulate pain fibres in the heart (Alaeddini and Shirani, 2015).

Angina is often described as a pressure or heaviness, tightness or a squeezing sensation (Carton, 2012). It is a type of visceral pain (Chapter 6) and is often referred. The referred pain is felt as radiating up the neck into the jaw and across the shoulders and upper arms. Angina may trigger nausea and sweating.

Angina is significant because it may be the first indication that a patient has advanced atherosclerosis. Atherosclerosis is often widespread through the arterial system and may be present in other arteries. The patient will then be at risk for other forms of cardiovascular disease including other forms of IHD, aortic aneurysm and stroke (Table 8.1).

Drugs used to treat stable angina

Treatments for angina fall into two categories. The first category is used to reduce risks of further cardiovascular disease. This would include non-drug, lifestyle measures such as exercise and smoking reduction. Drug measures to reduce risks would possibly include statins to reduce cholesterol and drugs to control hypertension. The second category includes drugs used to control symptoms. These include beta-blockers and calcium channel blockers which have been previously described. Another group of medicines, the nitrates, are also useful. Educating patients about what the medicines are for is very important.

Nitrates

In the scenario, GTN is being used to treat Angus's acute angina symptoms. GTN is an example of a nitrate. Nitrates work by releasing nitric oxide into the bloodstream. The nitric oxide works by relaxing the smooth muscles of veins and arteries. This leads to dilation of the blood vessels. As a result, coronary arteries, which are blocked in angina, open up and allow more blood to flow to the heart. This brings the extra oxygen the heart muscle needs and pain is relieved. Also by dilating blood vessels, the pressure in the vessels is reduced and this makes it easier for the heart to pump blood. This reduces the work the heart needs to do, which in turn reduces the amount of oxygen it needs.

GTN is given sub-lingually (under the tongue). It is absorbed rapidly from the blood vessels under the tongue and works very quickly. It is rapidly metabolised by the liver and has a very short half-life of only 1–3 minutes. This helps to explain why if it fails to work after 5 minutes, another dose should be tried. If the GTN does not relieve the pain it might be a sign that the patient is having a myocardial infarction and an ambulance must be called. GTN undergoes almost total first pass metabolism (Chapter 1) so would not work if it was given as a tablet to swallow. Other nitrates, such as isosorbide mononitrate, can be taken orally. Isosorbide mononitrate is usually taken two to three times a day, or as a long-acting preparation, once a day. Isosorbide mononitrate is taken to prevent angina attacks.

Common side-effects of nitrates

Side-effects are caused by the vasodilation nitrates cause. Patients may suffer from headaches and low blood pressure which might make a patient feel dizzy.

Acute coronary syndromes

Scenario

While you are working as a student nurse in A&E, Jeff, a 78-year-old man, presents with severe chest pain. His skin is cold, clammy and mottled and he complains of nausea. Following ECG monitoring, Jeff is found to have STEMI (ST-elevated myocardial infarction). During this time Jeff has blood taken for testing and morphine is given for his pain.

Jeff presents with acute coronary syndrome. Acute coronary syndrome (ACS) refers to the collection of syndromes resulting from the formation of a thrombus on a complicated atheromatous plaque (Figure 8.4). The syndrome ranges from unstable angina to transmural myocardial infarction. Patients usually present with severe chest pain of sudden onset, although it can develop more gradually. Pain is often accompanied by profuse sweating, nausea and vomiting. Patients may experience anxiety described as a feeling of 'impending doom'.

ACS is currently classified into main two groups:

- Unstable angina
- Myocardial infarction (MI).

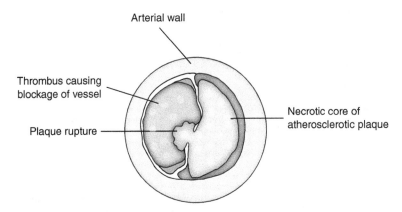

Arterial wall

Thrombus causing
blockage of vessel

Plaque rupture

Necrotic core of
atherosclerotic plaque

The figure shows an advanced atherosclerotic plaque whose cap has ruptured. Plaque rupture causes leakage of the contents of the core. A thrombus forms at the site of rupture. In the figure, the thrombus has completely occluded the artery.

Figure 8.4 Plaque rupture and thrombus formation

MI occurs when significant heart muscle tissue has been damaged (Figure 8.5). Unstable angina refers to an acute coronary event with no damage to the myocardium. This classification is based upon serum concentration of cardiac enzymes and markers. The presence of troponin T in the serum 12 hours after onset of symptoms indicates MI. Troponin T is released from damaged myocardial cells and indicates myocardial damage and injury. Jeff will have raised troponin T and/or creatinine kinase.

The immediate management of someone with an ACS depends upon the findings of their ECG. In particular is the presence or absence of 'ST segment elevation'. The presence of ST elevation indicates significant coronary artery occlusion with full-thickness damage to the heart muscle. This requires immediate reperfusion therapy. This is described below under treatment for MI with ST elevation (STEMI).

The thrombus can cause partial blockage of the coronary artery which can cause unstable angina or non-ST elevated myocardial infarction (NSTEMI) if associated with myocardial injury. A thrombus which completely occludes the coronary artery will lead to myocardial damage of full-thickness and STEMI. The ischaemic damage occurring during an MI is potentially reversible. It takes around 20 to 40 minutes of severe ischemia to cause irreversible cell death (Kumar et al., 2014). If the blood flow is restored within this time, for example by reperfusion therapy, it may be possible to reduce the extent of cell death. This is the rationale for prompt reperfusion treatment in MI.

The area of infarcted muscle depends upon the area supplied by the coronary artery. The area of infarcted tissue will eventually be replaced by scar tissue. Patients who have experienced an ACS are at high risk of further acute coronary events and the subsequent development of heart failure.

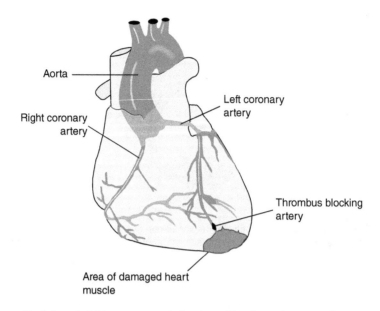

The figure shows the left and right coronary arteries branching from the ascending aorta. These supply oxygenated blood to the myocardium (heart muscle). A thrombus is shown blocking an anterior branch. The area of myocardium that is no longer supplied by the artery becomes damaged. Unless the blockage is reversed, the area of myocardium that is no longer supplied by the artery becomes damaged. Unless the blockage is reversed, the area of myocardium will die (myocardial infarction).

Figure 8.5   Coronary arteries and occluded vessel

Treatments for MI with ST elevation (STEMI)

Jeff was diagnosed with STEMI. To minimise damage to his heart he was given percutaneous coronary intervention (PCI) at his nearest specialist centre. This involves mechanically dilating coronary arteries and removing clots, for example with stents and angioplasty. There is evidence that intra-coronary stenting is more effective than angioplasty.

Patients will also receive acute treatment with medication. A common combination is sub-lingual GTN, intravenous morphine or diamorphine, an intravenous anti-emetic such as metoclopramide and oral aspirin. The opioid analgesic helps to control the pain and anxiety (Chapter 6). The GTN dilates coronary arteries and improves ischaemic pain by mechanisms already described. Metoclopramide prevents nausea and vomiting (Chapter 7). The aspirin is an antiplatelet drug which we shall now consider in more detail.

Antiplatelet medication

Platelets form part of the normal clotting mechanism. When they encounter injured tissue such as a wound or internal damage in blood vessels, they release chemicals which activate other platelets and cause them to stick together. A clot called a thrombus is formed. Antiplatelet drugs prevent platelets sticking together and reduce thrombus formation in arteries. Two drugs, aspirin and clopidogrel, are discussed below in their role as antiplatelets.

Aspirin

One of the chemicals released by platelets, which makes them stick together, is called thromboxane A2. Aspirin prevents the formation of this chemical by blocking an enzyme in platelets called cyclooxygenase. With no thromboxane, platelets cannot signal to each other to stick together. This can help to break up and prevent thrombus formation.

Much of the evidence supporting the use of aspirin in myocardial infarction comes from a large randomised controlled trial called ISIS-2 (1988). When aspirin was used deaths from strokes and re-occlusion of vessels were significantly reduced.

As well as acute treatment of MI, aspirin is also used to prevent strokes and MI in people who have CVD or who have had a stroke (i.e. they are used for secondary prevention). Lower doses of 75 mg are used. Aspirin has not been proved to be useful for primary prevention. This means that it probably will not stop you having an MI or stroke if you do not have cardiovascular disease.

Aspirin is metabolised to an active metabolite called salicylate. The half-life of both aspirin and salicylate are relatively short (aspirin 15–20 minutes, salicylate 2–3 hours). However aspirin blocks cyclooxygenase irreversibly. This means that once the enzyme is blocked that platelet will never be able to produce thromboxane and stick to others. The effect of aspirin therefore lasts for the life of the platelet which is 7–10 days.

Side-effects

As we saw in Chapter 6 on pain, blocking cyclooxygenase leads to side-effects. One of the most important for aspirin is gastrointestinal ulcers and bleeding. Aspirin causes direct irritation of the stomach lining. This can be reduced by giving aspirin with food or giving enteric coated tablets (aspirin e.c.). However, this will not completely solve the problem as when the aspirin is absorbed it will block cyclooxygenase which reduces prostaglandin synthesis. This systemic effect will lead to ulcers (Chapter 10). Aspirin can also cause difficulties in breathing in patients with asthma and allergies. Aspirin must be used with care in patients with renal impairment as it can cause further renal impairment (Chapter 6). It should also be avoided in severe hepatic impairment as the risk of bleeding is further increased.

Clopidogrel

Clopidogrel is another type of antiplatelet medication which works in a different way to aspirin. Adenosine diphosphate (ADP) is another chemical released by platelets that causes them to stick together. Clopidogrel blocks the binding of ADP to receptor sites on the platelet and stops platelets sticking together.

It is used in combination with aspirin to prevent thrombus formation after both STEMI and NSTEMI. It is also used with aspirin to prevent thrombus formation in patients with atrial fibrillation (AF) who cannot have warfarin.

Clopidogrel is actually a pro-drug (Chapter 1) and must be metabolised in the liver to produce the active ingredient. Like aspirin, its action is irreversible so lasts for the life of the platelet (7–10 days). Unlike aspirin, it does not work straight away. It can take 3–7 days to reach its full effect, so is less useful during an MI.

Side-effects

Increased bleeding is the most common side-effect of clopidogrel.

Activity 8.4   Communication

Angelique had an MI 6 months ago. She was treated with a stent and has recovered well with few residual symptoms. She is currently on ramipril 5 mg twice a day, aspirin 75 mg daily, clopidogrel 75 mg daily, atenolol 100 mg daily, atorvastatin 40 mg daily and lansoprazole 30 mg daily. You run a nurse-led clinic. At her appointment she confides in you that she is a bit 'hit and miss' with her medication. Since her heart attack she has been taking regular walks and has lost weight. She also feels her diet is much healthier. She does not think she really needs all this medication any more as she is much healthier than she was.

Can you describe to Angelique what all the medication is for and whether or not she should continue taking it?

An outline answer is given at the end of the chapter.

Activity 8.4 shows that people with CVD may be prescribed a number of different medications. Providing patient education and information is, therefore, an important aspect of the nursing role.

Heart failure

Scenario

As a heart failure nurse specialist you have known Florence, an 85-year-old woman, for several years. Florence was recently discharged from hospital. She has developed chronic heart failure following a previous MI. Florence lives with her family who support her on a practical level. She sees a close friend once a week for a short visit to the local park. Over the past four weeks Florence has developed a progressive increase in breathlessness, and ankle oedema. She now has difficulty breathing at night when lying down (orthopnea). She suffers from fatigue and has difficulty walking more than a few hundred yards without becoming breathless.

As part of your visit you assess Florence's condition and check her medication. She has been prescribed ramipril, furosemide and bisoprolol. You discuss with her how each of her drugs work, helping her to understand the importance of adhering to treatment. As part of your specialist role, you explain to Florence about her heart failure and explain the cause of her symptoms.

We can see from the scenario that heart failure has a significant impact on quality of life. Florence has quite severe heart failure with her poor capacity for exercise and shortness of breath on walking. The prognosis of heart failure is poor with mortality over 50% at five years. The incidence of heart failure in the UK is increasing probably due to increased survival rates of those patients with IHD, especially the treatment of MI. As with other cardiovascular diseases, heart failure shows an increased prevalence with age.

Heart failure occurs when the heart is unable to supply adequate blood flow to meet the metabolic needs of the body. Although the word 'failure' suggests that the heart may have stopped, this is not the case. The heart muscle has become weakened. Heart failure, in its chronic form, is often termed congestive heart failure, due to the build-up of fluid in the lungs, liver, gastrointestinal tract, and the arms and legs. However, congestion is not always present in chronic heart failure, and the term 'congestive' is not used in current literature.

There are a number of different forms of heart failure:

- acute or chronic heart failure
- systolic or diastolic heart failure
- right or left heart failure
- high output or low output heart failure.

The most common form of chronic heart failure is left ventricular failure.

The result of the weakening of the heart is a reduced cardiac output and low blood pressure. As a consequence, blood flow to organs and tissues is inadequate. This is described as underperfusion and triggers a number of compensatory changes to the heart and circulation which initially raise blood pressure (Figure 8.6). However, these compensatory mechanisms and raised blood pressure place greater pressure on an already weakened heart and exacerbate symptoms.

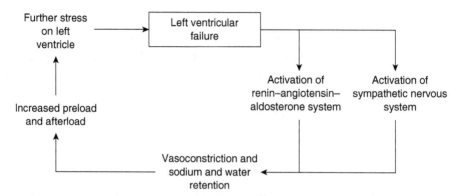

A fall in cardiac output from heart failure (left ventricular heart failure) causes a fall in blood pressure. The fall in blood pressure leads to activation of the renin–angiotensin–aldosterone system and activation of the sympathetic nervous system (see text under 'Normal blood pressure regulation'). These in turn cause vasoconstriction and sodium and water retention. However, these cause an increase in blood volume (preload), increased vascular resistance (afterload) and increased heart rate. These put further strain on the heart (Carton, 2012).

Figure 8.6   Compensatory mechanisms in heart failure

Loop diuretics

The loop diuretics furosemide and bumetanide are commonly used. They are called loop diuretics because they work on the Loop of Henle in the kidney. Usually 80% of the urine volume is reabsorbed from the Loop of Henle back into the blood. Loop diuretics inhibit the reabsorption of sodium, potassium and water from the Loop of Henle. This results in a large diuretic action, much larger than that of the thiazide diuretics. They also have a useful vasodilating effect. Together these actions reduce blood pressure and reduce stress on the heart.

If given by mouth the diuretic effect usually starts within an hour and lasts for four to six hours. Loop diuretics should, therefore, be given in the morning so a patient does not have to get up to urinate at night.

Common side-effects of loop diuretics

Low potassium (hypokalaemia) can occur as loop diuretics prevent potassium reabsorption from the kidney into the blood. Left untreated this can lead to disturbances in the rhythm of the heart and patients may complain of palpitations. This is because the heart muscle needs potassium for the conduction of electrical impulses. Other electrolyte imbalances can also occur, such as low sodium (hyponatraemia). Weakness and cramp in skeletal muscle can occur as a result of these electrolyte imbalances. Because they are powerful diuretics, dehydration and postural hypotension may occur, especially in elderly patients. Signs of dehydration include extreme thirst, dizziness and fatigue. It is important that nurses educate patients and carers to recognise these symptoms.

ACE inhibitors

The mechanism of action of ACE inhibitors has been explained under the treatment of hypertension. In heart failure, clinical trials have shown that they can increase life expectancy and reduce hospital admissions (Flather et al., 2000). When the heart fails the body attempts to compensate for the falling cardiac output by increasing vasoconstriction (Figure 8.6). This is mediated by an increase in angiotensin II. This increases strain in the heart. ACE inhibitors reduce strain on the failing heart by inhibiting angiotensin II formation and causing vasodilation.

Beta-blockers

Beta-blockers can also increase life expectancy. It used to be thought that, as beta-blockers reduce the rate and force of contractions in the heart, they would make heart failure worse. However, in heart failure, the fall in cardiac output and blood pressure stimulates the sympathetic nervous system which increases the strain on the heart (Figure 8.6). As beta-blockers block the effects of adrenaline and noradrenaline on the heart, they reduce strain on the heart. It is not known whether all beta-blockers are effective and only bisoprolol, carvedilol and nebivolol are licensed for this in the UK.

It is now time to review what you have learned within this chapter by undertaking some multiple choice questions.

Activity 8.5   Multiple choice questions

1. The build-up of fatty plaques within the wall of arteries is:
   a) Hypertension
   b) Atherosclerosis
   c) Ischaemic heart disease
   d) Heart failure

2. Consequences of atherosclerosis include the following except:
   a) Ischaemic heart disease
   b) Acute coronary syndromes
   c) Hypertension
   d) Stroke

(Continued)

(Continued)

3. Risk factors for atherosclerosis include all the following except:

   a) Advanced age
   b) Smoking
   c) Low levels LDL particles
   d) Hypertension

4. A blood clot within an artery is a:

   a) Myocardial infarction
   b) Thrombus
   c) Stroke
   d) Acute coronary syndrome

5. Hypertension of unknown cause is known as:

   a) Essential
   b) Secondary
   c) Angina
   d) Heart

6. Which of the following types of drugs is NOT used to treat hypertension?

   a) Thiazide diuretics
   b) ACE inhibitors
   c) Calcium channel blockers
   d) Nitrates

7. Glyceryl trinitrate (GTN) is administered sub-lingually to reduce pain in angina. It is not suitable for oral use because:

   a) It irritates the stomach lining and could cause significant peptic ulceration resulting in bleeds.
   b) It is destroyed by digestive enzymes in the stomach before it can be effectively absorbed.
   c) It would be almost completely metabolised by the liver before it reached the systemic circulation.
   d) It can cause side-effects such as headaches. Sub-lingual administration reduces the doses that are needed, which in turn reduces side-effects.

8. How do ACE inhibitors work?

   a) They block the liver enzyme 3-hydroxy-3-methylglutaryl-coenzyme A reductase
   b) They block the formation of the enzyme renin by the kidney
   c) They block the enzyme cyclooxygenase
   d) They block the conversion of angiotensin I to angiotensin II

9. Which of the following can interact with simvastatin to increase levels and cause potentially serious muscle toxicity?

   a) Erythromycin
   b) Flucloxacillin
   c) Trimethoprim
   d) All of the above

10. A patient who has experienced an acute MI may be prescribed the following medication long term: simvastatin, aspirin, ramipril and bisoprolol. Which of the following statements about these drugs is TRUE?

    a) Bisoprolol is being used to treat high blood pressure
    b) Aspirin is being used for ischaemic pain
    c) Simvastatin is being used for primary prevention
    d) Ramipril is being used to reduce the work of the heart

Chapter summary

Cardiovascular disease (CVD) is a leading cause of death in the UK and worldwide. CVD includes coronary heart disease (CHD) and stroke. Risk factors for CVD include those that can be modified (including hyperlipidaemia, hypertension, weight, exercise and smoking) and those that cannot (such as age and family history). Drug treatments such as statins for hyperlipidaemia and antihypertensive drugs such as calcium channel blockers, ACE inhibitors, thiazide diuretics and beta-blockers can help to reduce the risks of developing CVD. CHD occurs when there is a build-up of fatty plaques in the coronary arteries, a process known as atherosclerosis. This can lead to angina, myocardial infarction and/or heart failure. Drug treatments for these conditions aim to relieve symptoms, reduce further atherosclerosis and protect the heart.

Activities: Brief outline answers

Activity 8.1 Reflection (p204)

Risk factors for CVD include smoking, diet, blood pressure, age, sex, being overweight, exercise, high cholesterol and whether your family has a history of CVD. Special calculators are often used to add up the different risk factors. One example is QRISK2-2014 cardiovascular disease risk calculator. This enables clinicians to calculate the percentage risk that someone will develop cardiovascular disease over the next ten years. It takes into account many of the risk factors described above. More information about this risk calculator can be found at **www.qrisk.org/**

Activity 8.2 Critical thinking (pp211–12)

Erythromycin inhibits cytochrome P450 enzymes in the liver which metabolise simvastatin. As a result the levels of simvastatin in the blood will increase. The increased levels can cause muscle toxicity as described in the chapter. The simvastatin would have to be stopped. Tests would need to be carried out to see whether the muscle toxicity was mild, which would require no further treatment, or severe in which case further treatment might be needed. Once symptoms had subsided follow-up would be needed to ensure that Esther received further statin treatment if that was appropriate.

Activity 8.3 Evidence-based practice and research (p217)

Muhammed is on an appropriate treatment and is on stage 2 of hypertension treatment. This would mean that treatment with a single agent had not been effective. For the second patient you would start at stage one and choose a calcium channel blocker such as amlodipine. ACE inhibitors cause more angioedema in black people of African or Afro-Caribbean origin. Angioedema can be life-threatening, which is why they are not used (Vleeming et al., 1998).

Activity 8.4 Communication (p224)

Most of this medication is taken to prevent complications that can arise after an MI. Changes in the heart occur after an MI which can lead to heart failure and arrhythmias. Atenolol is a beta-blocker and many trials have shown that taking them long term after an MI reduces the risk of death and re-infarction. Ramipril is an ACE inhibitor which caused vasodilation and reduces the work of the heart. It should also be taken long term. Atorvastatin is a statin which lowers cholesterol and reduces the risk of another MI. Aspirin is an antiplatelet and reduces the risk of further clots forming which also reduces the risk of further MIs. Again it should be taken long term. Clopidogrel is also an antiplatelet – Angelique probably will not need this forever and it is usually stopped after a few months. The lansoprazole is to prevent GI bleeds that the antiplatelet agents may cause (Chapter 6). These treatments are all recommended by NICE CG 172. Angelique should be acknowledged for her diet, weight loss and exercise, as these are a very important part of rehabilitation and reducing further risks. Angelique must, however, continue her current drug regime.

Activity 8.5 Multiple choice questions (pp227–9)

1. The build-up of fatty plaques within the wall of arteries is:

    b) Atherosclerosis

2. Consequences of atherosclerosis include the following except:

    c) Hypertension

3. Risk factors for atherosclerosis include all the following except:

    c) Low levels LDL particles

4. A blood clot within an artery is a:

    b) Thrombus

5. Hypertension of unknown cause is known as:

    a) Essential

6. Which of the following types of drugs is NOT used to treat hypertension?

    d) Nitrates

7. Glyceryl trinitrate (GTN) is administered sub-lingually to reduce pain in angina. It is not suitable for oral use because:

    c) It would be almost completely metabolised by the liver before it reached the systemic circulation

8. How do ACE inhibitors work?

    d) They block the conversion of angiotensin I to angiotensin II

9. Which of the following can interact with simvastatin to increase levels and cause potentially serious muscle toxicity?

    a) Erythromycin

10. A patient who has experienced an acute MI may be prescribed the following medication long term: simvastatin, aspirin, ramipril and bisoprolol. Which of the following statements about these drugs is TRUE?

    d) Ramipril is being used to reduce the work of the heart

Further reading

Kumar, V, Abbas, A, Fausto, N and Mitchell, R (2014) *Robbins Basic Pathology* (9th edition). Philadelphia: Saunders Elsevier.

A comprehensive and detailed textbook on pathology. Chapter 10 gives details on atherosclerosis; Chapter 11 gives details on ischaemic heart disease and heart failure. Chapter 7 gives further information on familial hypercholesterolaemia.

Simonsen, T, Aarbakke, J, Kay, I, Coleman, I, Sinnott, P and Lysaa, R (2006) *Illustrated Pharmacology for Nurses*. London: Hodder Arnold.

A clearly written and well-illustrated pharmacology book aimed at nurses.

Tortora, G and Derrickson, B (2017) *Principles of Anatomy and Physiology* (17th edition). Oxford: Wiley.

A comprehensive and clearly written anatomy and physiology textbook.

Useful websites

http://cks.nice.org.uk/heart-failure-chronic#!topicsummary/

Evidence for heart failure treatment.

www.bhf.org.uk/

Website of the British Heart Foundation.

www.nhs.uk/conditions/high-blood-pressure-hypertension/

Information from NHS Choices on hypertension.

Chapter 9 Respiratory diseases

Chapter aims

After reading this chapter you will be able to:

- describe the risk factors, pathophysiology and clinical features of asthma and chronic obstructive pulmonary disease (COPD);
- relate the signs and symptoms of asthma and COPD to the underlying pathophysiology;
- explain how drugs for asthma and COPD exert their actions and can cause side-effects;
- describe the important drug interactions, cautions and contraindications of these drugs;
- explain how current guidelines are used to choose different drugs for patients with asthma and COPD.

Case study

Peter, a retired teacher aged 65 years, first developed symptoms of chronic obstructive pulmonary disease (COPD) five years ago. Prior to his diagnosis Peter smoked around 20 cigarettes per day. He started smoking cigarettes at school when he was 14 years old. Since his diagnosis of COPD he has managed to stop smoking.

Peter first noticed symptoms of breathlessness on exertion and a cough with the production of sputum (referred to as a productive cough). He initially put these down to the effects of ageing along with his smoking habit. As his breathlessness worsened his wife encouraged him to see his GP. The practice nurse completed a lung function test using a spirometer (see under 'Lung function tests'). This indicated mild COPD. Peter was also given a blood test to rule out anaemia as a cause of his breathlessness. He was prescribed a salbutamol inhaler to be used as required.

Introduction

Peter is typical of someone presenting with COPD. In this chapter we examine COPD and asthma, both of which are common lung disorders. Asthma often starts in childhood but COPD is predominantly diagnosed in those in their 50s or older. Both asthma and COPD are classified as **obstructive pulmonary disorders**. Obstructive pulmonary disorders are characterised by difficulties in breathing, especially breathing out (**exhalation**). There is an 'obstruction' to airflow which may be airway inflammation as is present in both asthma and COPD, or damage to lung tissue which is also characteristic of COPD.

Other common lung diseases can be classified as **restrictive**. Restrictive diseases include pulmonary fibrosis of which there are various types, including pneumonia and asbestosis (Chapter 2). Restrictive diseases are characterised by a 'restriction' on lung expansion causing a reduction in lung capacity. Restriction may be due to destruction of lung tissue, as is the case in pulmonary fibrosis where chronic inflammation and scarring destroys lung connective tissue. Restriction can also be due to problems outside the lung, including problems with the breathing muscles or the nerves supplying these. This is the case with, for example, Guillain–Barré and motor neurone disease. Other important respiratory conditions include upper and lower respiratory infections (such as the common cold, tuberculosis, influenza; Chapter 3); lung cancer; cystic fibrosis.

We begin this chapter by reviewing the structure and function of the respiratory system. We focus on aspects of anatomy and physiology which are needed to understand the clinical presentations of asthma and COPD. We then look at the risk factors, pathogenesis and clinical manifestations of asthma and COPD. We then examine the drugs used to relieve symptoms of asthma and COPD, and how different drugs are chosen for patients. We will also consider the side-effects, contraindications, cautions and interactions.

Review of the normal structure and function of the respiratory system

The respiratory system along with the cardiovascular system functions to deliver oxygenated blood to the cells of the body for **cellular respiration**. The two systems also function to remove carbon dioxide from the body to maintain the acid–base balance of the blood. The respiratory system draws air into the lungs in a process called inhalation, and removes air by exhalation. Together, the movement of air into and out of the lungs is known as **pulmonary ventilation**.

The upper respiratory tract includes the nasal cavity, pharynx and larynx (Figure 9.1). The lower respiratory tract includes the conducting airways making up the **tracheobronchial tree**. This is made up of the trachea, the bronchi and bronchioles. With the exception of the smallest bronchioles, these airways contain smooth muscle tissue in their walls. The smooth muscle regulates the diameter of the airways and plays an important role in the response to environmental allergens in asthma (see under 'Asthma', below). The airways are lined with a **ciliated epithelium** whose function is to trap inhaled dust particles and remove these from the airways. The ciliated epithelium contains goblet cells which secrete mucus. Inhaled dust particles entering the lungs during inhalation are trapped by the mucus. The cilia beat continually to move the mucus upwards and out of the lungs.

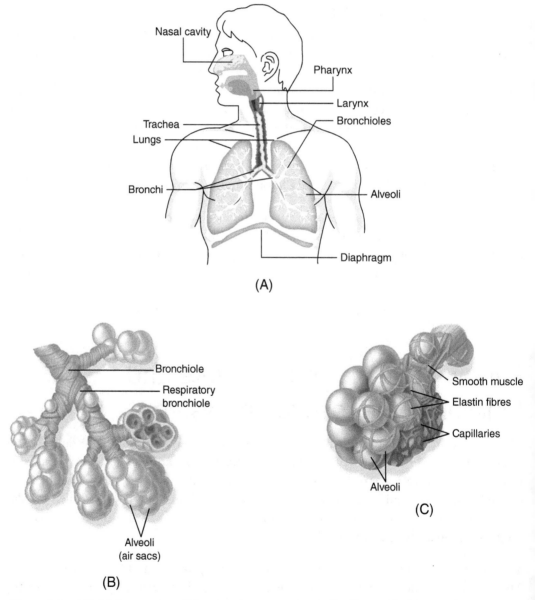

Figure 9.1 (A) Main organs of the respiratory system. (B) Bronchioles, respiratory bronchiole and alveoli. (C) Smooth muscle is shown in the walls of the bronchioles

Airway resistance and compliance are important terms needed to understand the difficulties in breathing experienced by patients with asthma and COPD. Airway resistance describes the resistance to airflow through the airways. The diameter of the airways is an important factor in determining airway resistance. Compliance is a measure of the ease with which the lungs and chest cavity can expand. Lung compliance is affected in patients with emphysema, one of the component diseases in COPD.

The smaller (respiratory) bronchioles and alveoli are the site of gas exchange. The alveoli are microscopic air sacs. These contain very thin walls made up of a single layer of epithelial cells lined with fluid. There are approximately 500 million air sacs in each lung, providing in total an extensive surface area for the exchange of oxygen and carbon dioxide. Each collection of air sacs is supplied with a network of blood capillaries from the pulmonary circulation.

The barrier or 'interface' between the air and the blood is known as the **respiratory membrane**. It consists of the wall of the alveolus and the wall of the blood capillary, each of which are only one cell thick (Figure 9.2). Between the two layers of cells is a thin layer of connective tissue called the interstitium. The respiratory membrane is extremely thin to allow oxygen to diffuse from the air in the lungs to reach the blood. Carbon dioxide diffuses in the opposite direction – from the blood into the air in the lungs to be exhaled. Any damage or thickening of the respiratory membrane will reduce the diffusion of gases and make gas exchange less effective. Gas exchange is driven by the concentration gradients of oxygen and carbon dioxide across the respiratory membrane. The role of breathing is to maintain these diffusion gradients (Tortora and Derrickson, 2017).

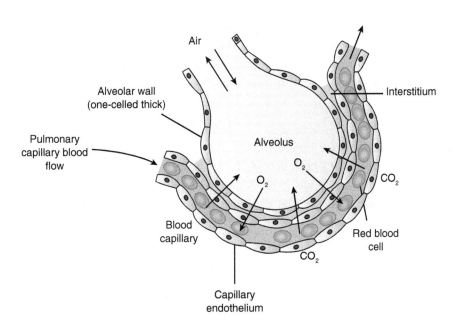

Figure 9.2 A single alveolus showing the structure of the respiratory membrane across which oxygen and carbon dioxide pass by diffusion

The lungs must also be effectively perfused. The pulmonary circulation supplies blood to the lungs for gas exchange. The pulmonary circulation is a low pressure circuit arising from the right side of the heart. Blood passing through the pulmonary capillaries becomes fully oxygenated. The pulmonary veins return oxygenated blood to the left atrium.

Many diseases of the lungs will affect the process of gas exchange. In turn, altered gas exchange can lead to alterations in blood gases such as hypoxaemia (low oxygen levels) and hypercapnia (elevated carbon dioxide levels). Gas exchange can be affected through reducing the volume of air moved during breathing, by altering the respiratory membrane to reduce the effectiveness of gas exchange or by reducing lung perfusion.

Breathing is regulated through the respiratory centres in the brainstem. The most important stimulus to increase breathing rate and depth is the acid–base balance of the blood. Respiratory acidosis evokes a strong stimulus to increase the breathing rate (Tortora and Derrickson, 2017). Retention of carbon dioxide due to difficulties in breathing is one of the main causes of respiratory acidosis. This is important to bear in mind when we consider asthma and COPD.

In the next section, we describe asthma, one of the most common respiratory disorders.

Asthma

Case study

Rachel, a 35-year-old musician, was admitted to the medical admissions unit with severe breathlessness for 2 hours. Rachel has a past history of asthma since childhood. Her asthma is normally reasonably well controlled with medication. Two days ago, she developed an upper respiratory tract infection which is a known trigger factor for her asthma.

On the medical assessment unit, she was unable to complete a whole sentence and her neck muscles were prominent when inhaling. Rachel was notably anxious. She struggled to produce a peak flow of 105 L/minute – her normal peak flow is 400 L/minute. Her heart rate was 132/minute and respiratory rate 30/minute. She had a distinct expiratory wheeze. Her oxygen saturation was 91%. Rachel was given oxygen therapy to maintain oxygen saturation at 94–98%, a short-acting β_2-agonist through a nebuliser and an oral corticosteroid.

Rachel has experienced a severe acute asthma exacerbation. Fortunately for her, these exacerbations are rare. Rachel has a good understanding of her asthma and the need for maintaining her regular medication. Her personalised asthma plan enables her to act appropriately when her asthma worsens and seek help quickly.

Asthma is a chronic inflammatory condition affecting the airways. Typical symptoms include breathlessness, tightness in the chest, coughing and wheezing. The prevalence of asthma is increasing and asthma is more common in developed countries. Some of the highest rates are found in New Zealand, Australia and the UK. The reason for this is not fully understood. In the UK, 5.4 million people are receiving treatment for asthma and 1.1 million of these are children. Asthma is estimated to cause 1000 deaths a year in the UK, with 90% of these attributed to preventable factors (BLF, 2018). Although the death rate from asthma is low, asthma causes considerable distress and contributes to days off school for children and days off work for adults. Anxiety and depression are up to six times higher in those with asthma than the general population.

At a physiological level, asthma has three characteristics.

- Airflow limitation which is normally reversible with treatment.
- Airway hyper-responsiveness to a number of stimuli or trigger factors. Bronchospasm occurs in response to a number of stimuli and is the sudden contraction of the smooth muscle in the wall of the bronchi. It results in narrowing of the airways and obstruction to breathing.
- Inflammation of the bronchi. Chronic inflammation of the bronchi is present in asthma. This is characterised by the presence of eosinophils (Chapter 4). These contribute to the long-term manifestations of asthma.

The aetiology of asthma is complex involving both genetic and environmental factors. Asthma is often provoked by exposure to environmental stimuli. Table 9.1 gives examples of possible environmental stimuli that can provoke asthma.

Stimulus
Environmental allergens, e.g. pollen, house dust, animal hair, latex
Respiratory tract infections
Exercise
Occupational sensitisers, e.g. isocyanates (from polyurethane varnishes)
Cold air
Ingestion of NSAIDs
Emotional stress
Exposure to bronchial irritants, such as cigarette smoke, perfume

Table 9.1   Environmental stimuli provoking asthma

In common with many conditions we have included in this book, including dementia, cancer and heart failure, asthma is seen as an 'umbrella' term for a range of different diseases. This reflects our increasing understanding of the different mechanisms by which the disease or condition arises.

In asthma there are many different immune mechanisms which can produce a clinical picture of asthma. Recent research has highlighted a number of different asthma 'phenotypes'. Asthma phenotypes represent different presentations of asthma, and include: early onset atopic, late onset atopic, obesity-related non-atopic and elderly (non-atopic) (Kuruvilla, 2018). If you remember from Chapter 4, 'atopic' or 'atopy' refers to the production of IgE antibodies in response to an allergen. Atopy is the hallmark of a type-1 hypersensitivity reaction, which is responsible for a wide-range of allergies. Atopy in turn, is driven by what was referred to in Chapter 4 as a Th2 response. For reasons not fully-elucidated, those people who develop allergies or asthma, produce T helper cells of type 2 (Th2) as opposed to T helper cells of type (Th1). It is the Th2 cells that cause production of IgE antibodies through the different cytokines they produce. The atopic/non-atopic distinction is one of the most important means of classifying asthma. This principle is important in choosing the most important treatment and management strategies for the patient. This has proved especially important in treating the patients with more severe forms of asthma in which monoclonal antibody therapy against IgE may be used (Eller et al., 2018).

For the purposes of this chapter we will focus on the pathogenesis of atopic asthma because it is one of the most common types of asthma and one of the best understood.

Pathogenesis

In atopic asthma, a sensitisation phase occurs in which exposure to an allergen causes the development of a Th2 response. Th2 cells release cytokines Il-4, -5 and -13. These in turn lead to B cell production of IgE antibodies, the recruitment of white blood cells called eosinophils. The IgE antibodies bind to mast cells. With respect to asthma there are many mast cells located within the lining (or mucosa) of the airways. The binding of IgE antibodies to mast cells lining the airways sensitises an individual to further exposure to the allergen.

On subsequent exposure to the same allergen, the allergen will be recognised and bind to the IgE molecules on the mast cells. This signals the immediate release of histamine – a potent inflammatory mediator and a range of other inflammatory mediators from the mast cells. Other mediators released include leukotrienes, prostaglandins and pro-inflammatory cytokines (Chapter 2). These mediators produce an *immediate allergic reaction* within seconds of exposure. This immediate reaction results in airway swelling and oedema, and stimulates the mucus glands and goblet cells in the airways to increase mucus secretion.

Bronchospasm is caused by a mixture of direct stimulation of the smooth muscle cells by the mediators and by reflexes involving the nervous system. The airways contain smooth muscle tissue which regulates the diameter of the airway. The contraction of the smooth muscle is under control of the autonomic nervous system. Nerve fibres from the sympathetic division of the autonomic nervous system cause **bronchodilation** – or widening of the bronchi – through relaxing the smooth muscle. Stimulation from the parasympathetic division causes bronchoconstriction through causing the smooth muscle to constrict. During an asthma attack, local sensory fibres (probably of type C; Chapter 6) are stimulated and cause a reflex firing of parasympathetic fibres. This causes the bronchospasm characteristic of asthma. We will return to the regulation of the airways by the autonomic nervous system when we discuss β_2-agonists in the section on pharmacological treatments of asthma.

The immediate allergic reaction in asthma results in the narrowing of the airways and increased resistance to air flow through three mechanisms.

- Airway swelling due to inflammation and fluid exudates (oedema).
- Increased mucus secretion which can form mucous plugs in the airways.
- Bronchospasm.

Narrowing of the airways increases the resistance to air flow and the clinical features of asthma (described below).

Following the immediate reaction, patients may experience a *late reaction*, 8–12 hours later. This involves the infiltration of immune cells including eosinophils, lymphocytes (especially Th2 cells) and neutrophils. Much focus has been made on the role of eosinophils in asthma. Eosinophil infiltration is characteristic of asthma and a key cause of chronic inflammation of the airways. Eosinophils release harmful proteins and reactive oxygen species which damage the lining of the airways. This causes airway 're-modelling' which describes the thickening of the walls due to mucous gland **hypertrophy** and the build-up of scar tissue. Chronic inflammation is also believed to make the airways hyper-responsive to other irritants.

Figure 9.3 illustrates the changes occurring in the airways in asthma during an asthma attack.

Clinical features

Rachel presented with typical symptoms of an asthma exacerbation. This included: wheezing, cough, chest tightness and breathlessness. The frequency and duration at which individuals experience asthma exacerbations varies greatly. Patients often experience prolonged expiration and hyper-inflation of the lungs may be visible. Nasal flaring and accessory muscle use are often evident. Children may show 'retraction' of the substernal, subcostal regions. Respiratory rate and pulse rate will be high. The reduced gas exchange brought about by the difficulties breathing can lead to low oxygen levels, raised carbon dioxide levels and low blood pH. These changes to blood gas levels and lowered pH in turn stimulate peripheral and central chemoreceptors to raise breathing rate and pulse (Tortora and Derrickson, 2017). The increased work of breathing may lead to exhaustion.

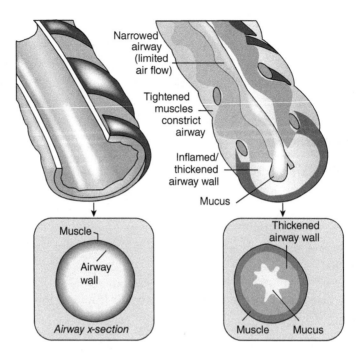

Figure 9.3 Changing occurring in the airways during an asthma attack

Asthma is characterised by the symptoms being intermittent and often worse at night. Symptoms will be provoked by the factors described in Table 9.1. However, some patients present without severe exacerbations but have chronic symptoms of cough and wheeze.

Management

An important aspect of asthma management is patient and family education. It is important for individuals with asthma to be taught the correct inhaler technique, to monitor their peak flow at regular intervals and, where possible, to avoid environmental triggers. Anyone with asthma needs to avoid exposure to tobacco smoke. NICE (2013a) recommends that everyone with asthma receive a written personalised action plan as part of structured education on asthma. This is where the educational role of the nurse is particularly important. Each person with asthma should be able to monitor and recognise when their symptoms deteriorate. They need to be aware of the actions to take should their asthma deteriorate. For some individuals, it will be appropriate for parents or a carer to be involved with review of the plan. This will be the case for children, those with learning difficulties and some older adults. In children, height and weight should be measured at least once a year because corticosteroid use can affect growth rate.

Before examining the drugs used to treat asthma, we examine the pathophysiology of COPD.

Chronic obstructive pulmonary disease (COPD)

COPD occurs following progressive lung damage and gradual worsening of lung function (NICE, 2018b). It is characterised by airflow obstruction which is not fully reversible. This absence of reversible airflow obstruction can help distinguish COPD from asthma. Most people with COPD are diagnosed in their fifties. NICE (2018b) state that there is an estimated 1.2 million people in the UK with COPD and many more people remain undiagnosed.

The main cause of COPD is smoking or exposure to environmental pollution. There is a rare genetic cause in those who inherit a faulty gene for α-antitrypsin (whose role in COPD is described below under 'Pathogenesis'). Despite the link with tobacco smoking, it is of note that only a minority of smokers develop COPD. Therefore it is likely that as yet unidentified genetic factors play a role in the development of COPD.

Clinical features

Peter in the case study at the beginning of the chapter had mild COPD. Peter presented with a productive cough and breathlessness on exertion. He is likely to have experienced chest tightness and a wheeze. Patients with COPD are susceptible to frequent lung infections which may cause exacerbations in symptoms. Severe COPD causes patients to be breathless even at rest, with a prolonged expiration ('out breath'). Patients will use their accessory muscles of breathing; chest expansion is poor and the lungs are likely to be 'hyper-inflated'. This can lead to a 'barrel-chest' appearance. The patient may sit forward in a hunched position to aid their breathing. There may also be peripheral and central cyanosis.

In advanced disease, there may be weakness and skeletal muscle wasting.

Diagnosis

A diagnosis of COPD is made based upon the patient's history. This will almost invariably include a history of smoking or exposure to environmental irritants. The following symptoms are likely to be present (NICE 2018b):

- exertional breathlessness
- chronic cough
- regular sputum production
- frequent winter 'bronchitis'
- wheeze.

A diagnosis will be supported by spirometry which is used to determine lung function. The lung functions measured by spirometry include lung volumes and the rate at which air can be exhaled from the lungs. Spirometry is used in diagnosing and monitoring a number of respiratory diseases. Its use is described under 'Lung function tests' in the box below.

Lung function tests

A spirometer is a device for measuring lung function. There are various makes of spirometer but they all have a mouthpiece into which the patient breathes (**http://patient.info/health/spirometry-leaflet**). The patient is asked to blow into the spirometer as hard and as fast as possible. A nose clip may be used to prevent air escaping through the nose.

The most important measurements for obstructive pulmonary disease are: forced expiratory volume in one second (FEV_1) – the maximum volume of air the subject can blow out within one second, and forced vital capacity (FVC) – the total volume of air the subject can blow out in one breath. It is of note that these measurements are taken after administration of a bronchodilator medication to ease airflow and give the optimum result (NICE, 2018b).

With COPD or other obstructive disease, FEV_1 is reduced due to airway obstruction. FVC on the other hand may be relatively normal, indicating that lung volume has not changed significantly. Restrictive diseases also produce a lowered FEV_1. However, the FVC is reduced as well indicating significant loss of lung volume. Due to this, the ratio FEV_1/FCV is important for diagnostic purposes.

Figure 9.4 shows a spirometry tracing from a normal healthy individual, an individual with an obstructive disease and one with a restrictive disease.

Those with COPD have an FEV_1 less than or equal to 80% predicted (for age, height, sex) and FEV_1/FVC is less than 0.7 (NICE 2018b). The following table categorises COPD from mild to very severe according to the percentage of predicted FEV_1. The degree of severity has implications for treatment and management.

Categorisation of COPD severity

Airflow obstruction	% of predicted FEV_1 (NICE 2018b)
Mild	≥ 80%
Moderate	50–79%
Severe	30–49%
Very severe	< 30%

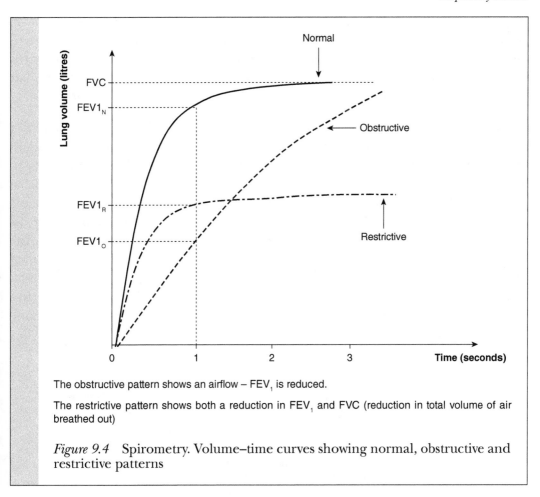

The obstructive pattern shows an airflow – FEV$_1$ is reduced.

The restrictive pattern shows both a reduction in FEV$_1$ and FVC (reduction in total volume of air breathed out)

Figure 9.4 Spirometry. Volume–time curves showing normal, obstructive and restrictive patterns

Pathogenesis

COPD is a diffuse inflammatory disease of the lung tissue and airways. 'Diffuse' means spread throughout the lungs. COPD has two elements: emphysema and chronic bronchitis. Most cases involve a combination of the two. Inflammation in the lungs, particularly the small airways, is part of the normal immune response to smoking. However, in those with COPD the response to inhaled smoke or other toxins is magnified and causes damage to the lung tissue. Chronic bronchitis can result, which is inflammation of the bronchial tubes and is characterised by a productive cough. There is increased mucus secretion from goblet cells lining the airways. There is in addition hypertrophy of the mucus glands within the wall of the airway. The increased mucus secretion causes the characteristic productive cough. Airway inflammation results in swelling and oedema and contributes to airway obstruction.

Emphysema is characterised by an enlargement of the airspaces beyond the terminal bronchioles. This is accompanied by destruction of the alveolar walls. There are different forms of emphysema according to the location of the alveolar destruction (Kumar et al., 2014). The one associated with smoking, centrilobular emphysema, causes damage to the respiratory bronchioles (Figure 9.5). This leads to the development of air spaces (or bullae) in the lungs. This reduces the total surface area available for gas exchange and may lead to reduced oxygenation of blood and reduced removal of carbon dioxide.

Current theory proposes that harmful chemical imbalances develop in the lungs of those with COPD: a protease/anti-protease imbalance; and an oxidant/anti-oxidant imbalance (Figure 9.6). These lead to the eventual tissue destruction characteristic of emphysema. Cigarette smoke and other environmental irritants activate the epithelial cells lining the airways and macrophages in the lungs to release chemotactic factors (Chapter 2). These factors attract CD8 lymphocytes and neutrophils from the circulation. Neutrophils and macrophages produce proteases. These are enzymes that break down proteins, particularly the elastic and collagen fibres of lung tissue. In normal lungs there is a significant presence of anti-protease enzymes, especially α_1-antitrypsin. The anti-proteases normally act to balance the proteases and limit their destructive effects. In emphysema, the balance is tipped in favour of the proteases partly because of the infiltration of a large number of neutrophils.

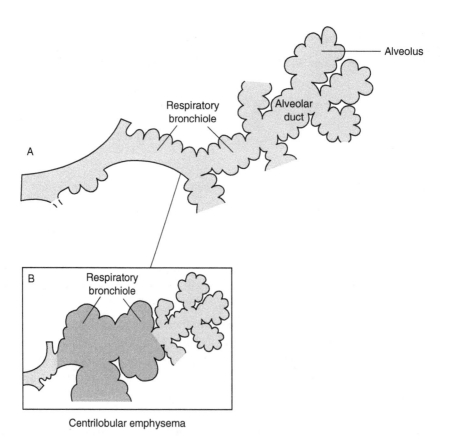

Figure 9.5 Damage to the alveoli shown in emphysema. (A) Shows the normal structure of the respiratory bronchiole and alveoli. (B) Centrilobular damage to the wall of respiratory bronchioles causing enlargement of the airspace

At the same time oxidants from smoke and reactive oxygen species released from inflammatory cells act to inactivate anti-proteases. This further contributes to tipping the balance in favour of the proteases. The excess of oxidants represents another imbalance. The lungs of healthy individuals normally contain antioxidants that minimise oxidative damage. Tobacco smoke contains a range of reactive oxygen species which outweigh the antioxidants. Activated neutrophils also release reactive oxygen species into the alveoli.

Pathophysiology

Airflow obstruction results from the inflammation and narrowing of the airways and the presence of inflammatory exudates. The loss of elastic tissue characteristic of emphysema causes the airways to narrow and collapse. The elastic tissue of the lungs normally provides a traction ('pull') force that keeps the airways open. In addition, following inhalation, elastic recoil of the lungs normally drives air out of the lungs. In emphysema elastic recoil is reduced. This makes the lung easier to inflate (i.e. increases lung compliance) but makes breathing out more difficult.

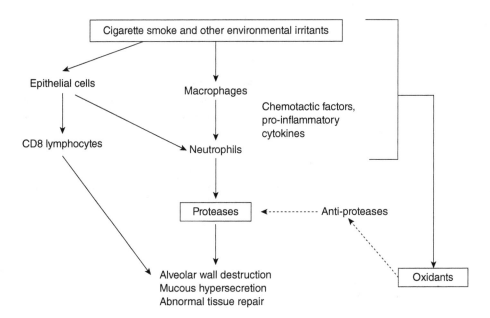

Summary of events leading to alveolar wall destruction

Cigarette smoke and other environmental irritants activate the epithelial cells lining the airways and macrophages in the lungs to release chemotactic factors. These factors attract CD8 lymphocytes and neutrophils from the circulation which produce proteases. In normal lungs, anti-proteases normally act to balance the proteases and limit their destructive effects. In emphysema, the balance is tipped in favour of the proteases. Oxidants from smoke and reactive oxygen species released from inflammatory cells act to inactivate anti-proteases. This further contributes to tipping the balance in favour of the proteases.

Figure 9.6   Pathogenesis of emphysema

During exhalation, airway obstruction traps air in the lungs. Airway obstruction and the loss of elastic tissue result in airway closure during exhalation. Air which should have been exhaled remains in the lungs. This results in hyperinflation of the lungs in which a larger than normal volume of air remains in the lungs following exhalation. Hyperinflation in turn reduces the volume of air that can be inspired. This can cause marked breathlessness in COPD, especially during exertion.

Airway obstruction and collapse can lead to arterial hypoxemia (low arterial blood oxygen levels) in advanced disease. Hypoxemia can present with or without hypercapnia (increased levels of carbon dioxide in the blood). Some patients are able to maintain blood oxygen levels by increasing their respiratory effort. Other patients fail to maintain respiratory effort and develop hypercapnia. This raised carbon dioxide (and associated respiratory acidosis) normally stimulates breathing rate. However, over time, patients with hypercapnia develop insensitivity to raised carbon dioxide levels in the blood. Low oxygen levels become the main stimulus for breathing. Low oxygen levels in the blood in turn stimulate red blood cell production (polycythaemia) and fluid retention. Patients appear cyanosed and 'bloated' due to fluid retention. Oxygen must be administered carefully to patients with hypoxemia and carbon dioxide retention. The main stimulus to breathe in these patients is the low oxygen level. If administered with too much oxygen, their drive to breathe decreases. Carbon dioxide levels then worsen as their breathing rate diminishes.

In advanced disease, patients may develop pulmonary hypertension. Blood vessels supplying parts of the lung which remain unventilated automatically constrict. This causes increased resistance to blood flow and raises the pulmonary blood pressure. Pulmonary hypertension can eventually lead to enlargement of the right ventricle (*cor pulmonale*) due to the increased work needed to pump blood through the pulmonary system. This results in weakness of the right ventricle and right ventricular failure.

Patients may experience exacerbations in COPD often due to lung infections. Increased airway inflammation and reduced gas exchange can lead to severe respiratory failure and death.

Activity 9.1   Reflection

Over the past five years, Peter has experienced a number of exacerbations of his COPD and his lung function has declined. He has been admitted to the respiratory ward where you work as a nurse. He is very breathless and wheezing. This causes great anxiety for him. How would you help to alleviate his anxiety?

A suggested answer is given at the end of the chapter.

Pharmacological treatment of asthma

Scenario

....

Rachel has recovered well from her asthma attack. Today she visits you in the nurse-led asthma clinic at the surgery. She tells you she is on a blue relieving inhaler and a brown inhaler for prevention. She uses the blue one only when it is needed but she uses the brown one every day. Her FEV_1 is 90% of that predicted. She has not had an asthma attack since her brown inhaler was increased three months previously. She also tells you that she generally has no 'wheeziness' or cough in the day or at night. You are happy with her progress and continue the treatment.

The scenario shows that Rachel's asthma is currently well controlled. Pharmacological treatments are the main treatment type for asthma. The blue 'relieving' inhaler mentioned by Rachel is a salbutamol inhaler. Salbutamol is a type of β_2-agonist. The brown 'preventative' inhaler is a corticosteroid inhaler. We will look at the differences in how these inhalers act to explain both their uses in asthma and their side-effects.

β_2-agonists

In the section on pathogenesis of asthma, we introduced the action of the two divisions of the autonomic nervous system: sympathetic and parasympathetic, which regulate the diameter of the airways. Most organs of the body receive a nerve supply from both divisions. As is the case with the airways, the two divisions usually work in opposite ways to regulate the organs they supply.

To understand how β_2-agonists work in asthma, and what their potential side-effects are, we need to examine the neurotransmitters released from the sympathetic and parasympathetic nerve endings. We also need to know the names of the receptors for these neurotransmitters and how they are distributed in the various body organs.

Sympathetic fibres release neurotransmitters adrenaline and noradrenaline. Adrenaline and noradrenaline are **adrenergic receptor** agonists (Chapter 1). There are two main types of adrenergic receptors: alpha (α) and beta (β). These are further divided into subtypes – α_1, α_2, β_1, β_2 – based on the response they produce and according to which drugs bind to them. By contrast, parasympathetic fibres release the neurotransmitter acetylcholine. Acetylcholine is a **muscarinic receptor** agonist. Table 9.2 summarises the effects of these neurotransmitters on various organs and tissues of the body.

Target	Effect of sympathetic stimulation (adrenaline/noradrenaline) (type of adrenergic receptor is given in brackets)	Effect of parasympathetic stimulation (acetylcholine) of muscarinic receptors
Lungs – bronchial smooth muscle	Relaxation causing bronchodilation (β_2)	Bronchoconstriction
Stomach and intestines – smooth muscle of wall	Decrease in motility and tone (α and β_2)	Increase in motility and tone
Heart – (cardiac) muscle	Increased rate and force of contraction (β_1)	Reduced rate and force of contraction
Arterioles – smooth muscle	Relaxation or contraction depending upon the organ: arterioles to kidney and gastrointestinal tract contract producing constriction and reduced blood flow; arterioles to skeletal muscle, heart, liver, adipose tissue relax producing dilation and increased blood flow (α and β)	No known effect
Liver	Synthesis and release of glucose (from glycogenolysis and gluconeogenesis) (Chapter 12) (α and β_2)	No known effect
Salivary glands	Little or no increase in saliva production	Increased secretion of a watery mucus
Eye – radial muscle of iris	Contraction leading to pupil dilation (α_1)	No known effect
Eye – circular muscle of iris	No known effect	Contraction leading to pupil constriction

Table 9.2 Effects of sympathetic and parasympathetic stimulation of various body organs and tissues

Side-effects and considerations for practice

β_2-agonists used in asthma, such as salbutamol and terbutaline, work directly to stimulate β_2 receptors on the smooth muscle of the airways causing bronchodilation. This reverses the bronchoconstriction seen in asthma. However, these drugs are often not completely specific for the lung or one type of β receptor. For example, salbutamol also activates cardiac muscle β_1 receptors to some degree which can lead to the side-effect of tachycardia.

Activity 9.2   Critical thinking

According to the World Anti-Doping Agency (2015), high doses of salbutamol are banned in sport. Use Table 9.2 to consider what unfair advantages salbutamol might provide for an athlete. Bear in mind that salbutamol activates both β_2 and β_1 receptors.

A suggested answer is given at the end of the chapter.

Activity 9.2 shows how stimulating the sympathetic nervous system with salbutamol can enable us to predict its actions and side-effects. It helps to explain why somebody who overuses their salbutamol inhaler might describe symptoms such as a 'racing heart'. Another important side-effect, unrelated to the effects on the nervous system, is hypokalaemia (low blood potassium). This is more commonly seen with higher doses from nebulised solutions. β_2-agonists must therefore be used with care with other medications, such as diuretics, which also cause hypokalaemia.

Using β_2-agonists with β-blockers (Chapter 8) can cause problems. β-blockers are β_2-antagonists and therefore block the action of β_2-agonists. β-blockers are contraindicated in asthma as they may actually precipitate asthma attacks. NSAIDs are also contraindicated in asthma (Chapter 6).

Salbutamol and terbutaline are short-acting β_2-agonists (SABAs) with a relatively short duration of action (salbutamol 4–6 hours). As a consequence they may need to be used up to four times a day to relieve symptoms. Long-acting β_2-agonists (LABAs) include salmeterol and formoterol. These take longer to work but have a longer duration of action (salmeterol 12 hours). They are able to relieve symptoms for much longer and are inhaled twice a day. Short-acting β_2-agonists are used for immediate relief of symptoms. Long-acting β_2-agonists are used as prophylactic treatments to prevent the development of symptoms. Their side-effects and drug interactions are similar to those described for short-acting β_2-agonists.

Corticosteroids

Corticosteroids have anti-inflammatory and immunosuppressant effects (Chapter 2). Corticosteroids are used in asthma to reduce inflammation, and have been shown to reduce the number of eosinophils in the circulation. This makes corticosteroids useful in asthma prophylaxis. They are not useful for symptoms of an acute asthma attack, where short-acting β_2-agonists should be used. Examples of corticosteroids used in inhalers are: beclomethasone, budesonide and fluticasone. There are many different inhaler types and strengths available. The current UK asthma guidance classifies the different strengths as very low (children's dose), low (usual adult starting dose), medium and high. The guidance contains a useful table outlining these different strengths (BTS/SIGN, 2016).

Activity 9.3   Critical thinking

You are a nurse on the ward. One of the junior doctors has just written up a drug chart for John who has been newly admitted. You notice that on the drug chart is written 'Beclometasone inhaler two puffs twice a day'. What other information would you need on the drug chart so that you can order it from the pharmacy?

A suggested answer is given at the end of the chapter.

Activity 9.3 shows the importance of being aware of different inhaler types, brands and strengths. Some inhalers also contain a mixture of drugs, such as a corticosteroid and a β_2-agonist. It is also very important that patients are using their inhalers correctly. Hickey (2014), listed in Further reading at the end of the chapter, gives advice on inhaler technique.

Side-effects and considerations for practice

You learned about the adverse side-effects of corticosteroids in Chapter 2. Steroid inhalers are used in asthma where possible, rather than oral medicines. This is to minimise absorption of the corticosteroid into the systemic circulation. This helps to reduce side-effects, although it does not completely eliminate them as some of the corticosteroid will be absorbed. The amount absorbed will increase as the dose of inhaler increases. High doses can cause adrenal suppression and, if a patient is on a high inhaled dose, a steroid card may be needed. Throat irritation and oral candidiasis can be a particular problem with corticosteroid inhalers. This is especially true if inhaler technique is poor as more corticosteroid is deposited in the mouth rather than the lungs. Rinsing the mouth after use or spacer devices can help.

Leukotriene receptor antagonists

Leukotrienes are inflammatory mediators released by mast cells, eosinophils and basophils during an inflammatory reaction (Chapter 2). In asthma, leukotrienes contribute to bronchospasm by directly stimulating contraction of the smooth muscle in the airways.

Blocking leukotrienes with leukotriene receptor antagonists can improve asthma symptoms and reduce exacerbations. They have an additive effect when used with corticosteroids. Examples include montelukast and zafirlukast. They are taken by mouth and are generally well tolerated. Side-effects include abdominal pain, headache, dizziness and sleep disturbance.

Xanthines

This group of oral medications includes theophylline and aminophylline which are related to caffeine. Aminophylline is a mixture of theophylline and ethylenediamine. They are usually given as slow release preparations, for example Phyllocontin Continus®, which is a slow release aminophylline preparation. They are only used if asthma control is poor despite inhaler therapy. Intravenous aminophylline preparations can also be used during severe asthma attacks.

The precise mechanism of action is unclear but they cause bronchodilation by relaxing smooth muscle in the bronchioles. They may also have some anti-inflammatory actions (Barnes, 2005).

Side-effects and considerations for practice

Xanthines stimulate the central nervous system and can cause tremor, nervousness and poor sleep as a result. They also stimulate the heart, causing tachycardia and palpitations, so must be used with caution in patients with cardiac arrhythmias or severe hypertension.

Aminophylline and theophylline have a narrow therapeutic range (Chapter 1). The concentrations in the blood must be carefully monitored. If the level in the blood is too high serious central nervous system and cardiovascular toxicity can result.

Activity 9.4   Research

In Appendix 1 of the BNF there is a section on drug interactions. Look up theophylline and note down some of the common drugs theophylline interacts with. How does the number of drug interactions compare with a drug like paracetamol?

A suggested answer is given at the end of the chapter.

The activity demonstrates that xanthines interact with many different medications. Xanthines are metabolised by cytochrome P450 enzymes in the liver (Chapter 1). Other drugs affecting cytochrome P450 enzymes will alter the rate of metabolism of xanthines. This is problematic because xanthines have a narrow therapeutic range. The interacting drugs cause a change in plasma level which can move the levels of xanthine out of its narrow therapeutic range. For example a cigarette smoker will need a higher dose of a drug like aminophylline because the cigarette smoke increases P450 enzyme action. The antibiotic erythromycin inhibits cytochrome P450 enzymes and will increase blood levels of xanthine.

Choosing drugs to treat asthma

As we have seen there are many drugs used in asthma to both prevent and relieve symptoms. Choosing which ones a patient needs depends on the severity of asthma. A stepwise approach is used (Joint British Thoracic Society/Scottish Intercollegiate Guidelines Network (SIGN) guidance, 2016). This is illustrated in Figure 9.7.

No preventer needed	• Short-acting beta agonist	Move down
Regular preventer therapy	• Add low-dose of inhaled corticosteroid (ICS)	the table as needed if symptoms deteriorate ↓
Initial add-on therapy	• Add long-acting beta-2 agonist (LABA)	
Additional add on therapy	• No response to LABA – stop LABA	
	• Partial response to LABA – increase ICS to medium dose OR consider additional treatment (LAMA, leukotriene antagonist or slow release theophylline)	Move up the table to maintain lowest controlling step↑
High-dose therapies	• Consider increase of ICS to high dose	
	• Consider adding a fourth drug	
Continuous frequent use of oral steroids	• Maintain high dose ICS	
	• Add lowest possible dose of oral steroid	
	• Consider other treatments to minimise steroid use	

Figure 9.7 Stepwise approach for selecting asthma treatment in adults (BTS and SIGN, 2016)

Activity 9.5   Critical thinking

A more detailed look at Rachel's inhalers shows us that she takes a salbutamol 100 microgram inhaler two puffs four times a day if needed. She is also on a Clenil 100 microgram aerosol inhaler and she takes this regularly at a dose of two puffs twice a day. What step is Rachel on in the asthma guideline? If her symptoms got worse what might be considered next in her treatment? What might happen if her symptoms continued to be well controlled?

A suggested answer is given at the end of the chapter.

The activity shows how the stepwise approach to treatment is applied to individuals to improve asthma control with the aim of achieving complete control. Asthma attacks can be fatal. For some people achieving control is very difficult. We can see from the table that these people are likely to be taking more medicines and may even be on oral corticosteroid tablets which can cause many side-effects.

Acute asthma attacks

Acute asthma attacks can be life-threatening and the patient may need admission to hospital. Hospital treatment would consist of a nebulised short-acting β_2-agonist (usually salbutamol), oxygen and an oral or IV corticosteroid. The short acting anti-muscurinic agent ipratropium might also be added as this will act together with the salbutamol to further improve dilation of the airways. Nebulisers deliver larger doses to the lungs than inhalers can. If you consider a salbutamol inhaler, the dose from one puff is 100 micrograms. The dose of a salbutamol nebule is 2.5 mg or 5 mg which is 25–50 times more. In the same way the corticosteroid given orally or IV will deliver a higher dose to the lungs than an inhaler can. Asthma attacks can occur if a person is not using their inhalers properly. Some people have poor inhaler technique. Others may be underusing their 'preventer' inhalers (corticosteroids) and overusing their 'reliever' inhalers (β_2-agonists). Nurses have a vital role to play in educating patients about the different types of inhalers, what they are for and how to use them.

Pharmacological management of COPD

Many of the inhalers used to treat COPD are the same as those used to treat asthma, but as we shall see, there are important differences. It should be remembered that the pharmacological treatments help to improve symptoms and reduce exacerbations but they do not prevent progression of COPD.

Bronchodilators

Irreversible airway obstruction occurs in COPD. Bronchodilators improve breathlessness and reduce hyperventilation. The use of bronchodilators will not return the airways to normal and may not improve the FEV_1 greatly. However the quality of life of many patients is often improved with these drugs.

Short-acting β_2-agonist (SABA) and long-acting β_2-agonist (LABA)

These bronchodilating drugs have already been introduced under asthma. Drugs such as salbutamol (a short-acting β_2-agonist) and salmeterol (a long-acting β_2-agonist) are used in COPD to relax smooth muscle in the lungs and cause bronchodilation.

Short-acting muscarinic antagonists (SAMA) and long-acting muscurinic antagonists (LAMA)

If we revisit Table 9.2 we can see that blocking (or antagonising) muscarinic receptors is another way of causing bronchodilation. This is how drugs such as ipratropium (a short-acting muscarinic antagonist) and tiotropium (a long-acting muscarinic antagonist) work. These drugs block the effect of acetylcholine on muscarinic receptors leading to bronchodilation. Theoretically these drugs could be used in the routine treatment of asthma but in practice they are less effective than β_2-agonists (Rodrigo et al., 2005). Muscarinic antagonists are sometimes used in acute asthma where other drugs have failed. They are, however, used very often for COPD, often in addition to β_2-agonists.

Side-effects and considerations for practice

Side-effects can be predicted from the pharmacology (see Table 9.2) and include dry mouth and constipation. Contact with the eyes, for example when nebulised solutions are used, can cause blurred vision and glaucoma.

Xanthines

Oral aminophylline or theophylline are also used in COPD that has not responded to other treatments. They are used for their bronchodilating effects in stable COPD. They are used for exacerbations only if nebulised bronchodilators have not worked (NICE, 2018b). They are not routinely used as they have a narrow therapeutic range so monitoring can be complicated. Also not all studies show they are effective for exacerbations.

Inhaled corticosteroids (ICS)

Inhaled corticosteroids can be used in the treatment of COPD but they are much less effective than in the treatment of asthma. Although COPD is also an inflammatory condition the pathophysiology is different. Neutrophils are implicated in COPD and these inflammatory cells are relatively insensitive to corticosteroids, unlike in asthma where eosinophils are implicated which are sensitive to corticosteroids. However many patients with COPD are prescribed corticosteroids inhalers and do appear to benefit from them (NICE, 2018b). They should not be used alone but in combination with a bronchodilator in a combination inhaler. An example of such an inhaler is Symbicort which contains budesonide (a corticosteroid) and formoterol (a LABA). They must be used with care as they cause a greater incidence of pneumonia.

Oxygen

As COPD progresses patients can become hypoxaemic (have low blood oxygen levels). Oxygen therapy can help to increase exercise capacity and provide relief of breathlessness. It can also be used during exacerbations of COPD. It should be started by a specialist as there are many risks that need to be considered. A full discussion is outside the scope of the book. Further information can be found in the full NICE guidelines (2018b).

Stepwise COPD treatment

The NICE guidelines (2018b) for COPD set out a stepwise approach to the treatment of COPD (see Further reading at the end of the chapter). Initial treatment choice would be a short-acting β_2-agonist (SABA) such as salbutamol or a short-acting muscarinic antagonist (SAMA) such as ipratropium. The next scenario helps to illustrate how such guidelines are used in practice.

Scenario

John is a 63-year-old ex-smoker with a diagnosis of COPD. He comes to see you at your nurse-led clinic. He is currently on an ipratropium inhaler and he takes two puffs four times a day. You check his FEV_1 and FVC and ask him questions about how his breathlessness affects his activities. You also check his inhaler technique. He tells you that he is currently feeling more breathless, especially when walking fast or uphill. You decide to move John onto the next stage of therapy. The next stage of treatment depends on whether a patient also has features of asthma, which means that their condition might be responsive to inhaled corticosteroids. You know that this is the case for John. You therefore suggest that his current inhaler is stopped and that Symbicort, a combination inhaler containing a LABA plus an ICS, is started. You ensure that John knows how to use his new inhaler before he leaves.

Acute exacerbations of COPD

Depending on the severity of symptoms, people with exacerbations of COPD may be treated at home or in hospital. The treatment for exacerbations include increasing the dose of short acting bronchodilators. This might be achieved by increasing the dose given by inhaler. In some cases nebulised ipratropium and salbutamol are used. This allows much larger doses to be given but requires specialised nebulising equipment. Short courses of systemic corticosteroid, usually prednisolone, are also used. The prednisolone would usually be prescribed for 7–14 days only, to minimise long-term side-effects of corticosteroids. An antibiotic would also be needed if a bacterial infection was suspected (NICE, 2018b).

It is now time to review what you have learned within this chapter by undertaking some multiple choice questions.

Activity 9.6   Multiple choice questions

1. 'Shortness of breath' is called:
   a) Asthma
   b) Dyspnoea
   c) Tachycardia
   d) Hypoxaemia

2. In a patient with COPD which clinical feature is *least* likely to be present?
   a) A history of smoking
   b) A slowly progressive disease

(Continued)

(Continued)

    c) Airway obstruction that is reversible

    d) Airway inflammation

3. Which of the following white blood cells is characteristic of the *chronic inflammation* in asthma?

    a) Eosinophil

    b) Neutrophil

    c) Monocyte

    d) Lymphocyte

4. Increased stimulation of sympathetic fibres to the airways brings about:

    a) Mucus secretion

    b) Bronchodilation

    c) Bronchoconstriction

    d) Swelling and oedema

5. According to NICE (2018b) COPD affects approximately how many people in the UK?

    a) 10.1 million

    b) 5.7 million

    c) 3.3 million

    d) 1.2 million

6. Corticosteroids should be delivered by which route in mild to moderate exacerbations of COPD?

    a) Inhaled via a dry powdered inhaler

    b) Nebulised

    c) Oral

    d) Intravenous

7. Which one of the following inhaled medicines is used to help prevent asthma attacks?

    a) Salbutamol

    b) Beclomethasone

    c) Ipratropium

    d) Salmeterol

8. Which one of the following inhaled medicines is used to help alleviate the symptoms of an acute asthma attack?

    a) Salbutamol

    b) Beclomethasone

    c) Ipratropium

    d) Salmeterol

9. Tiotropium is an inhaled medication used in maintenance treatment of COPD. It is an example of a:

   a) Short-acting β_2-agonist (SABA)
   b) Long-acting β_2-agonist (LABA)
   c) Short-acting muscarinic antagonist (SAMA)
   d) Long-acting muscarinic antagonist (LAMA)

10. Inhaled salbutamol can cause tachycardia as a side-effect, especially in higher doses. This occurs because:

    a) β_2 receptors on the heart muscle are blocked by salbutamol
    b) β_2 receptors on the heart muscle are stimulated by salbutamol
    c) Muscarinic receptors on the heart muscle are blocked by salbutamol
    d) Muscarinic receptors on the heart muscle are stimulated by salbutamol

Chapter summary

Asthma and COPD are obstructive pulmonary disorders. Asthma is a condition characterised by narrowing of the airways, hyper-responsiveness of the airways to triggers leading to bronchospasm and chronic inflammation. Airflow obstruction is reversible. COPD often develops later in life, is progressive and airflow obstruction is irreversible. Inflammation leads to damage of lung tissue, the development of air spaces and a loss of elasticity. Similar inhaled drugs are used in the treatment of both COPD and asthma. The smooth muscle in the walls of bronchi and bronchioles is controlled by the autonomic nervous system. Many drugs used in COPD and asthma cause bronchodilation by affecting the autonomic nervous system. β_2-agonists such as salbutamol act on β_2 receptors in the bronchi which leads to relaxation of smooth muscle. Muscarinic antagonists, such as ipratropium, block acetylcholine receptors to relax the smooth muscle. The xanthines, aminophylline and theophylline, are also bronchodilators used in the treatment of COPD and asthma. They are used less often as they have a narrow therapeutic range and are involved in many drug interactions. Corticosteroid inhalers are also used. They reduce inflammation in the lungs and are especially effective in asthma. They are less effective in COPD. Other drugs such as leukotriene receptor antagonists can also help reduce inflammation in asthma. Nurses have a vital role to play in educating patients, especially with so many different inhaler types.

Activities: Brief outline answers

Activity 9.1 Reflection (p246)

It is important that healthcare professionals acknowledge the effect that COPD may have on patients like Peter, and their psychosocial well-being. Patients with chronic respiratory diseases are often at high risk of developing symptoms such as anxiety and depression. Psychological symptoms may result from a patient's fear, which can be triggered by increasing breathlessness, anxiety over risk of acute exacerbations or concerns about lack of prognostic certainty.

Nursing strategies for managing breathlessness should adopt an integrated approach that does not separate psychological and physical aspects of breathlessness. Therapeutic interventions for reha-bilitation and supportive care may focus on helping patients (and their carers) to (1) increase their fitness and tolerance of restricted lung function and reducing functional disability by recognising/reducing triggers to breathlessness and managing their breathlessness; (2) manage their anxiety during an episode of breathlessness through, for example, breathing retraining techniques; and (3) acknowledging the meaning of breathlessness in the context of their life-limiting condition. It is therefore important that, alongside pharmacological interventions for breathlessness, health pro-motion advice including breathing control, activity pacing, relaxation techniques and information about their condition, as well as emotional support, is provided to patients and their careers.

Activity 9.2 Critical thinking (p248)

Salbutamol causes vasodilation and greater air passage in the lungs. This will increase gas exchange and lead to greater oxygen levels in the blood oxygen in the body. This will enable greater aerobic respiration, for example in active skeletal muscle of an athlete. Blood glucose levels are also increased as salbutamol increases glucose release from the liver. From the table we can also see that salbutamol increases heart rate and force and causes vasodilation. This would all potentially increase blood flow to skeletal muscles. All these factors could unfairly enhance sporting performance.

Activity 9.3 Critical thinking (p249)

You would need to know the type of inhaler the patient is taking. Both dry powder and aero-sol inhalers exist. In this case, the brand of inhaler is also important. Although it is often best practice for doctors to prescribe generically, sometimes this isn't the case. Clenil Modulite® and Qvar® are two different brands of beclomethasone aerosol inhaler. Qvar® has extra fine parti-cles and is twice as potent as Clenil Modulite® (BNF). If the brand is wrong you could overdose or underdose the patient. The type of inhaler device is also important. Qvar® comes as a stand-ard aerosol inhaler, an autohaler or a Salamol Easi-breathe inhaler. These other types can be useful for people who find it difficult to use inhalers correctly. It is also vital to know the strength of the inhaler. Clenil Modulite® for example comes in strengths of 50 micrograms, 100 micro-grams, 200 micrograms and 250 micrograms per metered dose inhalation (per puff).

Activity 9.4 Research (p251)

Examples include erythromycin, ciprofloxacin, antiepileptic drugs, calcium channel blockers and anti-fungals. Xanthines have a much longer list of drug interactions than that for many other drugs, for example paracetamol. It is therefore especially important to check for interac-tions if a patient is on aminophylline or theophylline.

Activity 9.5 Critical thinking (p252)

Rachel is currently on the regular preventer step of the asthma guidance. She is on a low dose of steroid inhaler. The next step would involve adding a long-acting beta agonist (LABA) such as salmeterol to her treatment. Combination inhalers are often used for this to ensure patients take the corticosteroid and the LABA. If a combination inhaler was used the corticosteroid would need to be changed as beclometasone isn't available in a combination inhaler. She could be started on a Seretide inhaler which contains fluticasone (corticosteroid) and salmeterol (LABA).

Activity 9.6 Multiple choice questions (pp255–7)

1. 'Shortness of breath' is called:
   b) Dyspnoea

2. In a patient with COPD which clinical feature is *least* likely to be present?
   c) Airway obstruction that is reversible

3. Which of the following white blood cells is characteristic of the *chronic inflammation* in asthma?
   a) Eosinophil

4. Increased stimulation of sympathetic fibres to the airways brings about:
   b) Bronchodilation

5. According to NICE (2018b) COPD affects approximately how many people in the UK?
   d) 1.2 million

6. Corticosteroids should be delivered by which route in mild to moderate exacerbations of COPD?
   c) Oral

7. Which one of the following inhaled medicines is used to help prevent asthma attacks?
   b) Beclomethasone

8. Which one of the following inhaled medicines is used to help alleviate the symptoms of an acute asthma attack?
   a) Salbutamol

9. Tiotropium is an inhaled medication used in maintenance treatment of COPD. It is an example of a:
   d) Long-acting muscarinic antagonist (LAMA)

10. Inhaled salbutamol can cause tachycardia as a side-effect, especially in higher doses. This occurs because:
    b) β_2 receptors on the heart muscle are stimulated by salbutamol

Further reading

BTS/SIGN (2016) *British Guideline on the Management of Asthma.* Available at: **www.sign.ac.uk/sign-153-british-guideline-on-the-management-of-asthma.html/**

This gives more information on the treatment of asthma including algorithms used to choose therapy.

Hickey, AJ (2014) Understanding the impact of inhaler technique on asthma and COPD. *Nurse Prescribing*, 12 (10): 492–6.

This article gives useful information on inhaler technique.

Kumar, P and Clark, M (eds) (2012) *Kumar and Clark's Clinical Medicine* (8th edition). Philadelphia: Elsevier Saunders.

A comprehensive textbook on pathology. Chapter 13 gives a detailed examination of the pathology of asthma and COPD.

NICE (2018b) NG114. *Chronic Obstructive Pulmonary Disease in Over 16's: Diagnosis and Management.* Available at: **www.nice.org.uk/guidance/ng115/**

This gives more information about treatment and diagnosis of COPD.

Useful websites

www.brit-thoracic.org.uk/

British Thoracic Society website. Provides information on asthma, COPD and other lung conditions.

www.asthma.org.uk/

A charitable organisation providing information and support for those with asthma.

Chapter 10 Disorders of the gastrointestinal system

Chapter aims

After reading this chapter you will be able to:

- describe the causes, clinical features and pathophysiology of constipation, diarrhoea, peptic ulcer and inflammatory bowel disease;
- relate the signs and symptoms of these conditions to the underlying pathophysiology;
- explain how drugs for constipation, diarrhoea, peptic ulcer disease and inflammatory bowel disease exert their actions;
- describe the important drug interactions, cautions and contraindications.

Introduction

Infectious intestinal diseases affect 1 in 5 people in the UK each year.

(Public Health England, 2018a)

In this chapter, we start by examining the range of gastrointestinal (GI) disorders and give examples of each. This will enable you to understand the wide range of conditions that can affect the GI system. We then focus on two common symptoms of GI disorders, constipation and diarrhoea, and their pharmacological treatments. We will look in detail at the pathophysiology of peptic ulcers and inflammatory bowel disease (IBD). Inflammatory bowel disease includes ulcerative colitis (UC) and Crohn's disease. We discuss both of these conditions and their pharmacological treatments.

Types of GI disorder

There are many types of GI disorders. This reflects the large number and diversity of digestive organs. A common method of categorising GI disorders uses a combination of anatomical and functional characteristics. Categories include 'infection and inflammatory disorders'; 'motility disorders'; 'malabsorption disorders' and 'cancers of the GI tract'. Examples of disorders in each of these categories are summarised in Table 10.1. As you will see, there can be overlap between categories.

'Infection and inflammation' is the largest category of GI disorders and, as indicated by Public Health England above, commonly experienced. Alterations in functioning of the GI system can have many consequences in a person's life. People can experience an acute infection where symptoms commonly improve within a few days without any medical treatment being required. In contrast, chronic GI disorders can severely limit a person's ability to maintain their physical and emotional health, their education and employment across their lifespan and can create difficulties with participating fully in social activities.

Category	Description	Clinical examples
Infection and inflammatory disorders	Alterations in the integrity of the GI tract may occur at any point along its length resulting from: • Infection (viral, bacterial, fungal, protozoan) • Irritating substances • Inflammatory process • Autoimmune diseases • Weakness of the intestinal wall Symptoms may include pain, bleeding and diarrhoea.	Infectious causes may include: Viral – Mumps virus, hepatitis A Bacterial – *Helicobacter pylori, Escherichia coli* Fungal – *Candida albicans* Protozoan – *Giardia lamblia* Infection and inflammatory disorders may include: *Oral cavity*: Mumps, thrush *Oesophagus*: Oesophagitis *Stomach*: Gastritis, peptic ulcer *Intestines*: Gastroenteritis Colitis including irritable bowel syndrome (IBS), inflammatory bowel disease (IBD) Pseudomembranous colitis Necrotising enterocolitis Appendicitis Diverticulitis *Accessory organs*: Pancreatitis, hepatitis
Motility disorders	Disorders of the GI tract that alter its regular propulsive ability, peristalsis, can affect the absorption of nutrients. Increased motility leads to nutrients passing through the GI tract too fast for adequate absorption. Blockage or constriction of the GI tract may lead to slow or absent motility. May be congenital, acute or chronic.	Intestinal obstruction – partial or complete blockage of intestinal lumen. Volvulus – twisting of bowel on itself causing intestinal obstruction and blood vessel compression. Intussusception – telescoping of a portion of bowel into an adjacent portion. Common in infants. Megacolon – congenital or acquired. Common cause prolonged constipation including in younger children. Hirschsprung disease – congenital disorder of the large intestine in which autonomic nerve ganglia in smooth muscle are absent.

Malabsorption disorders	Failure of the GI tract to absorb or normally digest one or more constituents of the diet – fat, protein, carbohydrate, vitamins, minerals. May be due to enzyme abnormality or infection. Can also occur following surgery in which portions of stomach or small intestine are removed.	Coeliac disease – autoimmune condition – reaction of the immune system to gluten found in wheat and wheat products. Immune system reacts by damaging the lining of the small intestine.
		Lactose intolerance – inability to digest lactose, a type of sugar mainly found in milk and dairy products due to inadequate lactase production. Lactase is an enzyme normally produced in the small intestine that digests lactose.
		Dumping syndrome – dumping of stomach contents into small intestine due to impaired gastric emptying. May occur following gastrectomy.
Cancer	Cancer can occur in every part of the GI tract. Types of cancer can vary depending on the cell type of origin.	Oesophageal
		Gastric
		Small intestine
		Carcinoid
		Lymphoma
		Sarcoma
		Colon

Table 10.1   Categories of GI disorder

Review of the GI system

The GI system consists of the GI tract and accessory digestive organs. Figure 10.1 identifies the main organs of the GI system. Ensuring that you understand the structure and function of these organs, including the processes of digestion, absorption and motility will help you as you progress through this chapter.

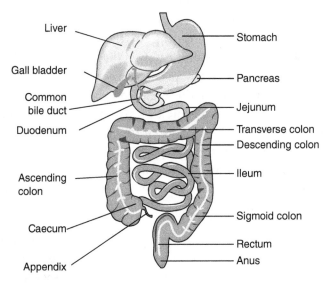

Figure 10.1   Organs of the GI tract

The GI tract is a hollow muscular tube divided into the oral cavity, pharynx, oesophagus, stomach, small intestine, large intestine, rectum and anus. Ingested food is propelled along the length of the GI tract by peristalsis, wave-like contractions of the muscular wall which create a squeezing action.

The wall of the GI tract is made up of four layers (Figure 10.2).

1. The innermost mucosa is a layer of epithelial cells supported by a connective tissue layer called the lamina propia. The lamina propia contains blood vessels, nerves, lymphoid tissue and glands. The epithelium is constantly shed and cells replaced – it is one of the most rapidly dividing areas of the body. Beneath the lamina propia is the muscularis mucosa. This thin smooth muscle layer can contract to change the shape of the lumen of the GI tract.

2. The submucosa layer surrounds the muscularis mucosa and consists of fat, connective tissue, blood vessels and nerves.

3. The muscularis comprises two smooth muscle layers and nerve connections that control the contraction, mechanical breakdown and peristalsis of food within the lumen.

4. The serosa or mesentery is the outer layer of the GI tract formed by fat and a layer of epithelial cells called mesothelium to create a fold of tissue which attaches the intestinal organs (including stomach, small intestine, pancreas, spleen) to the posterior wall of the abdomen.

The accessory digestive organs provide chewing, acids, enzymes and buffers that assist in the mechanical and chemical breakdown of food. The accessory organs include the teeth, salivary glands, liver, gallbladder and the pancreas. The salivary glands produce saliva – a lubricant containing the enzyme serum amylase. This starts the digestion of carbohydrates (starch) to sugars. The liver produces bile and metabolises nutrients. Bile is stored and concentrated in the gall bladder and released into the small intestine. Bile salts break down lipids (fat) into smaller particles for digestion by lipases. Lipases are enzymes that catalyse the breakdown of fats to fatty acids and glycerol in the small intestine. The pancreas secretes digestive enzymes amylase, lipases and proteases, important for the digestion of the three major food groups: proteins, carbohydrates and lipids. Proteases are enzymes that catalyse the breakdown of proteins into its constituent building blocks – amino acids. The three main proteases are pepsin, trypsin and chymotrypsin. Pepsin is produced in the stomach, while trypsin and chymotrypsin are produced in the pancreas. During the process of digestion, these enzymes work to break down dietary proteins into peptides and amino acids that can be absorbed by the small intestine.

The activities of the digestive system are controlled through a combination of local reflexes, autonomic nerve innervation and the release of gastrointestinal hormones such as gastrin (which stimulates secretion of gastric acid), secretin (which regulates water homeostasis and pH of the duodenum), and cholecystokinin (which causes

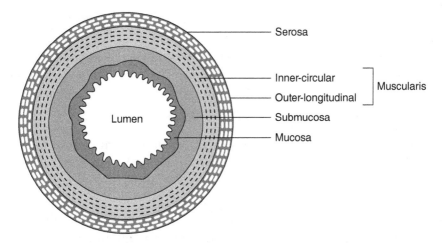

Figure 10.2 Layers of the wall of the GI tract

release of digestive enzymes and bile in duodenum for digestion of fat and protein). The main purpose of the GI tract is to break food down into smaller, soluble nutrients that can be absorbed into the body to provide energy.

Food must be ingested in the mouth to be mechanically processed and moistened with saliva. The stomach continues the mechanical breakdown of food and produces enzymes to begin the chemical digestion of proteins. Stomach acid (hydrochloric acid) is produced to destroy microorganisms. After the stomach, partially digested food – chyme – travels to the small intestine. Most chemical digestion occurs in the small intestine where macromolecules (proteins, fats and carbohydrates) are broken down into their basic building blocks (respectively amino acids, free fatty acids/monoglycerides, monosaccharides) by digestive enzymes. The enzymes in the small intestines work best in alkaline conditions. The acidic chyme from the stomach is made alkaline by pancreatic juice and bile – both of which are alkaline. Most absorption of these soluble food molecules occurs across the mucosal lining of the small intestine entering the epithelial cells.

Larger insoluble substances, such as fibre, remain undigested and cannot pass through the wall of the small intestine.

The small intestine is 6 metres in length and comprises the duodenum, jejunum and ileum compressed into many folds. Each fold has numerous villi and microvilli which increases the surface area for absorption. The villi contain blood and lymphatic vessels to carry away the absorbed food molecules. The duodenum provides a mixing function combining digestive secretions from the pancreas and bile salts from the liver and gallbladder with the contents, chyme, from the stomach. The jejunum is where most digestion and absorption takes place.

The large intestine consists of the appendix, caecum, ascending, transverse, descending and sigmoid colon and the rectum. Its main function is to form faeces, and reabsorb water and salts. Bacteria within the large intestines ferment any undigested sugars and proteins, releasing gas. Bacteria also produce vitamins, such as vitamin K, which may be absorbed through the colon. The mucosal surface of the large intestine is flat with glands lined by goblet cells that secrete mucus to lubricate faecal matter as it solidifies. The caecum receives material from the ileum and starts to compress food products into faecal material. The rectum expands to hold faecal matter before it passes through the anorectal canal and the anus.

Internal and external sphincters are thick bands of muscle that control the passage of faeces into the rectum and anus. These sphincters are usually constricted to ensure that faeces do not pass out continuously. The sphincters are controlled by the autonomic nervous system with sympathetic and parasympathetic nerves. The internal anal sphincter is controlled by parasympathetic nerves from the spinal cord that cause the sphincter to relax allowing faeces to pass through the anus when the rectum and anal canal contract. Sympathetic nerves cause the internal sphincter to contract/tighten. Internal anal sphincter control function is involuntary. This means that it is outside our conscious control and operates in a reflex manner responding to faecal content in the colon. In contrast, the external anal sphincter is controlled by spinal nerves and skeletal muscle that can be voluntarily (consciously) controlled. Once defaecation reflexes are triggered, peristalsis of the descending and sigmoid colon increases, faeces enter the rectum and the internal sphincter relaxes. This results in the urge to defaecate. Under conscious control of the external sphincter, undigested material and secreted waste products are squeezed from the body as faeces via defaecation. The process of defaecation should be painless, regular and under voluntary control. Repeatedly ignoring the natural urge to defaecate can, however, diminish the effectiveness of the defaecation reflexes and result in constipation. We discuss constipation and diarrhoea in more detail in the next section.

General symptoms associated with GI tract disorders

In this section, we focus on two of the general symptoms commonly experienced with a GI tract disorder. Alterations in bowel patterns, constipation and diarrhoea, may result from an infection or inflammatory condition, a change in GI tract motility or be part of a bowel disorder such as irritable bowel syndrome (IBS). Before reading further, undertake the activity to reflect on and research your understanding of constipation and diarrhoea.

Activity 10.1   Evidence-based practice and research

Consider:

- What is meant by the term 'constipation'?
- When might constipation occur?
- What is meant by the term 'diarrhoea'?

- When might diarrhoea occur?
- What nursing care and treatment might patients with constipation and diarrhoea require?

There is no model answer for this activity. However, you can compare your answer to the section 'General symptoms associated with GI tract disorders'.

Constipation

Constipation can be defined as small, infrequent or difficult defaecation. Fewer than three defaecations per week is often used as a guide for constipation. Normally, faeces are semi-solid with a mucus coating. Faeces contain water and solids including dead bacteria, undigested protein, carbohydrate or fibre, undigested fat and inorganic matter. The form of human faeces can vary in size, colour and texture according to the state of the digestive system, diet and general health. The Bristol Stool Chart classifies the form of human faeces into seven categories (Bladder and Bowel Foundation, 2016), the form of the stool being dependent on the length of time the faeces spends in the colon.

Cellulose, the carbohydrate component of dietary fibre, is indigestible and can be effective in promoting regular peristalsis, forming bulk in the intestinal lumen. Exercise also stimulates peristalsis. A lack of exercise contributes to the development of constipation. Dietary factors, for example a diet low in fibre or high in fat, slow the transit time of food. This reduces stimulation of peristalsis and increases water reabsorption leading to constipation. In older people, the rate of peristalsis is slowed due to the ageing process. Slowed peristalsis, in addition to a reduced level of physical activity, may lead to chronic constipation. Constipation can also result from a GI disease or condition. These conditions may include processes that alter the motility of the GI tract, for example intestinal obstruction, or processes that alter the integrity of the GI tract, such as diverticular disease, where diverticula (small pouches) have developed in the wall of the colon due to straining to pass the faeces. If the faeces or bacteria get caught in the pouches, diverticulitis can occur. As discussed earlier, repeatedly ignoring the natural urge to defaecate can reduce the effectiveness of the defaecation reflexes and result in constipation. Medication can cause constipation including opioid analgesics and tricyclic antidepressants.

Pharmacological management of constipation: laxatives

There are four main types of laxatives (Table 10.2). The type of laxative used depends on the cause of the constipation. In palliative care for example, constipation is often caused by opioids given for pain relief and regular laxatives can help prevent this. Laxatives that act as a softener plus a stimulant (co-danthramer) or lactulose plus senna are normally prescribed. Co-danthramer contains docusate, which has stimulant and softening actions, plus the stimulant danthron. Stimulant laxatives overcome the reduced peristalsis caused by opioid medication. The use of danthron is limited to elderly people or people who are terminally ill due to concerns that it is carcinogenic at high doses in animals (Waller and Sampson, 2018). Bulk forming laxatives are not recommended for opioid induced constipation in palliative care as they may cause abdominal colic and (rarely) bowel obstruction. Bulk forming laxatives act to distend the colon and stimulate peristalsis, but the opioids prevent the colon from responding with propulsive action (NICE, 2017b).

For other forms of constipation and, if lifestyle and dietary advice does not improve the symptom, guidance from the National Institute for Health and Care Excellence (NICE, 2017b) suggests starting with a bulk forming laxative. If ineffective, this can be changed to an osmotic laxative. If stools are soft, but the patient is still complaining of constipation, a stimulant laxative would be added.

Laxative type	Example	Notes on use	Action
Bulk forming	Ispaghula Husk (e.g. Fybogel®) Bran	Only required if fibre cannot be increased in the diet. Ensure adequate fluid intake. Avoid in intestinal obstruction.	These agents absorb water and soften stool mass. Also cause an enlargement of the stools that stimulates peristalsis in the GI tract and encourages the passage of intestinal contents.
Stimulant	Bisacodyl Dantron Docusate sodium Senna Glycerin	Often cause abdominal cramp. Avoid in intestinal obstruction.	Increase intestinal motility by being irritant to intestinal lining (senna) or stimulating nerves (bisacodyl).
Faecal softeners	Arachis oil	Given by enema.	Lubricate and coat stool with slippery lipids and slow colonic absorption of water to soften faeces and decrease intestinal transit time.
Osmotic	Lactulose Macrogols (e.g. Movicol®)	May take time to work. Avoid in intestinal obstruction.	Increase/retain water in colon by creating osmotic effect drawing water in from surrounding tissues and stimulating bowel peristalsis.

Table 10.2 Laxatives

Diarrhoea

Diarrhoea is defined as the passage of three or more loose or liquid stools per day, or more frequently than is usual for the individual (World Health Organization, 2018b). Normally, a healthy adult drinks 2 litres of fluid/day to which is added 1 litre of saliva, 2 litres of gastric juice, 1 litre of bile, 2 litres of pancreatic juice and 1 litre of intestinal secretions. These 9 litres of fluid are presented to the small intestine where all, but approximately 1.5 litres, is reabsorbed. The large intestine will absorb most of the remaining water minus about 100 mL. Normally, less than 200 grams of faeces are excreted per day, of which 65–85% is water. Diarrhoea may represent daily faeces production in excess of 250 grams containing 70–95% water. In severe cases, over 14 litres of fluid per day may be lost.

Diarrhoea can be an acute or chronic symptom. It can be accompanied by pain, urgency, perianal discomfort and incontinence. Acute diarrhoea can result from an infection, emotional stress or leakage around impacted faeces. Chronic diarrhoea is normally defined as a symptom lasting longer than four weeks. It can result from a chronic GI infection, alterations in the motility or integrity of the GI tract, malabsorption or certain endocrine disorders. Diarrhoea occurring episodically may be related to a food allergy, or follow ingestion of irritants to the GI tract such as caffeine. In children, diarrhoea often results from infection. Malabsorption, alterations in the structure of the GI tract and allergy are also possible causes.

Diarrhoea can be classified as:

1. *Osmotic diarrhoea*: A form of diarrhoea associated with water retention in the intestines that results from an accumulation of non-absorbable water-soluble substances. Osmosis is the movement of water from a less concentrated solution to a more concentrated solution through a partially permeable membrane. This means that, if a person drinks solutions with excessive sugar or excessive salt, water can be drawn into the intestinal lumen and cause osmotic diarrhoea. Sugar alcohols, such as sorbitol, are often found in sugar-free foods and these are difficult for the body to absorb. An excessive intake of sorbitol and mannitol, used as sugar substitutes in sweets, chewing gum and diet foods, can also result in slow absorption and rapid motility through the small intestine leading to osmotic diarrhoea. You may have noticed the warnings on sugar-free products.

   Osmotic diarrhoea can also arise due to malabsorption – as in lactose intolerance or coeliac disease where the nutrients are left in the GI lumen to draw in water. In lactose intolerance, lactose consumed, for example in dairy products, cannot be effectively broken down into glucose and galactose for absorption due to a deficiency in the enzyme lactase. Lactose is retained in the intestinal lumen where it draws in water, causing osmotic diarrhoea. As the unabsorbed lactose travels into the large intestine it is fermented by colonic bacteria producing distension of the colon with excessive gas. Osmotic diarrhoea can also be caused by osmotic laxatives that alleviate constipation by drawing water into the intestine. In most cases, osmotic diarrhoea stops when the causative agent (e.g. milk or sorbitol) is eliminated from the diet.

2. *Secretory diarrhoea*: As discussed above, large volumes of fluid are normally secreted into the small intestine to enable digestion. This fluid is usually reabsorbed on reaching the large intestine. Secretory diarrhoea occurs when the volume of fluid secreted is greater than the volume absorbed. This often results from viral

infection, for example, rotavirus. Rotavirus infects cells lining the mucosa of the small intestine. As these cells have a role in digestion of carbohydrates and the absorption of fluid and electrolytes, an infection with rotavirus can lead to malabsorption causing severe watery diarrhoea. Acute infectious diarrhoea is a major cause of morbidity in children and most frequently caused by viral infection. Bacteria, such as *Staphylococcus aureus*, also produce toxins that can cause secretory diarrhoea.

3. *Exudative diarrhoea*: Destruction of the intestinal epithelium that lines the mucosa causes exudative diarrhoea. This occurs when there are areas of inflammation and results in a fluid 'exudate' (Chapter 2) containing mucus, blood and protein. Water moves into the lumen across the epithelium by osmosis. In addition, if the surface of the intestine has been damaged by inflammation, less fluid will be absorbed. This reduction in fluid absorption contributes further to the fluid loss through diarrhoea. This is discussed further under 'Inflammatory bowel disease'.

4. *Diarrhoea related to motility disturbances*: Diarrhoea can result from a decreased contact time of chyme with the absorptive surfaces of the intestinal lumen. If inadequate absorption takes place in the small intestine large amounts of fluid will be delivered to the colon and may overwhelm its absorptive capability causing diarrhoea. In addition, if fatty acids and bile salts present in the chyme have not been adequately absorbed in the small intestine, they may induce secretory diarrhoea once they reach the colon. Diarrhoea associated with post-gastrectomy dumping syndrome is an example of this type of diarrhoea (Table 10.1). With dumping syndrome, ingested foods pass through the stomach too rapidly and enter the small intestine undigested. The small intestine expands due to the presence of these contents from the stomach and leads to fluid moving into the gut lumen, plasma volume contraction and acute intestinal distension. Osmotic diarrhoea, distension of the small bowel and hypovolaemia can result.

In order to provide the appropriate advice and nursing care to your patients, a detailed assessment of these symptoms is required to determine the cause and type of constipation or diarrhoea. Undertake Activity 10.2 to explore assessment of symptoms in more detail.

Activity 10.2   Critical thinking

Following a meal out the night before, Carol woke up early the next morning with crampy abdominal pain, nausea, aching limbs and diarrhoea. Carol recognised these symptoms as likely to be gastroenteritis. This is inflammation of the stomach and small intestine lining usually caused by an infection. Viruses, such as norovirus, and bacteria are common causes of gastroenteritis. Norovirus, also known as winter vomiting disease, causes gastroenteritis and is highly infectious (Public Health England, 2018b). The virus is easily transmitted through contact with infected individuals from one person to another. The virus is usually mild and lasts for 1–2 days. Symptoms include vomiting, diarrhoea and fever. Most people make a full recovery within a couple of days, but it can be dangerous for the very young and elderly people. Many bacteria causing gastroenteritis are from consuming infected food. This is more commonly known as food poisoning. Bacteria causing food poisoning include: *Campylobacter*, *Salmonella* and *Escherichia coli*.

Carol stayed at home from work and, after a few days, her symptoms of nausea and diarrhoea resolved as her immune system cleared the infection. To prevent dehydration, Carol sipped fluids, mainly water and, guided by her appetite, ate small amounts of food, gradually returning to her usual diet. Carol was careful to avoid spreading infection to others – washing her hands thoroughly and avoiding preparing food for others at home.

- Identify how norovirus, *Campylobacter*, *Salmonella* and *Escherichia coli* are spread.
- Which type of diarrhoea might Carol be experiencing?
- What advice would you give to Carol and your patients to reduce transmission of, for example, norovirus?
- What nursing actions can you take to reduce the risk of transmission of norovirus in care settings?

Compare your answers to the model answer at the end of the chapter.

Pharmacological management of diarrhoea

Anti-diarrhoeal medications include codeine phosphate, loperamide and diphenoxylate. These drugs reduce diarrhoea by slowing down the peristalsis of the GI tract so food takes longer to progress through the GI system. This slowing allows more time for the water produced by digestive processes to be reabsorbed by the colon and for faeces to be firmer and less urgent.

Opioids have an agonist action on the intestinal opioid receptors which when activated cause constipation (as briefly mentioned in the 'Constipation' section). Drugs such as morphine or codeine can be used to relieve diarrhoea this way. Codeine may also cause nausea and drowsiness as discussed in Chapter 6. Loperamide is an agonist of the mu opioid receptor in the large intestine and does not have an opioid effect in the central nervous system (CNS). This enables loperamide hydrochloride to be used to the same benefit as other opioid drugs but without the CNS side-effects.

Abdominal cramps and constipation can be side-effects of anti-diarrhoeal medication. Hard faeces may be formed which are difficult or painful to pass.

It is important to remember that the drugs identified manage the symptoms of constipation and diarrhoea. They do not address the cause(s). Patients may require additional investigations and treatment to address any underlying condition. For some patients, medication to manage constipation and diarrhoea may be contraindicated as discussed in the section 'Other pharmacological treatments for IBD'.

Infection and inflammatory disorders of the GI tract

Infection or the inflammatory process may affect the integrity of the GI tract. Integrity refers to an undamaged structure which functions normally. Alterations in integrity can adversely affect the functioning of the GI tract. These alterations may be acute and life-threatening, or chronic and disabling for the patient. We will discuss three examples including peptic ulcers, UC and Crohn's disease.

Peptic ulcers

Peptic ulcer refers to the development of an ulcer in the lower part of the oesophagus, the stomach (gastric ulcer) or the duodenum (duodenal ulcer) (Figure 10.3). An ulcer occurs where there is damage to the mucosa. This may be the result of exposure of the GI epithelium to the effects of pepsin and acidic gastric secretions of

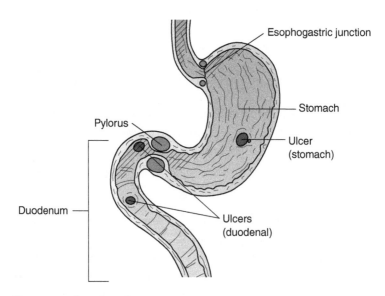

Figure 10.3 Common sites for ulcers

the stomach. Excessive gastric acid secretion is one factor in the development of peptic ulcer disease. Another factor is decreased mucosal protection against gastric acid. The integrity of the mucosa of the upper GI tract depends on the balance between 'hostile' factors such as gastric acid, *Helicobacter pylori (H. pylori)*, NSAIDs and pepsin, and 'protective' factors such as prostaglandins, mucus, bicarbonate and blood flow to the GI mucosa.

The risk factors for peptic ulcer include:

* Infection from *H. pylori* – a Gram-negative bacterium.
* Excessive consumption of alcohol and cigarette smoking.
* Excessive gastric secretions as a result of stress.
* Excessive use of NSAIDs and aspirin derivatives.
* Excessive consumption of caffeine.
* Familial history of peptic ulcer.

Mucus coats the lining of the GI tract and acts as a barrier against the acidic secretions of the stomach. Too little mucus production and excessive acid secretion leaves the mucosa vulnerable to acid erosion and ulceration. In the stomach, it is thought that a breakdown in the normally protective mucosa occurs. Substances such as aspirin, NSAIDs, alcohol and bile acids (regurgitated from the duodenum), can strip away the surface mucus and damage the gastric epithelial lining. Drugs, for example NSAIDs and aspirin, inhibit prostaglandin synthesis. We discussed the action of NSAIDs in Chapter 6. You will remember that prostaglandins promote inflammation, pain and fever as part of an inflammatory response. Prostaglandins protect the stomach and intestinal mucosa by inhibiting acid secretion, and stimulating mucus and bicarbonate secretion to protect against mucosal damage. Inhibition of prostaglandins by NSAIDs and aspirin will, therefore, reduce the effectiveness of these protective and healing mechanisms.

Studies suggest that the activity of the vagus nerve is increased in people with duodenal ulcer, particularly during a fasting state and at night. Part of the vagus nerve carries parasympathetic nerve fibres to the stomach and intestines. The parasympathetic nerve fibres stimulate epithelial cells in the pyloric antrum of the stomach and duodenum to release gastrin. Gastrin signals to cells in the stomach epithelium to secrete hydrochloric acid. Gastrin also binds to gastrin receptors on enterochromaffin-like cells (ECL) causing the release of histamine which stimulates the parietal cells to produce hydrogen (H+) ions. Hydrogen ions (or 'protons') create the very high acidity of gastric secretions. These details will be important for understanding drug treatments for peptic ulcer disease as discussed in section 'Pharmacological interventions for peptic ulcer disease' in this chapter.

H. pylori bacterial infection has a significant role in the development of gastric and duodenal ulcer formation. *H. pylori* is found in the mucus and on the inner surface of the epithelium. *H. pylori* is thought to survive the acidic conditions of the stomach by burrowing into the surface mucus where the pH is more neutral. *H. pylori* is able to neutralise the acid in the environment by producing the enzyme urease. Urease breaks down urea in the stomach to carbon dioxide (CO_2) and ammonia (NH_3). Ammonia is alkaline and acts to neutralise the stomach acid.

H. pylori may harm the stomach and duodenal lining by a variety of mechanisms and lead to inflammation. The ammonia produced by *H. pylori* to regulate pH (acidity of the stomach) is toxic to epithelial cells. Protease enzymes produced by *H. pylori* can also damage the epithelial cells. The inflammatory response, caused by the bacteria colonising the stomach, induces cells in the pyloric antrum to secrete gastrin. As described above, gastrin stimulates the parietal cells to secrete more stomach acid. The increase in acid causes further destruction of the mucosal lining and ulceration.

Other co-factors, including stress, caffeine, cigarette smoking and alcohol consumption, have been identified as possibly increasing acid production and the development of ulcers. The effect of stress on the GI tract is thought to decrease mucosal blood flow and suppress the production of mucus. As a consequence, stress is associated with mucosal erosions, particularly in the stomach. There is, however, limited evidence for the pathogenic role for alcohol, spicy food and caffeine.

Signs and symptoms of peptic ulcer include:

- dyspepsia
- epigastric pain
- heartburn
- nausea and vomiting
- blood in the vomit if the ulcer bleeds – known as haematemesis
- loss of weight
- eructation (belching).

Dyspepsia is the medical term for indigestion. Symptoms include feeling bloated, nauseous and having 'heartburn'. It is very common and can be caused by gastro-oesophageal reflux disease (GORD) or gastritis which is inflammation of the stomach lining. It can also be a sign that someone has a peptic ulcer or gastric cancer. This is illustrated in the scenario: Janette, below. Heartburn occurs when acidic stomach contents are forced into the oesophagus where they cause irritation.

Peptic ulcer usually responds to drug treatment but, if left untreated, can cause complications such as perforation of the GI wall, haemorrhage and stomach cancer. Pharmacological management is discussed in 'Pharmacological interventions for peptic ulcer disease'.

Scenario: Janette

Janette is a 45-year-old woman with a BMI of 30. She attends the GP surgery and mentions to you that she has been suffering from indigestion recently. Janette works part-time at a large teaching hospital as a pharmacist. Work has been very stressful. She explains that she has started to experience heartburn particularly at night. This is partially resolved by over-the-counter heartburn remedies and sleeping slightly elevated to prevent acid reflux. Janette also reports feeling sick which seems to improve once she has eaten. She is not on any NSAIDs or aspirin and has no features that suggest a serious condition such as cancer. After consultation with the GP it is suggested that she is suffering from dyspepsia. A full blood count (FBC) is taken to check there is no bleeding and her medicines are reviewed. Lifestyle factors are also considered. Initially she is started on an 'as required' antacid, but symptoms persist. It is decided that she may be suffering from an *H. pylori* infection and is tested for this. The test comes back positive and antibiotics are started to eradicate *H. pylori*.

Activity 10.3   Communication

The GP refers Janette to you, the practice nurse, to provide lifestyle advice for dyspepsia and additional information about *H. pylori*.

What information and lifestyle advice would you offer Janette?

A suggested answer is given at the end of the chapter.

Pharmacological interventions for peptic ulcer disease

We will now discuss some of the medication used to both prevent and treat peptic ulcers. Many of the drugs are also used to treat dyspepsia and GORD. As well as helping you to understand how these drugs work, it will help you to understand when and why such medicines are used. Medication encourages healing of the injured mucosa by reducing gastric acidity and helps to prevent recurrence.

Scenario: Akhtar

Akhtar is 85 years old, and lives in a nursing home where you work as a nurse. He is prescribed a number of drugs and he takes most of them as prescribed. He is prescribed aspirin 75 mg daily which he tells you is to 'protect his heart'. He also takes

(Continued)

(Continued)

Gaviscon when required which he tells you is for his indigestion. He is prescribed lansoprazole, but he often doesn't take it as he is not sure why he needs it. He remembers being told it is for his stomach, but he feels that his Gaviscon is working very well so he does not really need 'another pill'.

As his nurse, you suspect that lansoprazole is important, but want to check why before you speak to him.

Activity 10.4 Research and evidence-based practice

Find out about the action of lansoprazole and reflect on its importance to Akhtar's care.

Compare your answer with the section 'Proton pump inhibitors'.

Proton pump inhibitors (PPIs)

Lansoprazole, prescribed for Akhtar in the scenario above, is an example of a proton pump inhibitor. Other examples include omeprazole and pantoprazole. PPIs can be used to relieve dyspepsia and acid reflux symptoms. These drugs are also used to treat and prevent peptic ulcers. As we discussed above and in Chapter 6, both NSAIDs and aspirin can cause peptic ulcers as a side-effect. PPIs are commonly prescribed alongside such drugs to help prevent ulcers. You will have noticed that Akhtar is prescribed aspirin. The PPI is important to prevent peptic ulcers. It may be helpful to discuss this with Akhtar to promote understanding of his medication and concordance.

PPIs reduce acid secretion in the stomach by inhibiting the 'proton pump'. A proton pump is a cell membrane protein that transports hydrogen H+ ions (protons) across the membrane. The proton pump moves H+ ions from the gastric parietal cells into the lumen of the stomach. Although the stomach can protect itself from acid to a degree, acid (H+) can still damage the stomach lining and prevent the healing of lesions caused by aspirin. Also, as we saw in Chapter 6, both aspirin and NSAIDs reduce prostaglandin synthesis. The reduction in prostaglandin synthesis reduces the protection of the stomach to acid. Through the use of PPIs, a reduction in acid helps to promote healing and protect against the development of ulcers.

PPIs accumulate in the parietal cells in the stomach where they are activated. Their half-life is short but a single dose will reduce acid secretion for 2–3 days. They may take up to 5 days for their full effect to be achieved. This is another reason Akthar should take the medication as prescribed. Both omeprazole and lansoprazole are destroyed by stomach acid so are administered as enteric coated granules (Chapter 1).

Side-effects and implications for practice

Side-effects of PPIs can include headache, diarrhoea and rashes. There is concern that any drug that suppresses stomach acid can mask symptoms of gastric cancer and this should be investigated before treatment is started. Long-term treatment has been associated with an increase in the risk of fracture in those at risk of osteoporosis. It can also cause magnesium deficiency.

H_2 receptor antagonists

Another class of drugs that can be used to reduce stomach acid is the histamine (H_2) receptor antagonists such as ranitidine. As we discussed above, histamine acts to stimulate the parietal cells to increase acid secretion. Antagonising this effect with an H_2 receptor antagonist reduces acid secretion.

These drugs are no longer used as first line treatment as PPIs are more effective at reducing acid. However, they can be useful if PPIs are ineffective.

Side-effects and implications for practice

The H_2 receptor antagonists are well absorbed. Their absorption is not significantly affected by food or antacids. One of the first H_2 receptor antagonists developed was cimetidine. However, cimetidine is not frequently prescribed as it inhibits cytochrome P450 enzymes and can interact with other drugs (Chapter 1). Other H_2 receptor antagonists are usually well tolerated but side-effects include diarrhoea, dizziness, muscle pains and rashes.

In Activity 10.5, we consider another of the drugs Akhtar has been prescribed.

Activity 10.5   Critical thinking

Akhtar was also taking Gaviscon.

- What is Gaviscon and what is it used for?
- How do you think Gaviscon works?
- List other products of this type that you can think of.

A suggested answer is given at the end of the chapter.

Antacids and alginates

Having completed Activity 10.5, you will know that Gaviscon contains both an antacid and alginate. We will now discuss the difference between these.

Antacids

Antacids are the simplest medicines used to treat symptoms of increased acid secretion in that they are alkaline and neutralise acid. Examples include aluminium hydroxide, magnesium carbonate and magnesium trisilicate. Many antacid medicines also contain sodium bicarbonate and calcium carbonate which also neutralise acid. You may be more familiar with branded products such as Rennies. They are used when required to treat symptoms as they arise. It is important to note that they are not used to prevent ulcers or to promote the healing of ulcers.

Side-effects and implications for practice

Aluminium-based products tend to cause constipation whereas magnesium based products can cause osmotic diarrhoea as we discussed earlier in the chapter. Some products contain a mixture of the two to 'cancel' out these side-effects. For example Maalox. In patients with fluid retention, preparations containing large amounts of sodium should be avoided because this may increase fluid retention.

Antacids can impair the absorption of other drugs, for example anti-epileptic drugs, antipsychotics and antibacterials. They should not be taken at the same time. The full list of drug interactions can be found in the BNF. Antacids can also damage enteric coatings of tablets. These coatings would usually prevent tablets dissolving in the stomach so this effect would be lost.

Alginates

Alginates are used in combination with antacids. They increase the viscosity (thickness) of stomach contents as they absorb water. Some of them also form a 'raft' on top of the stomach contents. This makes them especially useful for acid reflux. Gaviscon is an example of a preparation containing an alginate.

Eradication of *H. pylori*

In Activity 10.3, we met Janette who presented with dyspepsia. You will remember that the test for *H. pylori* infection was positive and antibiotics were started to eradicate *H. pylori*.

The scenario demonstrates how *H. pylori* infection might be suspected and a test offered. *H. pylori* is a Gram-negative bacterium. Eradicating this bacterium can help reduce symptoms of dyspepsia, promote the healing of peptic ulcers and prevent reoccurrence of these ulcers. An *H. pylori* test might also be indicated for patients with peptic ulcer disease. A regime known as triple therapy, using three drugs including two antibiotics and a PPI, is used to eliminate the bacteria. A seven-day course is given. Two examples of triple therapy are given below.

1. Amoxicillin 1 g twice a day + clarithromycin 500 mg twice a day + lansoprazole 30 mg twice a day.

2. Clarithromycin 250 mg twice a day + metronidazole 400 mg twice a day + omeprazole 20 mg twice a day.

The choice of antibiotic will depend on a patient's allergy status and any recent use of antibiotics (NICE, 2014b). We discussed the side-effects and mechanism of action of these antibiotics in Chapter 3.

In the next section, we will discuss inflammatory bowel disease focusing on Crohn's disease and UC.

Inflammatory bowel disease (IBD)

IBD affects approximately 1 in 250 people in the UK (Crohn's and Colitis UK). Crohn's disease and UC are the two main forms of IBD. UC only affects the colon and rectum. Crohn's disease can affect the whole GI tract from mouth to anus. A combination of causative factors have been identified including genetic factors, which may predispose a person to developing IBD, and an abnormal reaction of the immune system to certain bacteria in the intestines. Viruses, bacteria, diet and stress have been implicated as environmental triggers but evidence is lacking. Crohn's disease and UC are managed as autoimmune diseases with anti-inflammatory drugs, immunosuppressants and biological therapies. As Crohn's and UC are managed differently in clinical practice, biopsies of the mucosa are taken to obtain a definitive diagnosis.

IBD is a chronic disorder characterised by periods of remission and exacerbations, and can, therefore, severely affect a person's quality of life. For example, people diagnosed with IBD may have concerns about the safety of drug therapies, the impact of the disease for their employment, concerns about access to toilets, and issues related to fertility and pregnancy. In order to provide the support and nursing care required by people with IBD and their families, you will need to have an understanding about these conditions, how they are managed and their acute and long-term impact on the daily lives of those affected.

Ulcerative colitis (UC)

UC affects the mucous membrane lining of the colon and rectum which become inflamed and ulcerated. The changes are normally most severe in the rectum and can extend around the colon. UC is also associated with a general inflammatory process that can affect many parts of the body.

Within the GI tract, the inflammatory process may begin in intestinal glands in the epithelial lining of the small intestine and colon, called colonic crypts or crypts of Lieberkuhn. The crypts are invaginations, meaning folds, in the epithelial inner surface of the colon. The inflammatory process in the colonic crypts may damage the crypt epithelium, bringing invasion of leukocytes and the formation of abscesses. Where multiple abscesses form close together large areas of ulceration develop. The inflammation may involve the whole colon up to the junction of the ileocaecal valve and, along with mucosal destruction, leads to oedema and bleeding. The ulceration may extend through the submucosa causing necrosis and sloughing of the mucosa. At the same time as this destructive process is occurring, attempts to repair damaged tissue are initiated with the development of fragile, highly vascularised granulation tissue.

For patients, mucosal destruction results in an increased need to defaecate – often many times a day. Patients may experience abdominal pain, diarrhoea and rectal bleeding. Exudative diarrhoea may result. Bleeding may result from mucosal destruction and ulceration as well as damage to the new granulation tissue. Those with UC may develop iron deficiency anaemia from poor absorption of iron. This can be exacerbated by blood loss in stools. Medication used for IBD, such as sulfasalazine and azathioprine, can also cause anaemia. In the later stages of the disease, the walls of the colon thicken, becoming fibrous. This leads to a narrowing of the lumen of the large intestine that may result in intestinal obstruction. Loss of large intestinal function can lead to complications such as dehydration and electrolyte imbalance alongside abdominal pain. An additional concern for patients with UC is the increased risk of developing colon cancer due to constant cell damage, cell renewal and cell adaptation which may result in metaplasia and dysplasia (Chapter 5). Patients may require regular endoscopy and biopsy to monitor for cell adaptation and early diagnosis of cancer. The presence of high-grade dysplasia may require prophylactic colectomy.

Case study

Jill is a 25-year-old woman who attends the specialist gastrointestinal clinic. When she was 18 years old Jill was diagnosed with UC and has normally managed her condition following lifestyle advice and prescribed treatment during intermittent exacerbations of her symptoms. She reports severe diarrhoea and opening her bowels up to five times a day. Her stools are dark and watery and she has noticed blood mixed in. She has no drug allergies and is not taking any medication except for the occasional ibuprofen for headaches. On examination, she appears pale with a temperature of 37.8°C and a pulse of 95 beats per minute. Her blood pressure is 105/62 mmHg. Her abdomen is tender. After further tests a diagnosis of moderate ulcerative colitis is made. Jill is started on mesalazine tablets. These help to alleviate her symptoms.

Activity 10.6   Critical thinking

Drawing on the information provided and using your understanding of UC, how might you explain the signs and symptoms Jill is experiencing?

A suggested answer is given at the end of the chapter.

Having looked at UC as one type of IBD, we will now consider Crohn's disease.

Crohn's disease

Crohn's disease is a chronic condition that can start at any age, usually appearing for the first time between 10 and 40 years. Unlike UC, Crohn's disease affects any part of the GI tract from the mouth to the anus, though often develops in the terminal ileum and/or the colon. For this reason the signs and symptoms may be different to those of UC depending on which area is affected. Inflammation of the GI tract may be patchy with sections of normal tissue in between. Patients may experience periods of remission and exacerbation of their symptoms throughout their lifetime.

Crohn's disease causes inflammation of the mucosa of the GI tract. This results in the development of deep ulcers in the GI wall. Eventually, all layers of the GI tract wall may become involved and the portion affected may become thickened by fibrous tissue. Deep fissures may develop into fistulas extending into adjacent tissue or other organs. Crohn's disease affects the body's ability to digest food, absorb nutrients and eliminate waste products.

While the exact cause is unknown, theories suggest that Crohn's disease may develop due to a combination of environmental, immune and bacterial factors in those who are genetically susceptible. Different theories have identified Crohn's disease as an autoimmune disorder that causes the immune system to attack normal, resident bacteria in the GI tract. Other theories suggest that Crohn's disease occurs due to an impaired innate immune response leading to a chronic inflammatory response. The body's immune system attacks the GI tract possibly directed at bacterial antigens. The increased incidence of Crohn's disease in industrialised countries also suggests an environmental component. Stress and smoking have been suggested as causing acute exacerbations in the condition (these are called 'flares').

In clinical practice, Crohn's disease may be categorised according to which parts of the GI tract are most affected. Terminal ileal Crohn's disease affects the end of ileum. Ileocaecal Crohn's disease affects the beginning of the large intestine. Patients may experience pain in the lower right side of the abdomen particularly after eating. Ileal Crohn's disease can make it difficult for the body to absorb bile salts and bile salts will irritate the bowel lining causing watery diarrhoea. Crohn's colitis affects the colon.

Due to inflammation, the colon cannot hold as much waste and patients may experience frequent bowel movements. Fistulae, fissures and abscesses, particularly around the anus, are common in Crohn's disease.

The signs and symptoms of Crohn's disease result from these pathological changes including diarrhoea, abdominal pain, weight loss and fatigue. Diarrhoea may be mixed with blood, pus or mucus as the bowel becomes incapable of adequately absorbing the intestinal contents. This may lead to weight loss. Iron deficiency anaemia is also common. Vitamin deficiency anaemia is caused by low intake or poor absorption of vitamins such as vitamin B_{12} (and folic acid). This may affect people with Crohn's disease who have had sections of the small intestine removed. Patients may feel generally unwell, with some experiencing a raised temperature due to the inflammatory response. In addition, patients can experience tiredness and fatigue due to the condition itself, from weight loss, from anaemia and also from lack of sleep due to pain and diarrhoea.

Other symptoms of IBD

UC and Crohn's disease may be associated with inflammatory-related conditions outside the GI tract. These include conditions affecting the joints, eyes or skin. Arthritis affects one in three people with IBD. Erythema nodosum is the most common skin problem causing painful red swellings usually on the legs. Episcleritis affects the white outer covering of the eye making it red, sore and inflamed. IBD may also lead to bone thinning, liver problems, blood clots and anaemia. Bone thinning can be due to the inflammatory process itself, poor absorption of calcium needed for bone formation, low calcium levels or the use of steroid medication. Some patients develop complications related to the liver and its function including the development of gallstones. Removal of the end of the small intestine or severe inflammation in this area can lead to poor absorption of bile salts that would normally help to digest fats during digestion. Primary sclerosing cholangitis causes inflammation of the bile ducts and may lead to liver damage in some people with Crohn's disease. Fever and mouth ulcers are also common.

Pharmacological treatment of IBD

In clinical practice, acute IBD can be life-threatening. Patients with severe symptoms will need admission to hospital. Most medication for IBD will be started by a specialist service but this will be monitored by the primary care team. Medication will not cure IBD but helps to relieve symptoms and reduce the risk of relapse. This can mean that patients are required to take drugs for many years. As these are inflammatory conditions, medicines with anti-inflammatory properties are used. The severity and areas of the GI tract affected will determine the types of drugs prescribed.

In the case study above we met Jill who was diagnosed with ulcerative colitis. The case study identifies a drug called mesalazine to treat UC. When Jill's symptoms are under control she will continue on this drug to prevent symptoms recurring. Mesalazine belongs to a group of drugs called aminosalicylates. We will look at these in more detail.

Aminosalicylates

These drugs are used in UC to achieve symptom control and remission of the disease. They are not very effective in Crohn's disease. Examples include sulfasalazine, mesalazine, olsalazine and balsalazide. Tablets are available but patients may also use suppositories, enemas or rectal foams, depending on which part of the GI tract is affected.

The active component of all these medicines is the drug 5-aminosalicylic acid (5-ASA). Because IBD affects the internal parts of the GI tract we need to deliver drugs to that area. Unlike other drugs, we do not want the drugs to be absorbed systemically. Sulfasalazine contains sulfapyridine joined to 5-ASA. The 5-ASA is liberated from the molecule by the action of bacteria in the GI tract. Mesalazine contains 5-ASA only. There are many different preparations, for example Asacol® and Pentasa®. These are all specifically formulated to release the 5-ASA in the distal lumen or colon where it is needed; otherwise the active drug would be absorbed too early in the duodenum.

These drugs are chemically related to aspirin and have anti-inflammatory and immunosuppressant actions that enable damaged tissue to repair and replace cells. The precise mode of action is unclear. It is thought that 5-ASA may inhibit neutrophil movement (chemotaxis) and reduce prostaglandin and leukotriene production.

Side-effects and implications for practice

Sulfasalazine can cause more side-effects than mesalazine because of the sulfapyridine part of the molecule which is absorbed. As a result its use is declining. Mesalazine causes many GI symptoms such as nausea, diarrhoea and bloating. It can also cause headaches and rashes. Patients should be encouraged to report signs of unexplained fever, sore throat, bruising or bleeding which can be a sign of more serious side-effects. These include blood disorders and kidney toxicity which are fortunately rare. If these do occur the medication must be stopped.

Corticosteroids

Corticosteroids are the usual treatment for acute exacerbations (often referred to as 'flares') in IBD. For severe exacerbations, intravenous drugs such as hydrocortisone are used. For milder flares a course of oral prednisolone may be used. Corticosteroids have anti-inflammatory effects (Chapter 2) and can help reduce redness, swelling and pain caused by the inflammation associated with an acute exacerbation of Crohn's disease or UC.

Activity 10.7   Reflection

Darragh is admitted to hospital with severe UC. He is treated with intravenous hydrocortisone 100 mg four times daily. After two days his symptoms resolve. You are his named nurse. He admits to you that he does not always take his medication as prescribed.

Is there anything you could do to help Darragh take his medication in the future?

Compare your answer to the suggestions at the end of the chapter.

Non-adherence is the most common cause of relapse in IBD (Hawthorne et al., 2008). In Activity 10.7, admission to hospital and administration of IV corticosteroid hydrocortisone were needed to bring the disease under control. If symptoms do not improve surgery might be needed. As discussed in Chapter 2, side-effects limit the long-term use of corticosteroids and courses are kept as short as possible. However, 10–20% of patients may become dependent on corticosteroids for control of their disease. This means that if the corticosteroid is stopped symptoms will flare up again. Long-term corticosteroids are needed for these patients. Examples of corticosteroids used are prednisolone, hydrocortisone, beclomethasone and budesonide.

Immunosuppressant drugs: thiopurines and methotrexate

Immunosuppressant drugs suppress the immune system. As we discussed in Chapter 4, the immune system is important for responding to infection but, in IBD, cells of the immune system attack the body's own tissues (autoimmune) and trigger chronic inflammation. Immunosuppressant drugs reduce this inflammation by damping down the over-activity of the immune system cells. These drugs may be used when treatment with steroids and aminosalicylates has not controlled inflammation, or when steroids cannot be withdrawn without causing a relapse. They can be used to reduce symptoms and maintain remission but it can be many months before patients report any benefits.

Examples of immunosuppressants include azathioprine, mercaptopurine and methotrexate. Azathioprine is metabolised to mercaptopurine. This drug is cytotoxic, inhibiting DNA synthesis in proliferating cells such as T cells and B cells of the immune system (Warner et al., 2016).

Side-effects and implications for practice

The side effects can limit the use of these drugs (Warner et al., 2016). These drugs are non-specific, so they will affect other rapidly dividing cells such as those in the skin and

GI tract. This can lead to skin rashes, nausea and vomiting. Patients may also experience suppression of bone marrow that can lead to reductions in red blood cell, white blood cell and platelet production. Regular monitoring of blood counts and liver function is required. Chapter 5 explains more about the side-effects of cytotoxic drugs. These drugs are all teratogenic which means that they can cause birth defects. Women are advised not to become pregnant while they are taking them.

Biological therapies

Biological therapies can be used to treat patients with IBD. There are different biological therapies used including, most commonly, infliximab and adalimumab. These are a type of monoclonal antibody (MAB) used to treat autoimmune diseases and may be referred to as 'anti-TNF drugs' (Chapter 4).

Infliximab and adalimumab target tumour necrosis factor (TNF). TNF is a pro-inflammatory cytokine (Chapter 2, Table 2.2). Over-production of TNF is implicated in the chronic inflammation of IBD. When infliximab or adalimumab bind to TNF this prevents TNF from attaching to its receptor in the cell and leads to a reduction in inflammation.

Other biological therapies have been developed for IBD including vedolizumab and ustekinumab. These may be used as a second line treatment when the patient's disease does not respond to TNF inhibitors. These target various components of the immune response in IBD and work in different ways to the 'anti-TNF' drugs. Vedolizumab is a type of monoclonal antibody called a 'gut selective integrin blocker' while ustekinumab is an 'anti-interleukin' – an immunosuppressant drug dampening down the activity of the immune system for patients with Crohn's disease.

Side-effects and implications for practice

Because biological therapies suppress the immune response they can make people more prone to infection and this must be monitored. Hypersensitivity reactions and blood disorders are other serious side-effects that need monitoring. A full list of side-effects can be found in the BNF. Clinical guidelines for the management of UC and Crohn's disease are available from NICE (NICE, 2013b; NICE, 2016b). Patient advice is also available at: Crohn's and Colitis UK under the Useful websites section at the end of the chapter.

Other pharmacological treatments for IBD

Other medication is sometimes used to manage the symptoms experienced by patients with IBD but these must be used with care. Paracetamol, for example, is the drug of choice for pain. NSAIDs may be associated with worsening of symptoms and should be avoided. Opioids are sometimes used under specialist supervision but can increase the risk of toxic megacolon (Table 10.1). This is a serious complication of IBD where inflammation causes gas to be trapped and the colon to become swollen. As a result sepsis can occur or the colon can rupture. Anti-diarrhoeal drugs are not usually used as they too can cause toxic megacolon. Bulk forming laxatives for constipation can be useful if dietary advice does not help. Antibiotics are sometimes used to treat complications of Crohn's disease such as abscesses and fistulas. Antibiotic use for treatment in IBD is based on the theory that, while the exact cause of IBD is not known, it may involve an abnormal reaction of the immune system to bacteria within the intestine. Antibiotics will reduce these bacteria and some antibiotics may have an immunosuppressant effect. Commonly used antibiotics include metronidazole and ciprofloxacin.

Other management and treatment options for IBD

This chapter has focused on the pharmacological management. However, the person with IBD may also need emotional and informational support to understand their disease and engage in decision-making about its management/treatment. They may also require instrumental support to meet their activities of daily living when the disease is in remission and during acute exacerbations/flares. Nutritional therapy (enteral feeding), for example, can be a useful treatment option in Crohn's disease especially for children. As IBD may be first diagnosed when a patient is in their twenties and thirties, concerns about fertility may also be expressed. Similarly, surgical options for IBD are beyond the scope of this book. You may wish to research these aspects of care, treatment and support in more detail.

Activity 10.8   Evidence-based practice and research

The chapter has focused on examples of infection and inflammatory disorders of the GI system. There may also be disorders in other categories that are of interest to you. Activity 10.8 gives you the opportunity to choose one GI disorder from a category other than 'infection and inflammation' in Table 10.1 which is relevant to your field of practice. Undertake research to:

1. Identify the aetiology and pathophysiology of the disorder.
2. Relate the pathophysiology to explain common symptoms experienced by patients.
3. Identify the drugs commonly used to treat the condition and explain how they act.

No model answer is provided as this is related to your own research.

Conclusion

Disorders of the GI system can affect people in many different ways. Symptoms of constipation, diarrhoea and indigestion are common in GI disorders and can be treated with laxatives, anti-diarrhoeal agents and antacids. However, it is important to understand the cause of the symptoms if care and treatment are to be effective. We have focused on examples of infection and inflammatory GI disorders and the drugs that reduce inflammation including corticosteroids, aminosalicylates, immunosuppressants and monoclonal antibodies. In doing this, the discussion has also highlighted content explored in other chapters. This should enable you to start to apply your learning to GI disorders.

It is now time to review what you have learned within this chapter by undertaking some multiple choice questions.

Activity 10.9   Multiple choice questions

1. The enzyme salivary amylase starts digestion of starch, a complex carbohydrate. Complex carbohydrates are finally broken down into:
   a) Sugars (monosaccharides)
   b) Fatty acids
   c) Glycerol
   d) Amino acids

2. Where is most of the water absorbed in the GI tract?
   a) Small intestine
   b) Large intestine
   c) Stomach
   d) Oesophagus

3. What do stool (faecal) softeners do?
   a) Lubricate and coat stools with lipids
   b) Create osmotic effect drawing water into colon
   c) Irritate intestinal lining
   d) Absorb water

4. A lesion that erodes the skin or a mucosa is termed:
   a) A fistula
   b) An exudate
   c) An ulcer
   d) An abscess

5. Which type of diarrhoea is associated with rotavirus infection?
   a) Osmotic
   b) Secretory

(Continued)

(Continued)

    c) Exudative

    d) Diarrhoea related to motility disturbance

6. Lactose intolerance can lead to which type of diarrhoea?

    a) Osmotic

    b) Secretory

    c) Exudative

    d) Related to motility disturbances

7. Hydrochloric acid secretion by the parietal cells of the gastric mucosa is inhibited by:

    a) Gastrin

    b) Proton pump inhibitors

    c) Histamine

    d) Parasympathetic vagal activity

8. What is the order of the four segments of the colon?

    a) Ascending, sigmoid, descending and transverse

    b) Transverse, ascending, descending and sigmoid

    c) Ascending, transverse, sigmoid and rectum

    d) Ascending, transverse, descending and sigmoid

9. Those with Crohn's disease may have a reduced ability to absorb vitamin B12 in the ileum. This can lead to:

    a) Gastritis

    b) Constipation

    c) Gallstones

    d) Anaemia

10. Which chemical mediator helps protect the stomach by stimulating mucus production?

    a) Hydrochloric acid

    b) Prostaglandins

    c) TNF

    d) Aspirin

Chapter summary

In this chapter we have:

- Described the causes, clinical features and pathophysiology of constipation, diarrhoea, peptic ulcer and inflammatory bowel disease.

- Related the signs and symptoms of these conditions to the underlying pathophysiology.
- Explained how medicines for constipation, diarrhoea, peptic ulcer disease and inflammatory bowel disease exert their actions.
- Described the important drug interactions, cautions and contraindications of the medicines.

Activities: Brief outline answers

Activity 10.2 Critical thinking (pp270–1)

Norovirus can be spread by eating food or drinking liquids contaminated with norovirus, and touching surfaces or objects with norovirus on them. For example caring for, or sharing food or utensils with someone with norovirus, and then putting your hand or fingers in your mouth. Norovirus can be found in the vomit and stools of an infected person.

Campylobacter bacteria may be present in uncooked or undercooked meat, particularly poultry, and unpasteurised milk.

Salmonella is spread by eating contaminated food that is undercooked or raw including poultry, eggs, meat products and untreated milk and dairy products. It can be spread by an infected person through inadequate handwashing after using the toilet or during food preparation.

Spread of *E. coli* infections are particularly food-borne occurring through consumption of contaminated meat. Other sources of infection include unpasteurised milk, contaminated leafy green vegetables and by swimming in or drinking contaminated water. *E. coli* can be spread by person-to-person contact from bacteria in loose stools. To prevent transmission of these good hygiene and regular handwashing are required.

Carol may be experiencing secretory diarrhoea. She does not require any medication to treat her diarrhoea.

Advice to Carol and your patients to reduce transmission of, for example, norovirus and the nursing actions you can take to reduce risk of transmission of norovirus in care settings can be found at: **www.gov.uk/government/collections/norovirus-guidance-data-and-analysis/**

Activity 10.3 Communication (p275)

Lifestyle advice for dyspepsia, peptic ulcers and additional information about *H. pylori*.

In addition to pharmacological interventions, nursing care will involve identifying any lifestyle factors that may be associated with dyspepsia, including stress, use of NSAIDs or aspirin, alcohol and coffee consumption, and smoking. While there is no conclusive evidence that any specific diet has a therapeutic effect, as a nurse you may provide informational support relating to stress management, smoking and alcohol cessation. Dietary advice may include small, regular meals and avoidance of spicy food to reduce irritation of the mucosa membrane of the stomach that may lead to inflammation and epigastric pain. Medication such as NSAIDs and aspirin should be avoided as these drugs irritate the stomach and inhibit the action of prostaglandins and can lead to gastrointestinal bleeding.

It may be useful to go through the following information with Janette: **www.nhs.uk/conditions/stomach-ulcer/diagnosis/**

Activity 10.5 Critical thinking (p277)

Gaviscon is a mixture of an alginate (sodium alginate) and sodium bicarbonate and calcium carbonate which are antacids. It is used for acid reflux and indigestion. Other examples include Peptac® and Gastrocote® (BNF).

Activity 10.6 Critical thinking (p281)

Fatigue is common in IBD especially during flare-ups. These symptoms could be due to dehydration, electrolyte imbalance or iron deficiency anaemia. Iron deficiency anaemia is caused by a lack of iron in the diet, poor absorption of iron from food and blood loss in the stools. Bowel movements might also be interfering with sleep. Pain and anxiety can also add to the problem. Chemicals produced by the body during inflammation, such as cytokines, can also cause fatigue. Blood in the stools occurs because the lining of the colon is damaged and ulcerated. The inflammation leads to diarrhoea and abdominal pain. As the body is less able to absorb water from the colon dehydration can occur. This could be the reason for a dry mouth and concentrated urine.

Activity 10.7 Reflection (p284)

Darragh is not unusual and a study showed that 40% of patients may not take their medication for preventing relapses (Horne et al., 2009). It might be useful to have a talk with Darragh and explore his health beliefs and understanding about both his disease and the medication he takes. The study found that some people do not take the medication due to side-effects, while others did not feel the medication was really needed. This is understandable as during remission a patient may have no symptoms but still be taking medicines every day. Some education about the disease and the role of drugs in preventing relapses like the one just experienced would be useful. Remember that mesalazine has also been shown to reduce cancer and this relapse could have led to the patient needing surgery.

Activity 10.9 Multiple choice questions (pp287–8)

1. The enzyme salivary amylase starts digestion of starch, a complex carbohydrate. Complex carbohydrates are finally broken down into:

    a) Sugars (monosaccharides)

2. Where is most of the water absorbed in the GI tract?

    a) Small intestine

3. What do stool (faecal) softeners do?

    a) Lubricate and coat stools with lipids

4. A lesion that erodes the skin or a mucosa is termed:

    c) An ulcer

5. Which type of diarrhoea is associated with rotavirus infection?

    b) Secretory

6. Lactose intolerance can lead to which type of diarrhoea?

    a) Osmotic

7. Hydrochloric acid secretion by the parietal cells of the gastric mucosa is inhibited by:

    b) Proton pump inhibitors

8. What is the order of the four segments of the colon?

   d) Ascending, transverse, descending and sigmoid

9. Those with Crohn's disease may have a reduced ability to absorb vitamin B12 in the ileum. This can lead to:

   d) Anaemia

10. Which chemical mediator helps protect the stomach by stimulating mucus production?

    b) Prostaglandins

Further reading

The following NICE websites are recommended for further reading. The NICE websites provide guidance for the assessment and management of dyspepsia, IBD for different patient groups and constipation. They offer guidance to inform your clinical decision-making through the implementation of evidence-based guidelines.

NICE (2014b) *Gastro-Oesophageal Reflux Disease and Dyspepsia in Adults: Investigation and Management.* **www.nice.org.uk/guidance/cg184**

NICE (2016b) CG 152. *Crohn's Disease: Management in Adults, Children and Young People.* **www.nice.org.uk/guidance/cg152/**

NICE (2013b) *Ulcerative Colitis: Management in Adults, Children and Young People.* CG 166.

NICE (2017b) *Clinical Knowledge Summary: Constipation.* **https://cks.nice.org.uk/constipation#!scenario/**

Useful websites

www.crohnsandcolitis.org.uk/

Crohn's and Colitis UK. A nationwide charity for IBD sufferers. Contains useful information about IBD.

http://s3-eu-west-1.amazonaws.com/files.crohnsandcolitis.org.uk/Publications/Infliximab.pdf/

Crohn's and Colitis UK information on Infliximab.

Chapter 11 Diabetes

Margaret Bannister

Chapter aims

After reading this chapter you will be able to:

- explain the pathophysiology of type 1 and type 2 diabetes;
- describe the risk factors and clinical manifestations of type 1 and type 2 diabetes;
- explain the pathophysiology of the acute complications of diabetes;
- explain the long-term complications associated with type 1 and type 2 diabetes and the reasons for the management of related risk factors;
- explain the action of oral hyperglycaemic agents and injectable therapies in the management of type 2 diabetes;
- describe the different types of insulin, the potential issues with insulin safety and strategies to prevent insulin errors.

Introduction

Diabetes is a complex and demanding condition with potentially debilitating complications. Effective management is largely dependent on how people care for themselves; this requires constant personal motivation and changes in behavior and routine. Not surprisingly, the impact of diabetes on emotional and psychological wellbeing can be profound.

(Diabetes UK, 2018)

As a nurse, it is likely that every day you will provide care to a person with diabetes. In 2017, 3.6 million people had a diagnosis of diabetes in the United Kingdom, and an estimated 1,000,000 people have the condition but do not know it (Diabetes UK, 2017). In 2017, 18% of hospital beds (1 in 6) were occupied by a person with diabetes (NaDIA, 2018). It is anticipated that by 2025, five million people will have been diagnosed in the UK. Diabetes will be the seventh leading cause of death worldwide by 2030. This increase will be largely due to type 2 diabetes resulting from the rapid rise in the number of people who are overweight or obese. In the UK, this is made worse by an ageing population.

Nurses in all fields need to understand the pathophysiology and management of diabetes as they are likely to encounter people at risk of developing, or diagnosed with, this condition. In addition, insulin is one of the top 10 'high alert' medications worldwide. This means that insulin is linked to potential drug errors and the possibility of causing harm. Implementation of an insulin safety campaign has been initiated in the UK in recent years. All nurses need to be aware of, and comply with, insulin safety policies within their field of clinical practice (Bannister, 2011).

We start this chapter by explaining the normal regulation of blood glucose. We then move on to explain the different types of diabetes, the clinical manifestations of type 1 and 2 diabetes and how they are diagnosed. We then examine the pathophysiology relating to acute and long-term complications of diabetes. Finally, we will discuss the management of diabetes, including oral and injectable treatments.

Throughout this chapter, we follow the case of Abida from when she first presents with symptoms of diabetes. This will illustrate how the underpinning pathophysiology informs the care people with diabetes should receive and the treatments, both oral and injectable, used to correct raised blood glucose levels.

Review of blood glucose regulation

Glucose is the main source of energy for most cells in the body. Blood glucose levels are maintained in normal healthy individuals between 3.5 and 6.5 mmol/L. Blood glucose levels are maintained within this narrow range through the action of the hormones insulin and glucagon. Regulation of blood glucose levels is an example of homeostasis (Chapter 1) and is regulated through negative feedback. Blood glucose levels rise following a meal rich in carbohydrates. Dietary carbohydrates will include starch, which is a complex carbohydrate made up from many thousands of glucose molecules, and simple sugars. Another name for this is a polysaccharide. Simple sugars include sucrose, lactose and glucose. Glucose is monosaccharide (made up from one glucose unit) and small enough to be absorbed directly into the bloodstream. Starch, by contrast, needs digesting into its component glucose units which can then be absorbed. The glycaemic index of a food type is a measure of the effect it has on a person's blood glucose level. The glycaemic index is related to how quickly the carbohydrate component of the food is digested and absorbed into the bloodstream. Food with a low glycaemic index causes a slower rise in blood glucose levels.

A rise in blood glucose levels triggers insulin release from beta cells in the pancreas. The pancreas contains clusters of endocrine cells called the islets of Langerhans (Figure 11.1).

The islets of Langerhans contain alpha and beta cells. Beta cells synthesise and release the insulin. Alpha cells synthesise and release glucagon. Insulin released into

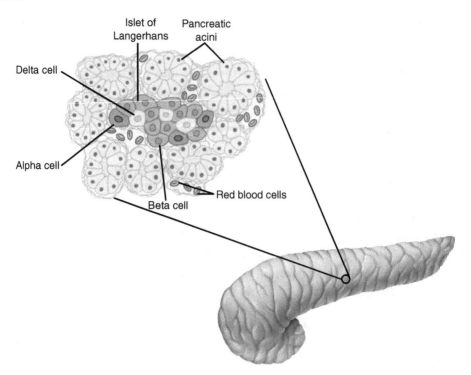

Within each islet, the beta cells synthesise and release insulin, and the alpha cells synthesise and release glucagon.

Figure 11.1   An islet of Langerhans in the pancreas

the bloodstream acts on the liver, skeletal muscle and adipose tissue. Insulin binds to insulin receptors on the cell surface. This opens up glucose transporter proteins in the cell membrane and glucose, from the blood, is transported into the cells. Overall, this results in a decrease in blood glucose levels. The reduction in blood glucose suppresses further insulin release leading to a fall in the levels of circulating insulin. This is an example of negative feedback. In skeletal muscle, the glucose is used to produce energy for muscle contraction, or it is stored as glycogen. In the liver, the glucose is stored as glycogen (Figure 11.2). In adipose tissue, the glucose is stored as fat.

By contrast, decreases in blood glucose levels and the resulting fall in circulating insulin, such as that which occurs between meals, trigger the release of the hormone glucagon from the alpha cells in the islets of Langerhans. Glucagon triggers the breakdown of glycogen into glucose by the liver (Figure 11.2). This breakdown is called glycogenolysis. Glucose is released into the blood increasing the blood glucose level. This rise in blood glucose levels suppresses the release of glucagon from the alpha cells and lowers the levels of circulating glucagon. This is also an example of negative feedback. Maintaining blood glucose levels within the normal range is continuous, achieved through a delicate balance of insulin and glucagon.

Insulin is released in two phases. 'First phase' insulin release occurs 2 to 10 minutes following a rise in the blood glucose level. This rapid release of insulin prevents the blood glucose level rising too high. 'Second phase' insulin release is much more controlled. The amount and speed of insulin release is determined by the actual rise in

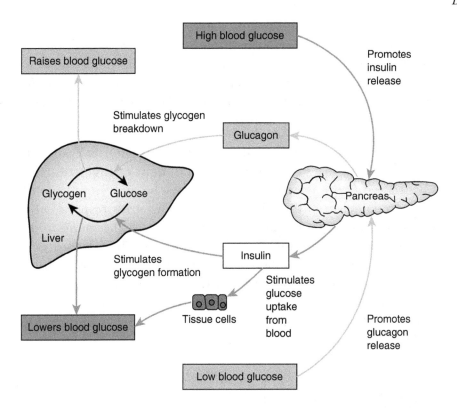

The hormones insulin and glucagon act to regulate blood glucose levels. The liver is an important store of glycogen.

Figure 11.2   Blood glucose regulation

blood glucose level and the rate that carbohydrate is digested. This rate is influenced by the quantity and glycaemic index of the ingested food. Second phase insulin secretion is maintained until blood glucose levels return to a level that no longer triggers insulin release.

First phase insulin release is stimulated by the hormone GLP-1 (glucagon-like peptide 1) which primes the beta cells in the pancreas to release insulin in response to a rise in the blood glucose level. GLP-1 is rapidly destroyed in the body by the enzyme DPP IV and, therefore, has a very short half-life. GLP-1 acts on the brain to cause a feeling of fullness (satiety). It also acts on the stomach to delay gastric emptying and on the alpha cells of the pancreas to suppress glucagon release. First phase insulin release is absent in type 2 diabetes as a result of low levels of the GLP-1 hormone (Holst, 2007).

Glucose should not be present in the urine. As blood passes through the kidney, glucose is filtered in the nephron (Tortora and Derrickson, 2017). One hundred percent (100%) of glucose and 99% of water are reabsorbed through a process of selective reabsorption. Glucose reabsorption occurs predominantly (90%) in the proximal tubule by a membrane transporter protein – the selective glucose transporter protein 2 (SGLT2). Water reabsorption follows passively by osmosis in the loop of Henle. The renal threshold (or maximum level) for glucose absorption is 10 mmol/L. If blood glucose levels in the filtrate exceed the renal threshold, glucose will remain in the filtrate. The presence of glucose in the filtrate causes an increase in the osmotic pressure in the tubule. This leads to retention of water within the tubule and a reduction in the absorption of water. As a result, glucose will appear in the urine, and large volumes of urine will be produced. This is known as osmotic diuresis. We will return to this when looking at the symptoms of a raised blood glucose level (hyperglycaemia).

Hypoglycaemia, which is a blood glucose level below the normal range, triggers a stress response. Part of the stress response is the 'fight or flight response' which is caused by triggering the sympathetic nervous system and the release of adrenaline and noradrenaline from the adrenal glands. The stress response also triggers the hypothalamic–pituitary–adrenal (HPA) axis (Chapter 2) leading to the release of the hormone cortisol. The increased levels of adrenaline, noradrenaline and cortisol in the blood prepare the body for 'fight or flight'. Key responses include: increased heart rate, peripheral vasoconstriction, increased sweating, release of glucose from the liver leading to raised blood glucose levels. We will return to hypoglycaemia and the stress response under 'Pathophysiology of the acute complications of diabetes'.

Types of diabetes

Diabetes mellitus develops when the body's ability to produce insulin declines or the body's response to insulin is impaired. Both result in an elevated blood glucose level.

- *Type 1 diabetes* is caused by autoimmune destruction of the beta cells. This results in an inability of the body to produce insulin. This destruction often occurs early in life and, at a critical level of destruction, can lead to rapid onset of symptoms. The aetiology of the autoimmune response is unclear but is thought to be associated with an environmental trigger such as a virus. Type 1 diabetes affects about 10% of those diagnosed with diabetes. Insulin therapy is initiated at diagnosis and it is an essential treatment for survival.
- *Type 2 diabetes* develops much more insidiously and is progressive in nature. In the majority of individuals, the main pathological abnormality is 'insulin resistance'. Insulin resistance occurs when the body produces insulin but is not able to use it effectively. Insulin resistance occurs because muscle, fat and liver cells do not respond to insulin as normal and, therefore, cannot take up as much glucose from the blood. The risk factors for insulin resistance are obesity, physical inactivity and ethnicity. Type 2 diabetes is up to six times more likely in people of South Asian descent and three times more likely in African and African-Caribbean people (Diabetes UK, 2015). As a result of insulin resistance, higher insulin levels are needed to help glucose enter cells. The beta cells of the pancreas try to keep up with this demand for insulin by increasing production. As long as the beta cells are able to meet this demand, blood glucose levels will be maintained in the normal range.

However, if the beta cells are unable to meet the demand, blood glucose levels will rise above the normal range. Raised levels of glucose can cause the development of beta cell failure. Beta cell failure refers to damage to the beta cell leading to an impairment and reduction in insulin production (Halban et al., 2014). Type 2 diabetes will occur when the beta cells can no longer produce enough to keep up with the increased demand for insulin arising from insulin resistance.

- A small proportion of people who develop type 2 diabetes, particularly the elderly and those with a BMI in the normal range, will have developed the condition due to beta cell failure alone. The treatment options for type 2 diabetes are numerous but, due to its progressive nature, 50% of people are likely to require insulin therapy during their lifetime (UKPDS Group, 1998). Insulin resistance has been linked with inflammation and the release of cytokines. Cytokines are thought to interrupt the action of insulin. Other risk factors for insulin resistance include steroid use, smoking and sleep problems (Kumar et al., 2014).
- *Gestational diabetes* describes diabetes present for the first time during pregnancy. Insulin resistance develops in women during pregnancy. However, some women are unable to produce sufficient insulin to maintain their blood glucose levels within the normal range. It is thought that the hormones produced during pregnancy can make it difficult for the body to use insulin properly and increases the risk of insulin resistance. Pregnancy, itself, places a heavy demand on the body, with some women less able to produce enough insulin to overcome this resistance, leading to gestational diabetes. It is essential that all women diagnosed with gestational diabetes have their glucose tolerance reviewed six weeks post-delivery to ensure that it has returned to normal. Gestational diabetes that requires treatment is a risk factor for type 2 diabetes in the future. It is essential that lifestyle advice is provided post-delivery to delay or prevent the development of type 2 diabetes and these women should be screened annually to promptly identify the development of type 2 diabetes.

In clinical practice, it is very important that, when caring for a patient with diabetes, you are able to correctly identify the type of diabetes they have. Activity 11.1 will ask you to think about a patient with diabetes you have nursed and reflect on whether you knew the type of diabetes they had.

Activity 11.1   Reflection

Think about a patient with diabetes that you have cared for. What type of diabetes did they have? What questions would enable you to correctly identify the type of diabetes?

An outline answer is available at the end of the chapter.

Having completed Activity 11.1, you should now be able to ask the appropriate questions to help you correctly identify the type of diabetes a person has. This is essential for the correct management of diabetes (as explained under 'Glycaemic management', below).

Clinical manifestations of undiagnosed/untreated diabetes

Symptoms of:

1. Type 1 diabetes

   - increased thirst
   - drinking lots of fluids
   - passing lots of urine
   - unexplained tiredness
   - weight loss
   - blurred vision.

2. Type 2 diabetes

   - genital itching
   - repeated episodes of genital thrush
   - slow wound healing.

Type 2 diabetes can be undiagnosed for many years as it is often symptom-free.

These symptoms will be explained below in the discussion of acute complications.

Diagnosing diabetes

In 2011, the World Health Organization (WHO, 2011) amended their diagnostic criteria to include the use of HbA1c measurement in the diagnosis of diabetes. HbA1c is a measurement of the quantity of haemoglobin that has been glycosylated (has glucose attached). Measurements of HbA1c enable clinicians to obtain an overall picture of average blood glucose levels over a period of weeks or months. The amount of glucose that combines with haemoglobin in red blood cells is directly proportional to blood glucose levels over the time period measured. It is an important longer-term gauge of blood glucose control (Diabetes UK, 2019). In a healthy person, the normal HbA1c range is 20–42 mmol/mol.

Diabetes can be diagnosed using either a fasting blood glucose (FBG), random blood glucose (RBG), HbA1c or an oral glucose tolerance test (OGTT). All must be laboratory tests.

It is essential in those who are symptomatic that an immediate random blood glucose level is used as a method of diagnosis. All other methods potentially delay the diagnosis of type 1 diabetes. In symptomatic adults and children, the first clinical action is to obtain a capillary blood glucose level and test a urine sample for ketones. Ketones can indicate insulin deficiency and the potential diagnosis of type 1 diabetes. Urgent telephone referral to a specialist diabetes team is indicated.

In asymptomatic people, two results in a diagnostic range are required to diagnose diabetes (Table 11.1). One method of testing HbA1c, for example, should be selected and repeated if it falls within the diagnostic range. If two different tests are performed and one is in the diagnostic range and one not, the test in the diagnostic range should be repeated.

Any person with an impaired glucose result is at high risk of developing type 2 diabetes. Type 2 diabetes can be prevented. Any individual found to be at high risk can reduce the likelihood of developing diabetes by making changes to their lifestyle, in particular losing weight and increasing their physical activity. Annual screening of high risk patients should be undertaken to ensure an early diagnosis of diabetes and to reinforce lifestyle advice.

Test	Impaired fasting glucose	Impaired glucose tolerance	Impaired glucose regulation	Diabetes
Fasting plasma glucose	6.1–6.9 mmol/L			≥7.0 mmol/L
OGTT 2-hour plasma glucose		≥7.8 and ≤11.0		≥11.1 mmol/L
Random plasma glucose				≥11.1 mmol/L
Laboratory HbA1c			42–47 mmol/mol	≥48 mmol/mol
In asymptomatic individuals two results in the diagnostic range are required to make a diagnosis. HbA1c should be repeated within two weeks.				
In symptomatic individuals one result in the diagnostic range is required.				

Table 11.1 World Health Organization diagnostic criteria (Diabetes UK, 2019)

Identifying people at high risk of developing or having diabetes, and undertaking the correct tests to ensure that diabetes is diagnosed quickly, are an important part of nursing. Activity 11.2 will ask you to think about Abida, identify what information you need, and what test should be requested to discover if she has developed diabetes.

Activity 11.2   Decision-making

Abida is a 38-year-old of Pakistani origin with a BMI of 32. She has three children. She has attended the surgery requesting treatment for

(Continued)

(Continued)

vaginal thrush. She is normally active, looking after her children, husband and parents. Abida's mother has type 2 diabetes. Abida has not had recent antibiotic therapy.

- What are Abida's risk factors for diabetes?
- What type of diabetes do you think she is most at risk of developing?
- What information do you need to obtain and which tests would you expect to be undertaken to confirm if she has diabetes?

A suggested answer is given at the end of the chapter.

Having completed Activity 11.2, you should be able to identify patients that may have diabetes that has not yet been diagnosed, and understand the tests that would help to correctly confirm this diagnosis.

Pathophysiology of the acute complications of diabetes

Diabetes is a manageable condition. Effective management requires balancing medication or insulin injections with food and activity. When this balance is affected, patients may experience either blood glucose levels which are too low leading to hypoglycaemia, or blood glucose levels which are too high resulting in hyperglycaemia. In this section, we discuss the acute complications of diabetes.

Hypoglycaemia

Hypoglycaemia, which we introduced above as a trigger of the stress response, can also be caused by the treatment of diabetes with hypoglycaemic inducing therapies (insulin or sulphonylureas). Hypoglycaemia is a blood glucose level below 4 mmol/L.

Hypoglycaemia is identified by symptoms of pallor, sweating, tremor, blurred vision, confusion, slurred speech and, ultimately, coma. These symptoms arise due to the raised levels of adrenaline and noradrenaline which are produced as a result of the 'fight or flight' response. Other symptoms, such as fatigue, confusion, memory loss, blurred vision and coma, are due to insufficient glucose being available to brain cells. These symptoms, whilst common, vary between individuals. It is important that patients are aware of their particular symptoms for hypoglycaemia.

Hypoglycaemia can be corrected by increasing the blood glucose level. The ingestion of rapid-acting glucose, such as glucose tablets, will return the blood glucose to within the normal range. As the blood glucose returns to normal, the symptoms of hypoglycaemia will resolve.

Mild hypoglycaemia is recognised by the individual and self-treated with 15 to 20 g of rapid-acting carbohydrate. Once symptoms have resolved and blood glucose levels have increased to above 4 mmol/L, some slow-acting carbohydrate needs to be eaten. This would be either the next meal if due, some fruit or a biscuit. If the blood glucose level has not increased to above 4 mmol/L after 15 minutes, the rapid-acting glucose should be repeated. Severe hypoglycaemia requires intervention by a third person and may require treatment with intramuscular glucagon or intravenous glucose (Joint British Diabetes Societies Inpatient Care Group, 2013). Capillary blood glucose levels should be checked after all hypoglycaemic episodes to ensure that the individual's blood glucose level is above 4 mmol/L.

Activity 11.3 will ask you to reflect on an occasion when a person with diabetes you were caring for experienced a hypoglycaemia episode.

Activity 11.3   Reflection

Think about the last patient you cared for who experienced a hypoglycaemic episode. What symptoms did they exhibit? What treatment was given? Was their blood glucose level checked after treatment had been given?

What would make you suspect hypoglycaemia in the future and how would you treat a hypoglycaemic attack?

If you have not cared for a patient that has experienced a hypoglycaemic episode, what would make you suspect hypoglycaemia and how would you treat the hypoglycaemic attack?

An outline answer is available at the end of the chapter.

Having completed Activity 11.3, you should have a clear understanding of the signs and symptoms of hypoglycaemia and be able to recognise and treat it appropriately.

Diabetic ketoacidosis (DKA)

DKA develops when the three elements of hyperglycaemia, ketonaemia and ketonuria present simultaneously (Table 11.2). They most commonly present in type 1 diabetes either if diagnosis is delayed, insulin is inappropriately omitted or insulin demand is significantly increased due to stress, such as an infection.

When insulin deficiency develops the body is unable to utilise glucose for energy. As a result fat stores are broken down and fatty acids released into the bloodstream as an

Ketonaemia 3 mmol/L and over or significant ketonuria (more than 2+ on standard urine sticks)
Blood glucose over 11 mmol/L or known diabetes mellitus treated with SGLT2i
Bicarbonate (HCO_3^-) below 15 mmol/L and/or venous pH less than 7.3

Table 11.2 Biochemical presentation of diabetic ketoacidosis (Joint British Diabetes Societies Inpatient Care Group, 2013)

energy source. In addition, excessive amounts of the regulatory hormones (adrenaline, glucagon and cortisol) are released which stimulate glycogenolysis – the breakdown of glycogen in the liver into glucose. Gluconeogenesis, production of glucose in the liver, also occurs.

The inability of the body to utilise glucose and the release of glucose from the liver result in significant hyperglycaemia. Hyperglycaemia results in glycosuria and osmotic diuresis with subsequent dehydration, hypotension and tachycardia (Figure 11.3). When levels of glucose in the blood rise, more glucose will be filtered by the kidneys and enter the kidney tubules (nephrons). As described above under 'Review of blood glucose regulation' above, there is a renal threshold for glucose reabsorption from the kidney tubules. The renal threshold for glucose will be exceeded in DKA leading to glucose remaining unabsorbed in the kidney tubules. The unabsorbed glucose causes water retention in the loop of Henle and causes osmotic diuresis. Osmotic diuresis refers to the production of large volumes of urine due to the presence of glucose in the kidney tubules. Unabsorbed glucose in the kidney tubules draws water into the tubules by osmosis. Both water and glucose remain unabsorbed and this leads to large volumes of urine (osmotic diuresis).

Free fatty acids are converted by the liver into ketones and are released into the bloodstream. Ketones, which include acetone, are acidic and lower the pH of the blood causing metabolic acidosis (ketoacidosis). Acidosis stimulates the respiratory centres in the brain and rapid shallow breathing (Kussmaul respirations) results. Ketones can cause nausea and vomiting that consequently aggravate fluid and electrolyte loss. Moreover, acetone produces the 'fruity breath' odour that is characteristic of ketotic patients. Ketonuria (ketones in urine) occurs as renal excretion of the ketones occurs.

Without treatment, dehydration, acidosis and increased plasma osmolarity may lead to coma and ultimately death (Figure 11.3).

The priority in the management of DKA is:

- correction of dehydration
- clearance of ketones
- correction of electrolyte imbalance.

To achieve this, rehydration using normal saline, a fixed rate insulin infusion and potassium supplementation are required. Parallel infusion of 10% glucose to maintain blood glucose levels may also be required to prevent hypoglycaemia and ensure sufficient insulin can be administered to fully correct acidosis and electrolyte imbalance (Joint British Diabetes Societies Inpatient Care Group, 2013).

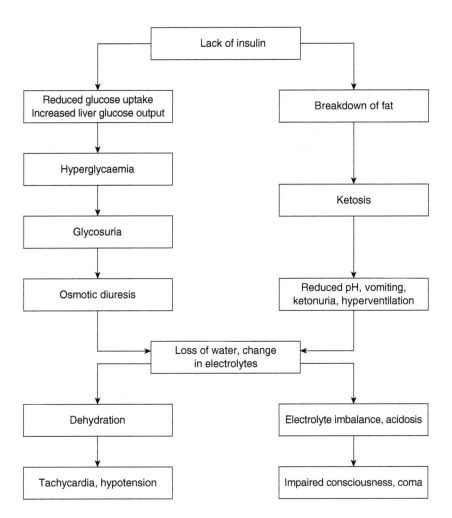

Figure 11.3   Diabetic ketoacidosis

The aim in the management of DKA is to:

- reduce blood ketones by 0.5 mmol/L per hour
- increase serum bicarbonate by 3 mmol/L per hour
- reduce blood glucose by 3 mmol/L per hour
- maintain serum potassium between 4 and 5 mmol/L.

Hyperosmolar hyperglycaemic state (HHS)

Hyperosmolar hyperglycaemic state is a medical emergency that presents in individuals with either undiagnosed type 2 diabetes, or type 2 diabetes complicated by a significant illness that leads to reduced fluid intake. Whilst DKA can develop in a matter of hours, HHS usually takes several days to develop. Although less common then DKA, HHS has a much higher mortality rate. Ketosis does not develop as individuals with type 2 diabetes continue to have significant levels of circulating insulin even if it is not sufficient to maintain blood glucose levels within the normal range.

The characteristics of HHS are hypovolaemia, marked hyperglycaemia (30 mmol/L or more) without ketonaemia (< 3 mmol/L) or acidosis (pH > 7.3, bicarbonate > 15 mmol/L) and an osmolality usually 320 mosmol/kg or more (Joint British Diabetes Societies Inpatient Care Group, 2012).

In patients with type 2 diabetes, a physiological stress such as a significant illness can cause a reduction in circulating insulin. The body's ability to utilise glucose drops dramatically. This leads to hyperglycaemia and hypovolaemia through the mechanisms described above for DKA and Figure 11.3. Although as noted, ketosis does not usually occur.

The goals in the management of HHS are to identify and treat the underlying cause while gradually and safely:

- normalising the osmolality (osmolality refers to the levels of circulating solutes in the blood. Hypersomolality results from increased blood glucose)
- replacing fluid and electrolyte losses
- normalising the blood glucose level.

Cautious rehydration is the initial management strategy for HHS with the aim to replace approximately 50% of fluid depletion within the first 11 hours. If there is no evidence of ketosis, insulin should not be commenced until the full impact of rehydration on blood glucose levels is established. A reduction of blood glucose of 5 mmol/L per hour is the aim. If ketones > 1 mmol/L are present or blood glucose levels ceased to fall and remain above 10–15 mmol/L following rehydration then a low dose (0.05 units/kg) of fixed rate insulin infusion should be commenced (Joint British Diabetes Societies Inpatient Care Group, 2012).

Cerebral oedema and central pontine myelinolysis are potential complications of HHS and more likely to occur if rehydration and/or reduction of blood glucose levels occurs too rapidly. Prevention of arterial or venous **thrombosis** and foot ulceration are also priorities in the management of HHS (Joint British Diabetes Societies Inpatient Care Group, 2012).

Activity 11.4   Decision-making

Abida, from our case study, has been diagnosed with type 2 diabetes and has completed a structured patient education programme. She has lost 3 kg in weight and made significant changes to her diet. She is walking every morning after dropping the children off at school with four other women around the local park.

Abida has contacted the surgery complaining of an abscess in her arm pit that is increasing in size, red and inflamed and very painful. She has not been commenced on any treatment for her diabetes.

In someone with diabetes, we have noted that infection can cause blood glucose levels to increase and put the person with diabetes at risk of either DKA or HHS.

Which acute complication is Abida most at risk of developing? What action needs to be taken when she contacts the surgery complaining of an abscess?

An outline answer is available at the end of the chapter.

Having completed Activity 11.4, you should have an understanding of the impact of illness on a person with diabetes.

Long-term complications of diabetes

The management of diabetes involves the correction of blood glucose levels to prevent the acute complications of hyperglycaemia but also the management of several risk factors to prevent the person with diabetes developing long-term complications.

Case study

Abida was diagnosed with type 2 diabetes 18 months ago. She has found the diabetes patient structured education course very beneficial and is happy that she is losing weight and her problems with thrush have resolved.

Microvascular complications

Microvascular complications affect the smallest of blood vessels in the body. The underlying cause of the damage that occurs to these microscopic blood vessels is hyperglycaemia although retinopathy and nephropathy development is accelerated by hypertension (Turner and Wass, 2007).

Retinopathy

The initial microvascular complications to be detected in individuals with type 1 diabetes is usually retinopathy with over 87% of individuals with type 1 diabetes having evidence of retinopathy 30 years post-diagnosis. Retinopathy is a disease of the retina in the eye which results in impairment or loss of vision. Retinopathy is detectable in 20–30% of individuals with type 2 diabetes at diagnosis and over 60% of individuals with type 2 diabetes show evidence of retinopathy 15 years post-diagnosis. Thickening of the capillary based membrane occurs and an associated accumulation of sorbitol, increased blood viscosity and abnormal fibrolytic activity leads to blockage of vessels. As a result of a capillary blockage and ischaemia new blood vessels form which are susceptible to leakage and formation of scar tissue (Turner and Wass, 2007). Diabetic retinopathy is a progressive condition with four clear stages: background retinopathy, preproliferative retinopathy, proliferative retinopathy and diabetic maculopathy. Diabetic retinopathy is the leading cause of blindness amongst the working population in the United Kingdom (Diabetes UK, 2014). All individuals with diabetes over the age of 12 should have a digital retinal photograph taken as part of their annual diabetes review.

Nephropathy

Diabetic nephropathy is a progressive kidney disease caused by damage to capillaries in the kidney glomeruli. Diabetic nephropathy develops as a result of thickening of the glomerular basement membrane, expansion of supporting tissues and fibrotic changes in renal arterioles. These changes result in the leakage of albumin into the nephric filtrate which presents as proteinuria (initially this will only be evident through laboratory testing). Proteinuria is usually first detected in individuals with type 1 diabetes 5 to 15 years post-diagnosis, but may be present at diagnosis in individuals with type 2 diabetes. Approximately 15% of all deaths in individuals with diabetes under the age of 50 are due to diabetic nephropathy (Turner and Wass, 2007). Diabetes is the most common cause of end-stage renal failure requiring treatment with dialysis or renal transplant (Diabetes UK, 2014). Annual screening of renal function by assessment of albumin creatinine ratio (ACR), serum creatinine and estimated glomerular filtration rate (eGFR) should be performed on all individuals with diabetes over the age of 12.

Neuropathy

Diabetic neuropathy is a type of nerve damage that can result from high blood glucose levels damaging the small blood vessels which supply the nerves.

Some abnormality in neurological sensation can be present at diagnosis but these usually resolve when blood glucose levels return to normal in individuals with type 1 diabetes. However, hyperglycaemia causes long-term damage resulting in nerve fibre loss with 50% of individuals with diabetes demonstrating some degree of impaired neurological function and, if evident in newly diagnosed type 2 diabetes, it is likely to be a long-term problem (Diabetes UK, 2014). Although a clear link to hyperglycaemia can be established the exact mechanism remains unclear; accumulation of polyol is evident and ischaemia is considered to be a contributing cause of the damage (Turner and Wass, 2007).

Diabetic neuropathy has several presentations. In some individuals, this will be peripheral sensorimotor neuropathy resulting in impaired sensation in their extremities predominantly affecting their feet. This is the leading cause of diabetic foot ulceration. Autonomic neuropathy has numerous presentations including erectile dysfunction, gastroparesis and loss of hypoglycaemic symptoms.

Microvascular complications, although affecting individuals with both type 1 and type 2 diabetes, are more commonly associated with type 1 diabetes. Diabetes Control and Complications Trial (DCCT) Research Group (1993) clearly demonstrated that optimum glycaemic control can reduce the risk of developing and delay progression of all micro-vascular complications. Epidemiology of Diabetes Interventions and Complications (EDIC) (1999) provided evidence that good glycaemic control from diagnosis protects against micro-vascular complications in later life and is referred to as the metabolic memory.

All individuals with diabetes over the age of 12 should have an annual diabetes risk assessment of their feet which includes sensation and circulation review and categorisa-tion of foot risk status.

Macrovascular complications

The macrovascular complications are more commonly referred to as cardiovascular disease (CVD) and include cardiac disease, stroke and peripheral vascular disease (Chapter 8). Individuals with diabetes have twice the risk of developing cardiovascular complications (Diabetes UK, 2014). Prevention of macrovascular complications requires much more than correction of hyperglycaemia and requires alterations to lifestyle and medication to address the modifiable risk factors for cardiovascular disease. These modifiable risk factors were dis-cussed in Chapter 8. It is important, therefore, that you look back to Chapter 8, to examine the modifiable risk factors and the ways in which these can be reduced. Cardiovascular dis-ease is a major cause of mortality and morbidity in people with diabetes accounting for 44% of deaths in type 1 diabetes and 52% in type 2 (Diabetes UK, 2017).

All adults with diabetes should have their blood pressure, cholesterol and smoking status reviewed annually. If their blood pressure is greater than 140/80 mmHg treatment should be commenced. The cholesterol target is a total cholesterol of less than 4 mmol/L and non-HDL cholesterol of less than 2 mmol/L. Statin therapy is recommended in all individuals with type 2 diabetes with a cholesterol above this level unless planning, or at risk of, pregnancy.

Glycaemic control is assessed by measurement of the individuals by HbA1c (glycosylated haemoglobin). The HbA1c target is individualised for each person. At the time of diagnosis this is generally 48 mmol/mol, and less than 59 mmol/mol when three or more therapies are required or when a treatment that has a risk of hypoglycaemia is used (insulin or sul-phonylurea). HbA1c and BMI should be assessed at least annually in all individuals with diabetes and 3–4 months after the introduction or removal of any new treatment.

All people with diabetes require regular reviews including an annual review to prevent the development of long-term complications. In Activity 11.5 you will be asked to iden-tify what tests should be performed or arranged for Abida, when she attends for her annual review appointment.

Activity 11.5   Evidence-based practice and research

Abida attends the diabetes clinic at the surgery for her routine appointment. What clinical parameters should be measured and discussed with Abida?

An outline answer is available at the end of the chapter.

On completion of Activity 11.5 you should understand which tests are performed annually as part of the diabetes review.

Glycaemic management

The aim of the glycaemic management of diabetes is to maintain blood glucose levels between 4 and 9 mmol/L and HbA1c between 48–59 mmol/mol without problematic hypoglycaemia. This is achieved in type 1 diabetes through the use of insulin and, in type 2 diabetes, through the use of a combination of oral and injectable treatments which include insulin (NICE, 2016c; NICE, 2017c).

Insulin

Insulin therapy is the only treatment for type 1 diabetes and is essential for the preservation of life. The majority of insulin used is biosynthetically engineered to replicate human insulin. Some insulin known as 'analogue insulin' has been further modified to alter the action profile of the insulin. Seven different types of insulin are currently available: very rapid-acting analogue, rapid-acting analogue, soluble, isophane, long-acting analogue, human premixed and premixed analogue (Table 11.3). Insulin preparations used in the United Kingdom are predominantly 100 units/mL in concentration, but stronger concentrations, e.g. 200 units/mL or 300 units/mL, are becoming available but only in disposable insulin pen devices.

The gold standard treatment for the management of type 1 diabetes is a combination of a long-acting analogue given once or twice daily and a rapid-acting analogue given immediately prior to food up to four times daily (NICE, 2016c). Alternatively, a rapid-acting insulin analogue can be given by continuous subcutaneous insulin infusion (CSII) more commonly known as an insulin pump.

The long-acting insulin analogue or basal insulin is administered at a regular time each day and a consistent number of units are injected. The rapid-acting analogue, or bolus insulin, is injected immediately prior to eating and the dose is calculated based on the individual's blood glucose level, expected level of activity and quantity of carbohydrate to be eaten. This insulin regime is commonly known as the basal bolus regime and is intended to closely mimic normal insulin secretion.

Insulin type	Generic names	Duration of action	Frequency of use
Very rapid-acting analogue	FiAsp	Onset 10 minutes Peak 2 hours Duration 4 hours	Three to four times daily with food
Rapid-acting analogue	Apidra Humalog Novorapid	Onset 30 minutes Peak 2 hours Duration 4 hours	Three to four times daily with food
Soluble	Actrapid Humulin S Insuman rapid	Onset 1 hour Peak 2–4 hours Duration 8 hours	Three times daily 30 minutes prior to food
Isophane	Humulin I Insulatard Insuman Basal	Onset $1\frac{1}{2}$ hours Peak 4–11 hours Duration 16–24 hours	Once or twice daily
Long-acting analogue	Abaslaglar Lantus Levemir	Onset 4 hours Peak–flat profile Duration 20–24 hours	Once or twice daily
Long-acting analogue	Tresiba Toujeo	Onset 4 hours Peak–flat profile Duration 20–36 hours	Once daily
Human pre-mixed	Humulin M3 Insuman comb 15 Insuman comb 25 Insuman comb 50	Onset 1 hour Peak 2–8 hours Duration 16–24 hours	Twice daily 30 minutes prior to breakfast and evening meal
Premixed analogue	Humolog Mix 25 Humolog Mix 50 Novo Mix 30	Onset 30 minutes Peak 2–8 hours Duration 16–24 hours	Two to three times daily immediately before food

Table 11.3   Commonly used insulins

Insulin is injected at 90° into the subcutaneous fat layer of the skin at recommended site (Figure 11.4). Insulin is predominantly administered using an insulin pen device and pen needle between 4 and 8 mm in length. Insulin must only be administered with an insulin syringe, reading in units, with insulin drawn up from an insulin vial or an insulin pen device. Insulin should never be withdrawn from an insulin cartridge or pen with an insulin syringe.

Which sites are recommended for insulin injection?

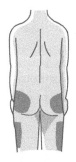 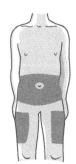

Abdomen
   quick insulin absorption

Upper thigh + buttocks
   slow insulin absorption

Figure 11.4   Recommended injection sites. From: www.bathdiabetes.org/images/pop-ups/needle%20image%203.png/

Non-insulin therapies

Glycaemic management in type 2 diabetes is much more complex due to the treatment options available and the progressive nature of the condition. The management of type 2 diabetes is a stepped approach (Table 11.4) with lifestyle modification underpinning all treatment options.

Step 1: Lifestyle modifications – healthy eating and physical activity
Step 2: One oral medication
Step 3: Two oral medications
Step 4: Three oral medications or addition of injectable therapy
Step 5: Oral medication and injectable therapy

Table 11.4 Stepped approach to type 2 diabetes

There are currently seven treatment options available for the management of type 2 diabetes: metformin, sulphonylureas (e.g. glimepiride and gliclazide), pioglitazone, DPP IV inhibitors (gliptins), SGLT2 inhibitors, incretin mimetic (GLP1) and insulin. The increased extracellular glycaemic pool that develops in type 2 diabetes is targeted in five different ways: digestion of glucose, hepatic glucose secretion, pancreatic insulin production, glucose uptake by the muscle and renal glucose excretion.

Metformin is the first line therapy after lifestyle modification in the majority of individuals with type 2 diabetes. Metformin's primary site of action is the liver where it suppresses hepatic glucose release, particularly overnight. Metformin should be taken after food to minimise gastrointestinal side-effects, and the dose should be commenced at 500 mg once daily, increasing in 500 mg increments over the 3 to 4 weeks until either the maximum therapeutic dose of 2 grams or maximum tolerated (no GI side-effects) dose is achieved. Metformin can be taken 2 to 3 times daily, but it is important to remember that increased frequency of medication can have a negative impact on concordance. If the lunch time dose is problematic a twice daily regime may be preferable. As metformin is excreted unchanged by the kidney, the dose should be amended in patients with renal impairment with a maximum recommended dose of 1 gram daily in individuals with an eGFR < 45 and discontinuation of metformin in individuals with an eGFR < 30. The accumulation of metformin does not cause any direct detrimental effect to the individual but increases the risk of lactic acidosis especially at times of dehydration.

In symptomatic patients presenting with type 2 diabetes, sulphonylurea should be commenced as first line therapy (NICE, 2017c). Sulphonylureas work by stimulating the beta cells to produce more insulin and, as a result, can cause hypoglycaemia if the resulting insulin secretion exceeds the level required by the individual.

DPP IV inhibitors also have a direct action on the pancreas. However, their mode of action is very different to that of sulphonylureas. DPP IV inhibitors enhance glucose-dependant insulin release, so they do not carry a risk of hypoglycaemia unless used in combination with a sulphonylurea. DPP IV inhibitors, which were introduced above under 'Review of blood glucose regulation', block the action of the DPP IV enzyme and as a result GLP-1 levels are increased and some degree of first phase insulin release is re-established. DPP IV inhibitors, with the exception of linagliptin, are excreted as an active metabolite by the kidney (Chapter 1) and therefore the correct dose is linked to the individual's eGFR. DPP IV inhibitors have very few side-effects but potentially do carry an increased risk of pancreatitis.

Pioglitazone works directly at a cellular level to target insulin resistance resulting in an enhanced response to insulin. Its mode of action means that it can take 6 to 12 weeks before the drugs impact on blood glucose levels is seen. Pioglitazone can cause fluid retention and should not be used in patients with heart failure. It has been associated with increased bone fractures and should not be used in patients with osteoporosis or osteomalacia. Pioglitazone is also associated with weight gain. To minimise this side-effect, it is important that the lowest therapeutic dose of the drug is used. The starting dose of 15 mg once daily can be increased to 30 mg daily if no impact on blood glucose levels is noted after 12 weeks. Although there is a 45 mg dose, this should not be used if no response to the 30 mg dose is noted. If a positive response to the 30 mg is seen, but the individual's HbA1c remains above target and the dose is increased to 45 mg, it should only be continued if further positive impact on the individual's HbA1c is noted.

SGLT2 inhibitors block the action of SGLT2 on the proximal tubule of the nephron reducing the renal glucose threshold, and reduce reabsorption of glucose present in the filtrate. As a result glucose is excreted in the urine. For SGLT2 inhibitors to have a positive impact on glycaemic control, good renal function is required and SGLT2 inhibitors will be ineffective in individuals with an eGFR of less than 60. SGLT2 inhibitors should not be commenced in patients with an eGFR less than 60 and the dose will either need to be reduced or the treatment stopped if the eGFR falls below 60 (depending on SGLT2 inhibitor prescribed). Due to the presence of glucose in the urine the side-effects of SGLT2 inhibitors are genital thrush and increased risk of urinary tract infections (UTIs). Glucose is an energy supply for the microorganisms (Chapter 3), and encourages growth of those microorganisms responsible for thrush and UTIs.

Incretin mimetics (GLP-1) mimic the action of the naturally occurring hormone GLP-1 (glucagon-like peptide 1, referred to under 'Review of blood glucose regulation') and, as a result, enhance glucose-dependant insulin release. This helps to re-establish first phase insulin release. The additional actions of the incretin mimetics are delayed gastric emptying and feeling of satiety which can result in reduced appetite and weight loss if food intake is reduced. The incretin mimetics can induce nausea, although this tends to be transient and resolves after 1 to 2 weeks. Occasionally, they cause vomiting which can also be transient, but may lead to the stopping of this treatment. The incretin mimetics are associated with a slight increased risk of pancreatitis.

Due to the progressive nature of type 2 diabetes, one treatment may initially achieve the level of glycaemic control required, but additional treatments will need to be added if deterioration in glycaemic control is noted by an increase in HbA1c.

A combination of three oral, or two oral and one injectable therapy, is considered to be the maximum combination of treatment in the management of type 2 diabetes. Incretin mimetics and insulin therapy can be used in combination but should be commenced and supervised by the specialist diabetes team.

It is essential when any treatment is commenced in the management of type 2 diabetes that its impact on glycaemic control is evaluated and if any of the oral treatment does not result in a fall of 6 mmol/mol, or incretin mimetic of 11 mmol/mol in 6 months, it should be discontinued and an alternative treatment commenced (NICE, 2017c). When commencing any treatment and reviewing its impact, it is essential that the individual's eGFR as well as HbA1c is reviewed as eGFR impacts on which treatments are suitable and the dose that is indicated.

Fifty per cent of patients with type 2 diabetes are likely to require insulin therapy within 10 years of diagnosis to achieve the required level of glycaemic control (UKPDS, 1998). Whilst the basal bolus regime is the gold standard treatment for the management of type 1 diabetes, a much wider variety of regimes are suitable in the management of type 2 diabetes. A basal isophane insulin (Table 11.4) once daily may initially be used, or a twice daily premixed insulin before breakfast and evening meal may be more suitable. The choice of insulin regime will depend on the individual's blood glucose profile, HbA1c, willingness to blood glucose monitor and self-inject.

All individuals treated with insulin are encouraged to know the name and dose of insulin they take. All adults treated with insulin should have an insulin passport with their name and NHS number on for each insulin that they take and be given a booklet explaining their use. Prior to an administration of insulin for the first time or when starting a new cartridge or device, the nurse should always check the insulin against the patient's insulin passport.

It is now time to review what you have learned within this chapter by undertaking some multiple choice questions.

Activity 11.6   Multiple choice questions

1. Insulin is produced by:
    a)   Beta cells in the pancreas when the blood glucose level falls
    b)   Alpha cells in the pancreas when the blood glucose level falls
    c)   Beta cells in the pancreas when the blood glucose level rises
    d)   Alpha cells in the pancreas when the blood glucose level rises

2. An increase in plasma blood glucose level results in:

   a) Increased insulin and increased glucagon secretion by the pancreas
   b) Decreased insulin and increased glucagon secretion by the pancreas
   c) Increased insulin and decreased glucagon secretion by the pancreas
   d) Decreased insulin and decreased glucagon secretion by the pancreas

3. Type 1 diabetes is caused by:

   a) Autoimmune destruction of the beta cells and insulin resistance
   b) Beta cell failure and over-eating
   c) Autoimmune destruction of the beta cells
   d) Insulin resistance and/or beta cell failure

4. Type 2 diabetes is caused by:

   a) Autoimmune destruction of the beta cells and insulin resistance
   b) Beta cell failure and over-eating
   c) Autoimmune destruction of the beta cells
   d) Insulin resistance and/or beta cell failure

5. The acute complications of diabetes are:

   a) Hypertension, hyperglycaemia and hypoglycaemia
   b) Retinopathy, nephropathy and neuropathy
   c) Hypoglycaemia, diabetic ketoacidosis and hyperosmolar hyperglycaemic syndrome
   d) Erectile dysfunction, peripheral neuropathy and macrovascular disease

6. The microvascular complications of diabetes include:

   a) Hypertension, hyperglycaemia and hypoglycaemia
   b) Retinopathy, nephropathy and neuropathy
   c) Hypoglycaemia, diabetic ketoacidosis and hyperosmolar hyperglycaemic syndrome
   d) Erectile dysfunction, peripheral neuropathy and macrovascular disease

7. The target blood glucose level in an individual with diabetes is:

   a) Between 3.5 and 6.5 mmol/litre
   b) Between 20 and 42 mmol/mol
   c) Between 6.5 and 7.5%
   d) Between 4 and 9 mmol/litre

8. Which statement is *false*:

   a) All individuals with diabetes are at risk of hypoglycaemia
   b) Individuals with diabetes treated with metformin only are not at risk of hypoglycaemia

(Continued)

(Continued)

   c) Individuals with diabetes treated with insulin are at risk of hypoglycaemia

   d) Individuals with diabetes treated with a sulphonylurea are at risk of hypoglycaemia

9. Type 1 diabetes is treated with:

   a) Insulin, metformin and diet

   b) Insulin, physical activity and diet

   c) Physical activity, diet and glimepiride

   d) Insulin, metformin and glimepiride

10. The 8 care processes that must be performed annually for all individuals living with diabetes include:

   a) HbA1c, blood pressure, cholesterol, eGFR, creatinine

   b) Blood glucose, blood pressure, BMI, cholesterol

   c) BMI, blood glucose cholesterol, eGFR, creatinine

   d) HbA1c, blood pressure, cholesterol, foot pulses

Chapter summary

Achieving excellent control of diabetes and preventing acute and long-term complications is hard work for everyone involved, but especially the individual with diabetes as 95% of diabetes management is patient self-care. In a 12-month period an individual with diabetes will have contact with a healthcare professional for approximately 4 hours but will self-manage for 8756 hours. Patient education is critical if individuals with diabetes are to develop the skills to self-manage their condition effectively, but equally, nurses supporting individuals with diabetes need to understand diabetes and maintain their knowledge and understanding of the disease to appropriately care for people with diabetes, ensure that all care requirements are fulfilled, and that people with diabetes are given the support to self-manage their condition.

Activities: Brief outline answers

Activity 11.1 Reflection (p297)

Ask the patient what type of diabetes they think they have, what age they were when they developed diabetes, how was it diagnosed, what treatment do they currently take and have they ever had any other treatment in the past.

They will either have had type 1 or type 2 diabetes; no other terminology is correct in terms of describing the type of diabetes someone is experiencing (unless the person was pregnant and they had gestational diabetes).

Patients with type 1 diabetes will be treated with insulin, are likely to have developed diabetes as a child or young adult (but it can develop at any age), will report marked symptoms at the time of diagnosis and will always have been treated with insulin.

Patients with type 2 diabetes may have been diagnosed as part of an opportunistic test and may have had no or vague symptoms. They will have been treated with oral medication in the past.

Activity 11.2 Decision-making (pp299–300)

Abida is at risk of developing type 2 diabetes, as she is of South Asian origin and is obese. A full history needs to be obtained, including the following questions: did she have any problems with her blood glucose levels in any of her pregnancies? Does she have any other symptoms of diabetes, e.g. tiredness, polyuria, polydipsia?

Abida has symptoms (thrush); capillary blood glucose and urinary ketones should be checked. Abida is symptomatic so only one abnormal laboratory result is required to confirm a diagnosis of diabetes. Ideally the test needs to be undertaken that day so a random blood glucose level (preferred choice if capillary sample in excess of 11.1 mmol/L) **or** HbA1c could be used.

It the ketones were positive, a telephone referral to the specialist diabetes team should be made as type 1 diabetes will need to be excluded.

Activity 11.3 Reflection (p301)

Typical hypoglycaemia symptoms are sweaty (cold and clammy), tremor, pallor, blurred vision, palpitations, slurred speech and confusion.

Treatment: 15–20 grams of rapid-acting glucose, e.g. 200 mL Lucozade, 4–7 glucose tablets depending on brand, 5 jelly babies; BGL rechecked after 15 minutes and re-treat if still < 4 mmol/L. Once BGL above 4 mmol/L, long-acting carbohydrate should be given, e.g. next meal if due, piece of fruit or biscuit.

Activity 11.4 Decision-making (pp304–5)

Abida has type 2 diabetes and an infection, therefore she is at risk of developing HHS.

Abida needs to be seen to have the abscess assessed and antibiotics prescribed if infected. She should also have her glycaemic control assessed by measuring her HbA1c and glycaemic treatment commenced if indicated. Self-blood glucose monitoring should be commenced if not previously performed by Abida, or she should be encouraged to check her blood glucose levels regularly to assess any impact on her diabetes control from the infection. Abida should be advised to contact the surgery if her BGL are elevated e.g. > 15 mmol/L.

Activity 11.5 Evidence-based practice and research (p308)

Annual reviews: They are known as the 8 care processes

Every person with diabetes must have as part of their annual review the 8 care processes completed and retinal screening booked.

The 8 care processes are: (1) measurement of their HbA1c; (2) blood pressure; (3) weight and height (BMI); (4) cholesterol; (5) eGFR; (6) creatinine; (7) albumin creatinine index (ACR); and (8) categorisation of the foot risk category. To enable the foot to be correctly risk-assessed, a foot assessment measuring sensation and pulses foot test is required.

To enable detection of diabetic retinopathy an annual retinal photography must be performed. The results of all these investigations and the potential need for any treatment change should be discussed with the person with diabetes.

Activity 11.6 Multiple choice questions (pp312–14)

1. Insulin is produced by:

    c) Beta cells in the pancreas when the blood glucose level rises

2. An increase in plasma blood glucose level results in:

    c) Increased insulin and decreased glucagon secretion by the pancreas

3. Type 1 diabetes is caused by:

    c) Autoimmune destruction of the beta cells

4. Type 2 diabetes is caused by:

    d) Insulin resistance and/or beta cell failure

5. The acute complications of diabetes are:

    c) Hypoglycaemia, diabetic ketoacidosis and hyperosmolar hyperglycaemic syndrome

6. The microvascular complications of diabetes include:

    b) Retinopathy, nephropathy and neuropathy

7. The target blood glucose level in an individual with diabetes is:

    d) Between 4 and 9 mmol/litre

8. Which statement is *false*:

    a) All individuals with diabetes are at risk of hypoglycaemia

9. Type 1 diabetes is treated with:

    b) Insulin, physical activity and diet

10. The 8 care processes that must be performed annually for all individuals living with diabetes include:

    a) HbA1c, blood pressure, cholesterol, eGFR, creatinine

Further reading

The Hospital Management of Hypoglycaemia in Adults with Diabetes Mellitus (Joint British Diabetes Societies Inpatient Care Group, 2018). This guideline explores the current evidence base for hypoglycaemia management and includes recommendations for hypoglycaemia management in hospital. Reading this document will help you understand the importance of prompt management of hypoglycaemic symptoms.

The Management of Diabetic Ketoacidosis in Adults (Joint British Diabetes Societies Inpatient Care Group, 2013). This guideline explores the current evidence base for diabetic ketoacidosis management and includes recommendations to be included in hospital guidelines for the management of DKA. Reading this document will help you understand the importance of accurate testing when caring for individuals admitted with DKA and the importance of effective communication with other clinical staff.

The Management of the Hyperosmolar Hyperglycaemic State (HHS) in Adults with Diabetes (Joint British Diabetes Societies Inpatient Care Group, 2012). This guideline explores the current evidence base for HHS management and includes recommendations to be included in hospital guidelines for the management of HHS. Reading this document will help you understand the importance of accurate testing when caring for individuals admitted with HHS and the importance of effective communication with other clinical staff.

Useful websites

www.nice.org.uk/guidance/conditions-and-diseases/diabetes-and-other-endocrinal–nutritional-and-metabolic-conditions/diabetes

National Institute for Health and Care Excellence – contains the national guidance and pathways for the management of diabetes in England and Wales.

https://www.diabetes.org.uk

Diabetes UK is the national diabetes charity in the UK and contains patient and healthcare professional information relating to type 1 and type 2 diabetes mellitus.

www.diabetesonthenet.com

This is a website that supports access to a range of diabetes-specific journals which provide current up-to-date information around diabetes management and research.

Chapter 12 Neurological conditions

Chapter aims

After reading this chapter you will be able to:

- describe the risk factors, clinical features and pathophysiology of Parkinson's disease, epilepsy and dementia;
- relate the signs and symptoms of Parkinson's disease, epilepsy and dementia to the underlying pathophysiology;
- explain how drugs used for Parkinson's disease exert their actions by increasing dopamine and how this leads to possible side-effects;
- explain how anti-epileptic drugs work, their main side-effects, drug interactions, cautions and contraindications, including their use in pregnancy;
- explain how drugs used in Alzheimer's work, their main side-effects and use in practice.

Case study

James is a 19-year-old man. Recently he went travelling and as a result got very little sleep. This triggered an epileptic seizure. He remembers very little except feeling vague and 'out of it'. The next thing he knew he was on the floor with a crowd of people watching him. The people watching him describe him going rigid and then falling to the floor. His whole body shook with convulsions. This lasted for about a minute and he came round soon afterwards. They tried to talk to him, but it took a while for him to respond as he seemed confused.

James, in the case study, experienced what is called a tonic–clonic seizure. We will return to this when we examine epilepsy which is the occurrence of recurrent seizures.

Introduction

The nervous system is a network of nerve cells and fibres which transmit signals between different parts of the body co-ordinating many of the body's actions. Many of the activities we take for granted such as walking, standing, thinking and feeling would not be possible without it. In humans, the nervous system is complex, consisting of billions of specialised cells called neurones. Because of this complexity, research is developing our understanding of the nervous system all the time, including how it works and how nervous system conditions arise. The branch of medicine that focuses on nervous system conditions is called neurology.

In this chapter we examine three neurological conditions: Parkinson's disease, epilepsy and dementia. We start with an overview of the nervous system. We move on to examine Parkinson's disease, including the risk factors for developing Parkinson's disease and its pathogenesis. This is followed by an explanation of how the drugs used in Parkinson's disease work and their possible side-effects. We then consider epilepsy and some of the different types of seizures that can occur. Management of seizures, including the mechanism of action of the anti-epileptic drugs, their side-effects and drug interactions, will be covered. Finally, we examine dementia and, in particular, Alzheimer's disease. We will look at the pathology and the action and use of drugs in Alzheimer's disease.

Overview of the nervous system

The nervous system is divided into the central nervous system (CNS), which comprises the brain and spinal cord, and the peripheral nervous system, which consists of nerves which connect the CNS to the rest of the body. In Chapter 1, we identified that the nervous system is made up of highly specialised cells called neurones. These cells can transmit messages, in the form of electrical impulses, to other cells. Neurones are highly branched and connect with many other neurones. Where the neurones join there is a gap called a synapse. In order for messages to be transmitted across this synapse a chemical called a neurotransmitter is needed. Some of the main neurotransmitters in the body are serotonin, noradrenaline, dopamine, glutamate and GABA (gamma-aminobutyric acid). Many drugs that work on the nervous system act by affecting the balance of these neurotransmitters.

We recommend looking at Chapter 1 in the section on 'Cellular communication'; and Chapter 6 on pain where we discussed synaptic transmission in more detail. Parkinson's disease and epilepsy are disorders of the central nervous system. Parkinson's disease primarily involves the loss of dopamine pathways in the brain. It is, therefore, useful at this point to examine the synthesis and metabolism of dopamine in the brain.

Neurones that use dopamine as a neurotransmitter are described as dopaminergic. Dopamine, along with noradrenaline, adrenaline and serotonin are 'monoamine neurotransmitters'. This refers to their chemical structure which contains one amino group. Dopamine is synthesised from the amino acid L-tyrosine in dopaminergic neurones (Figure 12.1). Tyrosine is converted to levodopa by the enzyme tyrosine hydroxylase. Levodopa is converted to dopamine by the enzyme dopa decarboxylase. In dopaminergic neurones, dopamine is stored in synaptic vesicles ready for synaptic transmission (Chapter 6; Figure 6.3). Dopamine is inactivated by the enzyme monoamine-oxidase in the nerve cell terminal where it is oxidised. The synthesis and metabolism of dopamine will be important in your understanding of the drugs used to treat Parkinson's disease.

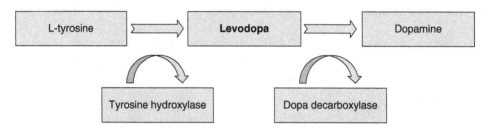

Dopamine is synthesised from the amino acid L-tyrosine in dopaminergic neurones by the enzyme tyrosine hydroxylase. Levodopa is converted to dopamine by the enzyme dopa decarboxylase.

Figure 12.1 Pathway of the synthesis of dopamine

Parkinson's disease

Parkinson's disease is one of the most common neurological disorders. It usually affects those over the age of 65 years, where its prevalence is estimated as 1%. The cause (aetiology) is unknown, but risk factors include genetic and environmental factors. Infection and exposure to neurotoxins are thought to be involved. Parkinson's disease is a neurodegenerative disorder which means that it leads to the progressive loss of neurones or loss of neurone function (Kumar et al., 2014).

Scenario

George is a 72-year-old man who comes to your clinic for a check-up. He was diagnosed with Parkinson's disease five years ago. He tells you that his symptoms came on gradually. He started with a tremor in his right arm, which was worse when he was relaxed and he also felt a 'bit slower' than usual. As you speak to him you notice that he speaks quietly and that his facial expressions are diminished. When he walked into the room he had a 'shuffling gait'. He tells you he feels 'down' and is worried that his memory is not as good as it was. He also has occasional trouble sleeping.

The scenario illustrates the most common symptoms of Parkinson's disease: tremor, rigidity and hypokinesia.

- *Tremor.* This occurs at rest and is sometimes described as a 'pill rolling' tremor as this is what a person's hands appear to be doing.
- *Rigidity.* Muscle tone is increased and a patient may complain of stiffness.
- *Hypokinesia.* This refers to reduced movement of the body. Movements are often slow (bradykinesia) and a patient may experience difficulty in initiating movement (akinesia).

Tremor often affects one side of the body first. Patients can find fine movements difficult which can lead to reduced facial expressions. They may speak quietly and find writing difficult. This can also affect their ability to self-care. Chewing and swallowing can become difficult. Patients may complain of feeling stiff because of muscle rigidity. Postural reflexes are also affected. This can result in stooping and falls as balance is affected. Sleep disturbance, memory loss and depression may also occur and it is important that these symptoms are not overlooked.

Diagnosis

Diagnosis can only be made with certainty at post-mortem by finding Lewy bodies in the substantia nigra (see 'Pathogenesis'). Diagnosis has improved, but 10% of cases may still be misdiagnosed (Hughes et al., 2002). The use of brain imaging can help to rule out other causes of movement problems. Some drugs, for example antipsychotics, can cause symptoms that resemble Parkinson's disease. Antipsychotics are dopamine antagonists which block dopamine receptors. Antipsychotics are useful when dopamine is blocked in areas of the brain which are believed to be involved in hallucinations. However, they also block dopamine in brain areas involved in movement leading to parkinsonian symptoms, that is, symptoms which resemble Parkinson's disease.

Pathogenesis

Parkinson's disease affects parts of the brain called the basal ganglia (Figure 12.2). The basal ganglia are important in controlling learned, voluntary movement. In Parkinson's disease a specific part of the basal ganglia, called the substantia nigra, is affected. Nerve fibres from the substantia nigra send signals to the striatum to co-ordinate and control movement. The striatum also co-ordinates aspects of cognition, such as action planning, decision-making and motivation. These aspects also appear to be affected for people diagnosed with Parkinson's disease. In Parkinson's disease dopaminergic neurones in the substantia nigra die. As part of this degenerative process Lewy bodies appear in the nerve cells. Lewy bodies are abnormal, microscopic collections of a protein called a-synuclein and are the diagnostic feature of Parkinson's disease. Death of these neurones results in problems with controlled movement which leads to the symptoms of Parkinson's disease we identified earlier.

As more and more of the dopaminergic neurones die, the symptoms a patient experiences worsen. For example, a mild tremor may progress to a situation where walking is impossible. Parkinson's disease typically progresses over 10–15 years until end-stage disease is reached. Pneumonia is a common cause of death. It is estimated that 10–15% of patients with Parkinson's disease develop dementia. Dementia in some of these patients is associated with wide distribution of Lewy bodies in the cerebral cortex (Kumar et al., 2014).

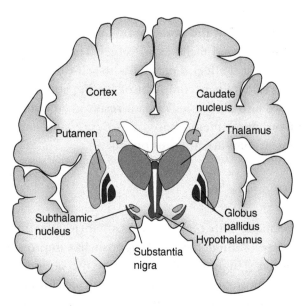

Figure 12.2   Basal ganglia and related structures

Drugs used in Parkinson's disease

The symptoms of Parkinson's disease are caused by degeneration of dopaminergic neurones and a lack of the neurotransmitter dopamine. The drugs used in Parkinson's disease counteract this by increasing dopamine levels in the brain. However, the neurones will continue to degenerate and eventually the drugs stop working. This means that, although the drugs help to control symptoms, none have been shown to delay progression of Parkinson's disease. However, drug therapy can improve the quality of life for most patients.

Drugs increase dopamine in different ways and people with Parkinson's disease are often prescribed a variety of drugs to help control their symptoms. Initially, low doses are used. As the disease progresses, however, higher doses and a combination of drugs are needed.

Levodopa, co-careldopa and co-beneldopa

The most obvious way to increase dopamine would be to give dopamine itself. However, dopamine cannot cross the blood–brain barrier and enter the brain where it is needed (Chapter 1). Instead, levodopa is given. Levodopa can cross the blood–brain barrier. As illustrated in Figure 12.1 levodopa is converted into dopamine by the enzyme dopa decarboxylase.

Levodopa enables the lost dopamine to be replaced which, in turn, helps control the motor symptoms of Parkinson's disease. However, levodopa is also converted to dopamine in the rest of the body. This is a problem because it leads to side-effects such as nausea, vomiting and cardiovascular effects (Chapter 7). Try Activity 12.1 to understand why these side-effects occur.

Activity 12.1   Critical thinking

Many drugs used to treat Parkinson's disease cause side-effects of nausea, vomiting and hallucinations. Why do you think these side-effects arise and what can be done to reduce them?

A suggested answer is given at the end of the chapter.

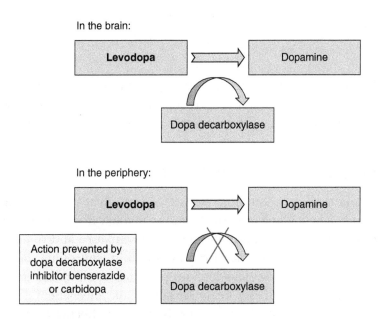

Peripheral dopa decarboxylase inhibitors are administered with levodopa to prevent conversion of levodopa to dopamine in the periphery (outside the brain). Peripheral dopa decarboxylase inhibitors cannot cross the blood–brain barrier so do not inhibit dopa decarboxylase activity in the brain.

Figure 12.3   Action of dopa decarboxylase inhibitors

To prevent the conversion of levodopa to dopamine in the rest of the body, yet enable it to exert its effect in the brain where it is needed, levodopa is usually administered with a second drug. These are known as peripheral dopa decarboxylase inhibitors.

Dopa decarboxylase inhibitors do not cross the blood–brain barrier. Because of this, they prevent the action of dopa decarboxylase in the rest of the body but not the brain (Figure 12.3). This means that dopamine is produced from levodopa in the brain where it is needed, but not the rest of the body, where it could cause side-effects. There are two such peripheral dopa decarboxylase inhibitors available called carbidopa and benserazide. Co-careldopa (trade name Sinemet) contains levodopa and carbidopa. Co-beneldopa (trade name Madopar) contains levodopa and benserazide. Controlled release preparations of these drugs are also available.

Activity 12.2   Decision-making

Joan is a 73-year-old woman with Parkinson's disease on your ward. You are administering drugs. Her drugs include some for Parkinson's disease. She is prescribed co-beneldopa 25/100 at 8 am, 1 pm and 8 pm. In the drug trolley you only have some co-beneldopa CR 25/100 medication. Explain what these tablets contain and whether you could use the co-beneldopa CR for your patient.

An outline answer is given at the end of the chapter.

As Activity 12.2 shows, the number and types of preparations available can be confusing. It is important to be clear that the correct preparation is being administered. If the incorrect preparation is given, a patient's symptom control can be seriously affected.

Side-effects and considerations for practice

Nausea and vomiting are common side-effects of drugs containing levodopa. Co-careldopa and co-beneldopa are usually started at a low dose and increased in small steps. Giving the drug with food can also help reduce nausea and vomiting. The antiemetic drug domperidone (Chapter 7) can be useful in controlling these side-effects. Sometimes, in advanced disease, levodopa preparations are administered before food to maximise absorption. It is, therefore, important to ask your patient if they are taking the drug before food (Burn, 2000). Levodopa is the most effective drug for controlling the symptoms of Parkinson's disease. However, when used long term, levodopa can cause movement problems and neuropsychiatric symptoms such as hallucinations. For this reason, doses are kept as low as possible and patients may choose to try a different drug first.

Dopamine agonists (non-ergot derivatives)

Examples of these types of dopamine agonists include pramipexole, rotigotine and ropinirole. Dopamine agonists work by stimulating dopamine receptors mimicking the effect of dopamine. In general, they are less effective than levodopa and patients report more side-effects initially. In the longer term, dopamine agonists cause fewer motor complications than levodopa. They can be used alone or in combination with levodopa. If used in combination, the dose of levodopa can be reduced which can improve motor complications.

Side-effects and considerations for practice

Common side-effects include nausea and vomiting, postural hypotension, hallucinations and confusion. Some patients report that they find it difficult to control their impulses when taking these drugs. This can lead to pathological gambling, binge-eating and increased sexual urges. Patients and their carers should be warned about these potential effects. Excessive drowsiness has also been reported which can be made worse by alcohol and other sedatives. Again, patients should be warned about these risks when driving.

Dopamine agonists (ergot derivatives)

Examples of these types of dopamine agonist include bromocriptine, pergolide and cabergoline. These drugs also act to stimulate dopamine receptors. They are derived from a fungus called ergot which explains their name. Side-effects and uses are similar to the non-ergot derivatives. In addition, they can cause pulmonary fibrosis, so these drugs are rarely used today.

Monoamine-oxidase B inhibitors

Examples of monoamine-oxidase B inhibitors include selegiline and rasagiline. Monoamine-oxidase is an enzyme which breaks down monoamine neurotransmitters including dopamine, serotonin and noradrenaline. The effect of inhibiting this enzyme in the striatum is to slow the breakdown of dopamine. This leads to an increase in dopamine and improved motor control. These drugs can be used alone during early treatment of Parkinson's disease. They can also be used with levodopa to reduce 'end of dose' deterioration, where progressively short duration of benefit from levodopa occurs.

Side-effects and considerations for practice

Side-effects include nausea, changes in blood pressure, abnormal movements, hallucinations and confusion.

Catechol-O-methyltransferase (COMT) inhibitors

Examples of COMT inhibitors include entacapone and tolcapone. COMT inhibitors inhibit the enzyme COMT. This prevents the peripheral breakdown of levodopa which allows more levodopa to reach the brain. They are not used alone in Parkinson's disease. They are used in addition to levodopa to reduce 'end of dose' deterioration.

Side-effects and considerations for practice

These drugs increase levodopa. This results in the side-effects expected with increased levodopa levels, including unwanted movements, nausea, vomiting and hallucinations. Other common side-effects include sleeping problems, dizziness, diarrhoea, falls, headache, confusion and dry mouth. Urine may also be discoloured a reddish brown.

Case study: Long-term Parkinson's disease treatment

Haidar is an 82-year-old man with advanced Parkinson's disease. He has been admitted to your ward after a fall. He was diagnosed with Parkinson's disease 12 years ago. He tells you that initially his symptoms were well-controlled with selegiline. After five years his symptoms deteriorated and his tremor and stiffness returned. Co-careldopa was added to his treatment and once again his symptoms improved. The dose was gradually increased to keep his symptoms under control. A controlled release preparation was added at night because he found it difficult to get up in the morning. His current medication is co-careldopa four times a day plus selegiline. He says that sometimes his symptoms are well-controlled but, at other times, the tremor and rigidity returns and he can feel himself 'freezing up', even though he has taken his drugs as prescribed. It is during these times that he has fallen. At other times he experiences involuntary, jerking movements in his legs.

The case study illustrates the problems that many patients with long-term Parkinson's disease face. Despite treatment, symptoms continue to worsen. The response to levodopa begins to fluctuate; at times symptoms are well controlled but at other times less so. The 'freezing' that Haidar describes is one of the movement problems associated with long-term levodopa therapy (treatment with co-beneldopa or co-careldopa) and is often referred to as 'on–off' symptoms. The jerking movements are known as dyskinesias. 'End of dose' deterioration can also occur whereby a dose of levodopa does not seem to last as long as it used to. Some of these problems are due to progression of the disease. However, the neurones in the brain also change in response to levodopa therapy. For this reason initial treatment is often not started until symptoms cause significant problems for a person. Overall, levodopa has been shown to increase life expectancy in Parkinson's disease.

Activity 12.3   Reflection

It is very important that patients with Parkinson's disease are administered their drugs on time when they are admitted to hospital. There are reports that this does not always happen (see Parkinson's UK website available at the end of the chapter). The consequences for patients can be very serious and include hallucinations and an inability to move. A patient may be unable to drink or get out of bed. It can take days or weeks for the condition to re-stabilise.

As a nurse on a ward, what steps could you take to ensure this does not happen?

A suggested answer is given at the end of the chapter.

Epilepsy

More than half a million people in the UK have epilepsy. This is around 1 in 100 people. Anyone can develop epilepsy; it happens in all ages, ethnic groups and social classes (Epilepsy Society, 2018).

The Epilepsy Society defines epilepsy as a common neurological condition where there is a tendency to have seizures that start in the brain. However, not all seizures are due to epilepsy. Seizures can happen for other reasons such as diabetes or a heart condition. Epileptic seizures always start in the brain.

The neurones of the brain usually transmit electrical impulses to each other in a co-ordinated way. As a result messages are sent to other neurones and the rest of the body which help to control its actions. In epilepsy, a sudden burst of electrical activity occurs. Large groups of neurones spontaneously fire electrical activity in an unco-ordinated way which results in an epileptic seizure. The symptoms that a patient experiences depends on where this electrical discharge occurs and whether it spreads to other parts of the brain.

James, who we met at the start of the chapter, experienced the type of seizure that people are most familiar with and it is the most common type. It is called a tonic–clonic seizure. The tonic phase refers to the rigidity that James experiences as a result of the electrical discharge in his brain which causes his muscles to contract (it increases muscle tone). This causes James to fall to the floor and can cause injury. The clonic phase refers to James's rhythmic jerking which occurs when his muscles contract and relax. During the seizure breathing may be affected and James may go pale or blue particularly around the mouth. He may also bite his tongue and lose control of his bladder.

Aetiology (causes) of epilepsy

Seizures can be caused by a variety of conditions. In some cases, if the cause is removed, the seizures will improve. Causes include low sodium, low glucose, low oxygen levels, low calcium levels, drug and alcohol abuse and fever. Epilepsy is only diagnosed if the seizures are recurrent, which means they happen repeatedly, and if they are not provoked by other illnesses. A person with epilepsy usually needs to have had at least two unprovoked seizures before a diagnosis is made (Fisher et al., 2014). Damage to the brain can also cause epilepsy. This might be caused by a tumour, meningitis, a stroke or a brain injury. Seizures are also common in people with a learning disability if the brain has not developed as expected or has been damaged. In many cases the cause of epilepsy is unknown. The condition can be life-long but for some people the seizures may disappear.

You might notice that James had a period without sleep before his seizure. In people with epilepsy, seizures can be brought on by triggers including poor sleep and flashing lights. In most people their first seizure occurs before the age of twenty. An electroencephalogram (EEG) is often used to help diagnose epilepsy. This shows the electrical activity of the brain. It can however be normal between seizures, even in a person who has epilepsy.

The pathophysiology of epilepsy remains unresolved. As discussed at the start of this chapter, neurones normally communicate using electrical and chemical signals which cause depolarisation (Chapter 6). Sometimes neurones send out an abnormal message which can be excitatory and cause a larger than normal depolarisation. If many neurones from the same part of the brain send out these abnormal messages at the same time, seizures may occur. The part of the brain where the disruption starts is called the 'epileptic focus'. Abnormal messages may arise from:

- damaged neurones
- an excess or insufficiency in neurotransmitters
- slow-responding ion channels.

This is explained further under 'Mechanism of action of anti-epileptic drugs'.

Activity 12.4   Reflection

The NICE (2012 updated 2018) guidance on epilepsy states that 'Healthcare professionals have a responsibility to educate others about epilepsy so as to reduce the stigma associated with it'.

How do you think an understanding of the physiological nature of epilepsy can help you to do this?

A suggested answer is given at the end of the chapter.

As demonstrated in Activity 12.4, an understanding of epilepsy can help you to reduce the stigma associated with it. In the next section, we examine the different types of seizure in epilepsy.

Types of epilepsy

Epilepsy describes a range of conditions and classifying seizures can be complicated. Classification depends on where the seizure starts, where in the brain the electrical discharge spreads, what causes the epilepsy and the age of the person affected. If the electrical activity starts in a well-defined area of the brain they are called focal (or partial) seizures. This electrical activity can spread. If the electrical activity affects all of the brain immediately it is known as a complex seizure. There are different types of seizure within each category and some examples are given here. The type of epilepsy can dictate which drug therapy is prescribed for the seizure.

The following are different types of seizure (National Clinical Guideline Centre, 2013).

Focal (partial seizures)

Simple focal seizure: electrical discharge starts in a localised part of the brain and does not impair consciousness.

Complex focal seizure: electrical discharge starts in a localised part of the brain and consciousness is impaired.

Focal seizures evolving to secondary generalised seizures: electrical discharge starts in a localised part of the brain and consciousness is impaired. The electrical discharge then spreads to the whole brain.

Generalised seizures (convulsive or non-convulsive)

Absence seizures: patient loses consciousness for a short time and looks blank and is unresponsive.

Myoclonic seizures: patient may or may not lose consciousness. Muscles jerk.

Tonic–clonic seizures: electrical discharge affects the whole brain.

Drugs used to treat epilepsy

Drug treatment is the treatment of choice for epilepsy. There are many different drugs that can be used. The drugs are known as anticonvulsants or anti-epileptic drugs. The choice of treatment will be informed by patient factors such as age, gender, type of seizure, other medication and co-morbidities. Examples of older drugs used to treat epilepsy include sodium valproate, carbamazepine, phenytoin and phenobarbitone. These can be very effective and up to two-thirds of patients with epilepsy can be seizure free with medication (NICE, 2012). However, these drugs can have many side-effects. Newer drugs have been developed to try and improve this. Examples include gabapentin, levetiracetam, oxcarbazepine, lamotrigine and topiramate. These are often only licensed as 'add-on' therapy where a single drug fails to work. They also have their own side-effects.

Case study

James has a second seizure and an EEG reveals epileptic activity. He is diagnosed as having generalised tonic–clonic seizures. After consultation with James and his family he is offered a trial of the anti-epileptic drug sodium valproate in line with NICE guidance. Unfortunately, his seizures are not controlled. Lamotrigine is prescribed and valproate is slowly withdrawn. His seizure control is now improved, and he remains on lamotrigine.

James has been started on the anti-epileptic drug sodium valproate as this is the choice of drug for generalised epilepsy. The NICE Guidance on Epilepsy (2012) is a useful source of information for treatment choice in different epilepsy types. As in the above case study, treatment would start with one anti-epileptic drug (known as monotherapy). A low dose is usually started and slowly increased. If this did not work or the patient experiences severe side-effects, a second drug would be added and the first slowly withdrawn. Where possible, monotherapy is used. This means treatment with one drug only. If monotherapy does not control the epilepsy, a combination of drugs would be used.

Evidence

Sodium valproate is useful for most types of epilepsy. For generalised seizures sodium valproate is the drug of choice (NICE, 2012) with lamotrigine a useful second alternative if sodium valproate does not work or is poorly tolerated. Marson et al. (2007) carried out a drug trial which compared older and newer anti-epileptic drugs. In the trial arm for patients with generalised epilepsy, they compared valproate, lamotrigine and topiramate. Valproate was the most effective. Fewer patients discontinued lamotrigine because of side-effects. Topiramate was the drug most likely to cause problematic side-effects. The results of this trial have helped to shape the NICE guidance. For people whose epilepsy does not respond to one drug, the choice of which drug to add is difficult as there are few trials to help guide the choice. The NICE guidance (2012) offers some suggestions.

Brand name prescribing

Some anti-epileptic drugs, such as phenytoin and carbamazepine, should always be prescribed by brand name. This is because different brands might have differing bio-availabilities (Chapter 1). This can lead to differences in blood concentrations which can affect seizure control and have catastrophic consequences for a patient. For other drugs, such as lamotrigine and sodium valproate, the issue is less clear cut and patients should be consulted. It is, therefore, always helpful to check before making a change. A full list of which drug brands can be switched is available from the MHRA (Medicines and Healthcare Products Regulatory Agency) website in the Further reading list at the end of the chapter.

Mechanism of action of anti-epileptic drugs

Anti-epileptic drugs do not cure the epilepsy but control symptoms by reducing the chance that the neurones will discharge randomly. The precise mechanism of action of many drugs is unknown but three main mechanisms are thought to be important:

1. Blocking calcium channels.

2. Blocking sodium channels. Calcium and sodium channels are both ion channels in nerve cell membranes. In order for nerve cells to conduct electrical impulses (also called action potentials; Chapter 6) ions must enter the cells through these channels. Blocking the channels reduces the excitability of the cell membranes of neurones. This means that the cells are less likely to generate a burst of electrical activity and cause a seizure. The drugs are more effective at doing this for cells that are particularly excitable. They can reduce seizures but do not block the usual lower level of electrical activity that is needed for the brain to function.

3. Enhancing the action of gamma-aminobutyric acid (GABA). GABA is an inhibitory neurotransmitter which means that it generally works to reduce the excitability of neurones. Increasing the action of GABA can therefore help reduce bursts of electrical activity and reduce seizures.

Side-effects of anti-epileptic drugs and considerations for practice

As might be expected with drugs that reduce excitability of neurones in the brain, they can result in drowsiness, fatigue and problems with thinking clearly. Co-ordination and balance can also be affected. This can be more of a problem with older drugs such as phenobarbitone, phenytoin and carbamazepine. Higher doses are more likely to cause the problem.

Some anti-epileptics, notably carbamazepine, oxcarbazepine and lamotrigine, can cause skin rashes. In some cases these skin rashes can be severe. Lamotrigine, for example, can cause a severe skin hypersensitivity reaction called Stevens–Johnson syndrome which can be life-threatening. Starting the drug slowly can help reduce this complication. Reduced blood cell counts are another potentially serious side-effect caused by carbamazepine, oxcarbazepine, phenytoin and lamotrigine. Patients prescribed anti-epileptic drugs that cause skin and blood problems should be advised to report symptoms such as fevers, rash, mouth ulcers, bruising or bleeding which can be caused by low blood counts.

Osteoporosis, which can lead to bone fractures, is another side-effect of some anti-epileptic drugs. The cause is thought to be an increase in the rate at which vitamin D is excreted from the body. It is suggested that patients at risk, who are on long-term carbamazepine, phenytoin or sodium valproate therapy, take vitamin D supplements (MHRA, 2009).

Some anti-epileptic drugs, notably sodium valproate, can also cause weight gain.

A full list of side-effects for each drug can be found in the latest edition of the BNF.

> ## Activity 12.5 Critical thinking: Adherence and anti-epileptic drugs
>
> Poor control of epilepsy can lead to increased seizures and death. Despite this some patients do not take their medication as prescribed. Why do you think this is? How do you think you could help improve adherence?
>
> *A suggested answer is given at the end of the chapter.*

Research suggests that between 30–50% of people do not take their medication as prescribed (Dillorio et al., 2004). As we can see from Activity 12.5, there are many factors that affect adherence to anti-epileptic drugs. However, people may be more likely to be adherent to medication if they are involved in decision-making about managing their epilepsy.

Anti-epileptics in pregnancy

Women on anti-epileptic drugs during pregnancy have a two to three times higher risk of their baby being born with major congenital malformations compared to the general population (where the risk is 1–2%). Malformations caused include cleft palate, spina bifida and heart problems. This risk increases with higher doses and where more than one drug is used. Sodium valproate is a particular risk (Gedzelman and Meador, 2012). As a result, women of childbearing potential may not be given sodium valproate. Women on epileptic drugs should seek advice before pregnancy. It is also important to note that stopping anti-epileptic drugs, or changing them during pregnancy, is very risky. Seizures may occur resulting in harm or death to mother and foetus. Women need to be informed of the risks. Before pregnancy, women on anti-epileptic drugs should take folic acid 5 mg daily as this helps to reduce risks. The dose of some anti-epileptic drugs may also need to be adjusted during pregnancy.

Drug interactions involving anti-epileptic drugs

We saw in Chapter 1 that some drugs speed up the metabolism of specific drugs while others slow it down. Many anti-epileptic drugs have these effects, so it is a good idea to check interactions for a patient prescribed these drugs. A full list of the interactions can be found in Appendix 1 of the BNF.

Carbamazepine, oxcarbazepine and phenytoin are enzyme inducers. They speed up specific cytochrome P450 liver enzymes. This increases metabolism of drugs such as warfarin, other anti-epileptic drugs, oestrogens and progesterones, resulting in reduced concentrations. The effect on hormones means that contraceptive choice can be complicated. Progesterone-only contraceptives, for example, should not be used as the interaction can result in lower progesterone levels and the contraceptive not working. To further complicate matters, oestrogen can reduce lamotrigine concentrations and reduce seizure control. Further advice on contraception and anti-epileptic drugs is available in the BNF.

Sodium valproate is an enzyme inhibitor. It can increase concentrations of the anti-epileptic drug lamotrigine. Using these drugs together can be complicated and the BNF has some specific dosing instructions on this.

Some medication can make it more likely that a person with epilepsy has seizures because they lower the seizure threshold. Some antidepressants and antipsychotics can cause this problem.

Status epilepticus

Activity 12.6   Decision-making

You are a nurse waiting for a train. On the platform you see a woman fall to the ground and begin shaking. You recognise that the woman is having an epileptic fit. What should you do?

A suggested answer is given at the end of the chapter.

Sometimes a seizure lasts a long time or one seizure follows another without a long gap in between. This is called status epilepticus. In Activity 12.6 it may well be that you are witnessing a seizure that may be normal for that person. However, if it lasts for more than 5 minutes, it may be a sign of status epilepticus. Status epilepticus is a medical emergency and an ambulance should be called or treatment given. Midazolam is the drug of choice to stop the seizures. It is administered as drops into the nose or between the cheek and gum. Midazolam belongs to a group of drugs called the benzodiazepines. It acts to increase the action of GABA. As we saw in the section on how anti-epileptic drugs work, GABA is an inhibitory neurotransmitter and increasing its action can stop convulsions.

Dementia

Case study

Rose is an 85-year-old woman. Her daughter became concerned with her mother's increasing forgetfulness and made an appointment to see the GP. Blood tests were done by the GP but these all came back normal suggesting there was no reversible cause for the memory impairment. She was referred to the specialist memory services for assessment. Cognitive and behavioural and psychological issues were explored with both Rose and her daughter. She was also given a cognitive screening test. After assessment she was diagnosed with mild Alzheimer's dementia and started on done-pezil 5 mg daily. After a month the dose was increased to 10 mg.

In the case study above, Rose has been diagnosed with Alzheimer's disease, which is currently the most common type of dementia. Dementia is a term used to refer to a range of cognitive and behavioural symptoms. Symptoms include memory loss, problems with reasoning and communication and change in personality. Along with this, there is likely to be impairment in activities of daily living.

Cognitive functions refer to 'intellectual' activities that involve information processing, such as planning and problem solving. These activities involve symbolic operations and mental representations of the world (Naish et al., 2018). Cognition involves memory, executive attention and language. Cognitive functions are considered as separate from affective or emotional functions which involve mood states and emotions. However, it is important to note that dementia affects a person's mood and behaviour as well as their cognitive functions.

A report published by the Alzheimer's Society (2014) found that in 2013 there were approximately 815,000 people living with dementia in the UK. If current trends continue, this number is expected to increase to 1,143,000 by 2025. The main risk factors for dementia is age and family history.

There are many different types of dementia, classified according to the cause of the disease and/or the pattern of injury to the brain. Table 12.1 gives some of the main types of dementia.

Alzheimer's disease is the most common type of dementia, accounting for 50–70% of cases. In patients with Alzheimer disease, semantic memory is affected early. Problems with semantic memory include difficulty in 'finding words', failure to recognise or identify people or objects and being unable to navigate through familiar surroundings (Naish et al., 2018). Alzheimer's disease is often noticed first by relatives who may become concerned by a loss of memory in their relative, as was the case with Rose.

Degenerative Alzheimer's disease Frontotemporal dementia Parkinson's disease with dementia Dementia with Lewy bodies Huntingdon disease
Vascular Vascular dementia
Metabolic Uraemia Liver failure
Toxic Alcohol related dementia Solvent use Heavy metals
Vitamin deficiency B12 and thiamine
Infectious HIV dementia Prion-associated disorders (e.g. Creutzfeld–Jacob disease)
Endocrine Hypothyroidism
Psychiatric 'Pseudo-dementia' in depression

Table 12.1   Types of dementia

Vascular dementia is the second most common form of dementia, accounting for around 20% of dementia cases. Vascular dementia is due to damage to the blood supply to the brain. There may be evidence of small vessel disease on brain imaging. There may be a history of transient ischaemic attacks (TIAs), or evidence of cerebral infarction.

Frontotemporal dementia often presents in people below 65 years of age and has a distinct presentation. There may be a change in personality with emotional blunting or apathy, or a disinhibition. Memory is usually preserved at this stage. Alternatively, frontotemporal lobe dementia may cause a progressive difficulty with the meaning of words whilst speech remains fluent.

Pathology of Alzheimer's disease

Advanced Alzheimer's disease is associated with extensive neurone death throughout the cortex. There is both cortical and subcortical atrophy and enlargement of the ventricles (Figure 12.4).

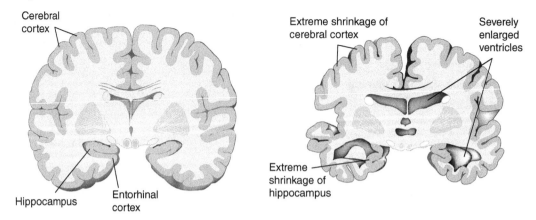

Cerebral cortex

Extreme shrinkage of cerebral cortex

Severely enlarged ventricles

Hippocampus

Entorhinal cortex

Extreme shrinkage of hippocampus

Figure 12.4 Comparison of a normal aged brain (left) and the brain of a person with Alzheimer's (right). In advanced Alzheimer's disease, extensive neurone death throughout the cortex and subcortex leads to cortical and subcortical atrophy and enlargement of the ventricles

There is degeneration of subcortical monoaminergic and acetylcholine 'projections' to cortical cells. Monoamine 'projections' (sometimes called 'fountains' or 'diffuse regulatory systems'; see Chapter 13) are discrete bundles of nerve fibres within the brain which secrete monoamine neurotransmitters onto neurones of the cortex. The monoamines include serotonin, noradrenaline and dopamine. Cholinergic projections to the cortex, in particular, show marked degeneration. Cholinergic fibres secret the neurotransmitter acetylcholine. It is hypothesised that the neurodegeneration of the monoamine and cholinergic projections may be due to an absence of neurotrophic factors which they would normally receive from their target cells in the cortex. The role of monoamines and neurotrophic factors is explored in more detail in the chapter on depression.

At a microscopic level, two distinctive brain lesions are found in Alzheimer's disease: amyloid plaques and neurofibrillary tangles. Amyloid plaques are extracellular deposits of amyloid – which is made up of microscopic fibrils of a protein called amyloid beta (Aβ). Aβ is believed to elicit an inflammatory response which may cause damage to neurones.

Management of Alzheimer's disease

As the case study above demonstrates, Alzheimer's disease is diagnosed at specialist memory clinics. You can read more about the assessments and screening tests used in the NICE guidelines on dementia (2018c). Depending on the severity of the condition, different drug treatments may be offered. It should be noted that these drugs are used for Alzheimer's and not for other types of dementia such as vascular dementia. The disease mechanisms are different in the different types of dementia. The drugs for Alzheimer's disease work specifically to alleviate the neurodegenerative effects specific to Alzheimer's. The drugs do not cure the disease and the aim of therapy is to improve symptoms and delay further decline. The effects of the disease are different for every patient and the benefits of treatment are therefore also different for every patient. It is not only memory that is improved. Other signs and symptoms such as loss of confidence, communication, cognition, activities of daily living and behaviour may also improve. Some people may improve significantly. For other people the effect is minimal and the drug should be stopped as the side-effects and cost of treatment outweigh any benefit.

The case also demonstrates that the dose should be increased to the maximum tolerated dose to achieve maximum benefit. This differs from other drugs where we often aim to use lowest possible dose.

Activity 12.7   Research

The case study of Rose mentions that the GP carried out some checks to rule out reversible causes for the memory impairment. List some possible reversible causes of memory problems. What blood tests can be done to rule out these causes?

A suggested answer can be found at the end of the chapter

Cholinesterase inhibitors

As discussed earlier in the chapter, in Alzheimer's disease there is a reduction in the number of cholinergic neurones in the brain. These neurones are very important in memory. We cannot increase the number of neurones with medication, but we can increase the amount of acetylcholine available at the cholinergic receptors that remain. Acetylcholinesterase is an enzyme which breaks down acetylcholine in the synapse. If this enzyme is blocked with a cholinesterase inhibitor, the levels of the neurotransmitter in the synapse are increased. This might improve cognitive or behavioural symptoms such as memory, motivation and concentration. They can also improve the ability of people to get on with daily activities such as washing, dressing, eating and drinking. For some patients, this improvement is maintained for a time (usually for 6 to 12 months) before declining again. For others, there may be no obvious improvement, but the current level of functioning is maintained for a period before declining. In others the drugs have no noticeable effects and the person continues to decline.

The cholinesterase inhibitors available are donepezil, galantamine and rivastigmine. They are all licensed for the treatment of mild to moderate Alzheimer's disease. NICE (2018c) recommends that, where possible, the drug with the lowest cost is tried first. The formulations available differ, for example only rivastigmine is available as a patch, and for a patient with swallowing difficulties this might be the first choice despite the increased cost.

Side-effects and considerations for practice

The side-effects can be predicted by considering the normal function of the **parasympathetic nervous system** (PNS) which relies on acetylcholine as a neurotransmitter (see Chapter 9). Potentially, these effects would be increased by a cholinesterase inhibitor which increases acetylcholine at the synapse. For example, the PNS reduces heart rate. Cholinesterase inhibitors can cause bradycardia and, in rare circumstances, cause heart block. They can also cause gastric and duodenal ulcers due to increased hydrochloric acid production. Some of the actions of the PNS and implications for cholinesterase inhibitor use are shown in Table 12.2.

	Action of parasympathetic nervous system (PNS)	Implications for cholinesterase inhibitor use
Cardiovascular	Decreased heart rate	Can cause bradycardia and heart block. Can cause dizziness and syncope.
Respiratory	Constriction of bronchioles	Caution in asthma and COPD as it may make these conditions worse
Gastrointestinal	Increased hydrochloric acid and GI motility	Increased risk of developing ulcers. Diarrhoea.
Bladder	Contracts smooth muscle, relaxes sphincter	Incontinence

Table 12.2   Action of PNS and side-effects of cholinesterase inhibitors

Other side effects include nausea and vomiting, agitation, hallucinations, insomnia and seizures.

Memantine

Memantine is an N-methyl-D-aspartate (NMDA) receptor antagonist. The NMDA receptor is a glutamate receptor; this means that the neurotransmitter glutamate usually acts as an agonist here. Glutamate is the main excitatory neurotransmitter in the brain (see Chapter 6). An increase in glutamate can lead to over-activation of glutamate receptors. This causes calcium to flow into the neurones. Increased calcium levels can lead to the death of neurones. Blocking the NMDA receptor is believed to protect neurones. Memantine is recommended for patients with moderate Alzheimer's disease who cannot tolerate cholinesterase inhibitors, or for those with severe Alzheimer's disease (NICE, 2018c). It can also be used in addition to a cholinesterase inhibitor in moderate or severe Alzheimer's.

Side effects include constipation, hypertension, dizziness, headache and tiredness. Less commonly it can also cause vomiting, confusion, seizures and hallucinations.

Behavioural and psychological symptoms of dementia (BPSD)

As dementia progresses, a patient's behaviour can be adversely affected. BPSD includes symptoms and signs such as agitation, wandering, repetitive behaviour, aggression and sleep disturbance. It is important to try and understand these behaviours from the patient's point of view and modify the environment where possible. In some cases, when patients are distressed, medication can be helpful alongside these environmental interventions. Antipsychotic medications such as risperidone may be used. In the past, antipsychotics were overprescribed. It was discovered that antipsychotics could triple the risk of stroke (MHRA, 2004). As a result antipsychotics are only used in special circumstances. Non-pharmacological interventions should be explored and other causes affecting a patient's behaviour, such as delirium and untreated pain, should be assessed and managed first. Carers should be involved in decision-making where possible. It is also important to regularly review the need for treatment as a person's presentation will change over time. You can read more about dementia care strategies in the NICE (2018c) guidance.

It is now time to review what you have learned within this chapter by undertaking some multiple choice questions.

Activity 12.8   Multiple choice questions

1. Many drugs used in the treatment of Parkinson's disease act to increase which neurotransmitter?
   a) Acetylcholine
   b) Dopamine
   c) Serotonin
   d) Glutamate

2. Symptoms of Parkinson's disease are caused by the degeneration of which part of the brain?
   a) Motor cortex
   b) Cerebral cortex
   c) Basal ganglia
   d) Amygdala

3. Which of the following are symptoms of Parkinson's disease? For each symptom choose TRUE or FALSE.
   a) Bradykinesia
   b) Dystonia
   c) Stiffness
   d) Stooped posture

4. Which of the following statements about co-beneldopa is TRUE?
   a) It contains the dopa decarboxylase inhibitor carbidopa
   b) It is generally reserved for use in end stage Parkinson's disease

(Continued)

(Continued)

    c) Long-term treatment can lead to movement problems such as dyskinesias

    d) Another name for co-beneldopa is co-careldopa

5. Which of the following is NOT an anti-epileptic drug?

    a) Sodium valproate

    b) Lamotrigine

    c) Topiramate

    d) Cabergoline

6. Absence seizures are a type of:

    a) Tonic–clonic seizure

    b) Generalised seizure

    c) Simple focal seizure

    d) Partial seizure

7. The following are statements about status epilepticus. Decide whether each statement is TRUE or FALSE.

    a) Status epilepticus is a medical emergency

    b) It can be treated with buccal carbamazepine

    c) People should be restrained during status epilepticus so they don't hurt themselves

    d) Status epilepticus can be caused by sodium valproate

8. A patient prescribed Tegretol brand of carbamazepine should be continued on this brand because:

    a) It is the cheapest form of carbamazepine

    b) Different brands have different bioavailabilities

    c) Different brands contain different anti-epileptic drugs

    d) Different brands are metabolised differently

9. A patient has been started on sodium valproate and asks you to let them know what side-effects they might experience. Which of the following are likely side-effects? Answer TRUE or FALSE for each.

    a) Drowsiness

    b) Osteoporosis

    c) Weight gain

    d) Skin rashes

10. Which ONE of the following statements about donepezil is TRUE?

    a) It stops the progression of Alzheimer's disease

    b) It is a glutamate antagonist

    c) It acts to increase acetylcholine in the brain

    d) It is used in all types of mild to moderate dementia

Chapter summary

Parkinson's disease is one of the most common nervous system disorders. It is a degenerative disorder and symptoms include tremor, stiffness and hypokinesia. Symptoms are caused by a lack of the neurotransmitter dopamine in brain areas responsible for controlling movement. Drug treatments such as co-beneldopa act to increase dopamine in the brain where it is needed, but not in the rest of the body where it leads to side-effects such as vomiting. Dopamine can also be increased with drugs such as selegeline which inhibit enzymes that break dopamine down. Dopamine receptors can also be stimulated directly using dopamine agonists such as pramipexole. In hospital, it is important that patients receive their drugs on time, as failure to do so can result in patients losing motor control.

Epileptic seizures are caused by spontaneous and uncoordinated electrical activity in the brain. There are many different types of epileptic seizure. The symptoms experienced depend on the area of the brain affected by electrical activity. Tonic–clonic seizures are generalised seizures affecting the whole brain, causing loss of consciousness and rhythmic jerking of muscles. Seizures may be triggered by stress and fatigue but, in many cases, the cause is unknown. Anticonvulsant drugs are used to control seizures. Examples include sodium valproate and carbamazepine. Their precise mechanism of action is unknown but they are thought to block ion channels, which reduces electrical impulses, and enhance the action of inhibitory neurotransmitters. Patients may need more than one drug to control seizures. The choice of drug will depend on the seizure type and how well a patient can tolerate the side-effects. Side-effects of each drug are different but may include drowsiness, skin rashes, weight gain and osteoporosis. Healthcare professionals have a vital role in educating patients about their medication as people often adhere poorly to anti-epileptic drugs. By understanding the condition nurses can also help to reduce stigma by educating the public.

Dementia is a term used to refer to a range of cognitive and behavioural symptoms. These include memory loss and problems with reasoning and communication which often lead to impairment in activities of daily living. Alzheimer's is the most common form of dementia and is associated with neurone death throughout the cortex. Two distinctive brain lesions are evident, amyloid plaques and neurofibrillary tangles. Cholinergic nerve projections show particular degeneration. The cholinesterase inhibitors donepezil, rivastigmine and galantamine act to increase acetylcholine in the brain. They cannot cure Alzheimer's disease, but can improve symptoms and delay worsening of symptoms in some but not all patients. Memantine, an NMDA receptor antagonist, can be useful in more severe dementia or in people who cannot tolerate the acetylcholinesterase inhibitors. Non-drug measures are very important in dementia, and many behavioural issues, which may occur in later stages of dementia, can be helped by altering a patient's environment and trying to understand experiences from a patient point of view.

Activities: Brief outline answers

Activity 12.1 Critical thinking (p323)

Dopamine is a neurotransmitter in other areas of the brain as well as those which control movement. Parkinson's drugs are not specific to movement centres and also increase dopamine in other areas which leads to side-effects. For example if dopamine is increased in the vomiting centre, nausea and vomiting result (see Chapter 7). Increasing doses slowly and giving drugs with food can help. At times anti-emetics can be helpful, for example domperidone. However these must be chosen with care as some, such as metoclopramide, can make movement disorders worse because they block dopamine.

Increased dopamine can also lead to hallucinations. Contrast this with drugs that are used to reduce hallucinations in schizophrenia, the antipsychotic drugs, which act by reducing dopamine. Antipsychotic drugs can cause movement disorders and we often call these parkinsonian symptoms. Treating hallucinations in patients with Parkinson's disease can be very difficult. Doses can be reduced but this can make the movement problems worse. Antipsychotics are sometimes used but again these can make movement disorders worse.

Activity 12.2 Decision-making (p324)

Co-beneldopa 25/100 contains 25 mg benserazide which is peripheral dopa decarboxylase inhibitor and 100 mg levodopa. Co-beneldopa CR 25/100 is a controlled release preparation also containing 25 mg benserazide and 100 mg levodopa. These preparations are not interchangeable as the duration of action and peak concentration of each will be different. Administering the wrong one could result in a deterioration of Parkinson's disease symptoms.

Activity 12.3 Reflection (pp326–7)

There are many suggestions given on the website. Some things you might have considered are setting timers to remind staff, allowing patients to self-medicate, educating other healthcare professionals, ensuring medication is ordered and there are sufficient stocks and carrying out audits to ensure best practice.

Activity 12.4 Reflection (p328)

Many people can feel stigmatised by a diagnosis of epilepsy but this is not true for everyone and there may be cultural differences (Baker et al., 2000). An understanding of how electrical discharges in the brain give rise to seizures and that treatment is available can help reduce the stigma by demystifying the condition. It has been hypothesised that feelings of stigma can arise because people with epilepsy worry about the impact of their condition on others. Educating others to understand why seizures occur and what to do about them can be useful.

Activity 12.5 Critical thinking (p332)

Non-adherence may involve taking more or less than prescribed and changing dosage intervals. It may be intentional or non-intentional. Reasons can include lack of knowledge that medication is needed long term and forgetting medication, especially if dose regimes are complicated. Some people may have difficulties swallowing tablets, for example those with learning difficulties. Side-effects may also put people off. The stigma of epilepsy can also reduce adherence. Education about the medication and illness is important but studies have shown that this in itself does not improve adherence. Patients with epilepsy should be asked about adherence in a non-judgemental way and the reasons explored. It has been shown that if people are encouraged to talk to a professional who listens, concordance can be achieved more readily and that this should be part of an annual review (Packham, 2009).

Activity 12.6 Decision-making (p333)

The epilepsy society has this advice:

Stay calm.

Look around – is the person in a dangerous place? If not, don't move them. Move objects like furniture away from them.

Note the time the seizure starts.

Stay with them. If they don't collapse but seem blank or confused, gently guide them away from any danger. Speak quietly and calmly.

Cushion their head with something soft if they have collapsed to the ground.

Don't hold them down.

Don't put anything in their mouth.

Check the time again. If a convulsive (shaking) seizure doesn't stop after 5 minutes, call for an ambulance (dial 999).

After the seizure has stopped, put them in the recovery position and check that their breathing is returning to normal. Gently check their mouth to see that nothing is blocking their airway such as food or false teeth. If their breathing sounds difficult after the seizure has stopped, call for an ambulance.

Stay with them until they are fully recovered.

Activity 12.7 Research (p337)

Blood tests such as U&Es, calcium, thyroid function, full blood count and liver function tests would be carried out to rule out reversible causes of confusion and fatigue (which may cause cognitive slowing).

Activity 12.8 Multiple choice questions (pp339–40)

1. Many drugs used in the treatment of Parkinson's disease act to increase which neurotransmitter?

   b) Dopamine

2. Symptoms of Parkinson's disease are caused by the degeneration of which part of the brain?

   c) Basal ganglia

3. Which of the following are symptoms of Parkinson's disease? For each symptom choose TRUE or FALSE.

a)	Bradykinesia	True
b)	Dystonia	False
c)	Stiffness	True
d)	Stooped posture	True

4. Which of the following statements about co-beneldopa is TRUE?

   c) Long-term treatment can lead to movement problems such as dyskinesias

5. Which of the following is NOT an anti-epileptic drug?

   d) Cabergoline

6. Absence seizures are a type of:

   b) Generalised seizure

7. The following are statements about status epilepticus. Decide whether each statement is TRUE or FALSE.

   a) Status epilepticus is a medical emergency   True

   b) It can be treated with buccal carbamazepine   False

   c) People should be restrained during status epilepticus so they don't hurt themselves   False

   d) Status epilepticus can be caused by sodium valproate   False

8. A patient prescribed Tegretol brand of carbamazepine should be continued on this brand because:

   b) Different brands have different bioavailabilities

9. A patient has been started on sodium valproate and asks you to let them know what side-effects they might experience. Which of the following are likely side-effects? Answer TRUE or FALSE for each.

   a) Drowsiness   True

   b) Osteoporosis   True

   c) Weight gain   True

   d) Skin rashes   False

10. Which ONE of the following statements about donepezil is TRUE?

   c) It acts to increase acetylcholine in the brain

Further reading

NICE (2017d) *Parkinson's Disease in Adults.* NG71: Available at: **www.nice.org.uk/guidance/ng71/**

MHRA (2017) *Anti-Epileptic Drugs: Changing Products.* Available at: **www.gov.uk/ drug-safety-update/antiepileptic-drugs-updated-advice-on-switching-between-different-manufacturers-products/**

NICE (2012) *The Epilepsies: The Diagnosis and Management of the Epilepsies in Adults and Children in Primary and Secondary Care.* CG137. Available at: **www.nice.org.uk/guidance/cg137/**

NICE (2018c) *Dementia: Assessment, Management and Support for People Living with Dementia and Their Carers.* Available at: **www.nice.org.uk/guidance/ng97/**

Useful websites

www.parkinsons.org.uk/

Parkinson's Disease Society. Lots of useful information including booklets on drugs and symptoms.

www.epilepsysociety.org.uk/

The National Society for Epilepsy. The topic 'seizures: the role of neurones' is particularly informative.

www.epilepsy.org.uk/

Epilepsy Action. Advice and information for people living with epilepsy.

www.alzheimers.org.uk/

Alzheimer's Society. For information and advice about all types of dementia.

Mental health conditions: depression

Chapter aims

After reading this chapter you will able to:

- describe how depression is diagnosed;
- explain the monoamine theory of depression including its limitations;
- describe the importance of the stress response in depression;
- describe the role of inflammation in depression;
- describe the different types of antidepressant used to treat symptoms of depression including their mechanisms of action and side-effects.

Introduction

One in four adults experience at least one diagnosable mental health problem in any given year. People in all walks of life can be affected and at any point in their lives, including new mothers, children, teenagers, adults and older people. Mental health problems represent the largest single cause of disability in the UK. The cost to the economy is estimated at £105 billion a year – roughly the cost of the entire NHS.

(Independent Mental Health Task Force to the
NHS in England, 2016, p4)

There are many different mental health diagnoses. These can include anxiety, phobias, depression, obsessive-compulsive disorder, eating disorders, bipolar disorder, schizophrenia and personality disorders (Mind, 2018; NICE, 2011b). As identified in the quote above, mental health problems can occur to people across the age spectrum. One in ten children aged 5–16 is identified as having a diagnosable mental health problem with half of all mental health problems established by 14 years and rising to 75% by aged 24 years. One in five mothers have been identified as experiencing depression, anxiety or psychosis during pregnancy or in the first year following childbirth. People with long-term physical illnesses experience more complications if they also develop mental health problems, whilst people with severe, prolonged mental illness are at risk of dying 15–20 years earlier than other people (Independent Mental Health Task Force to the NHS in England, 2016). Whatever your field of practice or care setting, you will care for patients experiencing mental health conditions. It is important that you have the knowledge and skills to recognise and assess the needs of these patients and their families. Depending on your level of knowledge and skill, this may involve seeking advice from, or referral to, specialist colleagues or services for further assessment and management.

This chapter focuses on depression. Depression is a serious health issue worldwide. Globally, depression is identified as the predominant mental health problem, followed by anxiety, schizophrenia and bipolar disorder. A recent UK survey found that 20% of people questioned had symptoms of possible anxiety or depression (Mental Health Foundation, 2016) and other studies show that 1 in 4 people will experience depression in their lifetime (Spiers et al., 2016). Depression has been identified as a leading cause of years lived with disability. Clinical depression is a medical condition that goes beyond what we might describe as a transient low mood. It is a clinical syndrome, termed a depressive episode, where people can experience changes in mood, appetite, sleep, thoughts and psychomotor activity for weeks or months. In milder forms people might be able to get on with their lives but it might feel like a struggle. In its most severe form depression may contribute to death by suicide.

We start the chapter by describing how depression is diagnosed. We will then examine some of the biological theories that attempt to explain depression. We will consider the stress response, the monoamine theory and inflammation. The pharmacological treatments for depression will be explained including their place in patient-centred care. We will discuss the different types of antidepressants, mechanisms of action and important side-effects. Finally, the factors governing the choice of antidepressants for patients will be considered. It is important to acknowledge that there are a number of biological, psychological and social theoretical explanations about what depression is, how it is caused and how it should be treated. Our focus on biological theories is because an understanding of the biological changes occurring in the brain of those vulnerable to depression, and the changes seen during an episode of depression, can provide insights into the symptoms, causes and treatment of depression.

Diagnosis

Case study

George is a 30-year-old man. He is admitted to the ward after he attempted to overdose on his medication. He was found by a neighbour and taken to the Emergency Department where he was treated. He was then admitted to an acute inpatient mental health unit. He was diagnosed with cancer 3 months ago. George described feeling a complete loss of hope and belief in himself and the future. Although he used to enjoy watching television and reading he now finds it difficult to concentrate and does not enjoy either any more. He felt his family would be much better off without him as he is useless and feels tired all the time. He has lost a stone in weight over a month and hardly sleeps all night. While speaking to George, you notice that he takes time to respond and, at several points, had to be reminded of the question you have asked.

Depression is classified as a mood, or affective, disorder. It is characterised by low mood, the absence of positive affect, a loss of interest and enjoyment and a range of emotional, cognitive, physical and behavioural symptoms (NICE, 2018d). Persistent sadness/low mood and loss of interest or pleasure (anhedonia) in most activities are key symptoms of depression. Whilst, for some patients like George, their mood remains low throughout the day and is unreactive to circumstance, others may experience diurnal variation, with gradual improvement in their mood throughout the day returning to a low mood on waking. There can be cognitive symptoms such as slowed thinking, poor concentration and attention. Pessimistic and recurrent negative thoughts and rumination about the past and future can also feature. A loss of interest and enjoyment in everyday life, and feelings of guilt and worthlessness are commonly experienced alongside loss of self-esteem, feelings of helplessness and suicidal ideation. Behavioural and physical symptoms may include 'circadian dysregulation' and appetite changes. 'Circadian dysregulation' means that a person can experience disturbances in their body clock that can disrupt sleep patterns. Most commonly, people sleep less and wake up very early feeling at their lowest at this time. Other people may find themselves sleeping excessively. Appetite may be lowered leading to weight loss whilst, for some, appetite may be increased. Behavioural symptoms may include tearfulness, irritability and social withdrawal. People can also suffer from a general slowing down and reduction in energy levels, experience exacerbation of any pre-existing pain and lack of libido. These symptoms may lead patients to believe that they have a physical illness. Some patients may also experience agitation and/or anxiety (NICE, 2018d).

These signs and symptoms of depression fall into four overlapping domains (Figure 13.1): mood change, cognitive impairment, motor deficits and circadian dysregulation (Mayberg, 2003). Different neurobiological processes and brain regions are thought to underlie the different symptomatic domains. Cognitive impairments, for example, represent changes in brain areas and pathways in the frontal cortex of the brain responsible for cognition. Mood changes represent alterations to areas and pathways in the limbic system responsible for mood and emotions (Bear et al., 2015). We will discuss these brain areas and pathways later in the chapter. It is important to acknowledge that depression is more than a disorder of mood and thought (cognitions).

The individual presentation of depression can vary. Mayberg's (2003) conceptual framework encourages links to be made between the different symptoms experienced by patients and the areas of the brain that may be responsible for these symptoms.

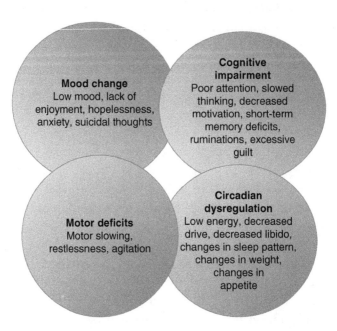

Figure 13.1   Overlapping domains of depression (developed from Mayberg, 2003)

The symptoms of depression are considered to occur on a continuum of severity. Depression is often divided into mild, moderate or severe. This division can help healthcare professionals to offer appropriate treatments (see 'Stepped care for depression' in this chapter (NICE, 2018d)). Identification and diagnosis of depression is based not only on the severity of these symptoms, but also on their persistence, the presence of other symptoms and the degree of functional and social impairment (NICE, 2018d). A diagnosis of depression is made following a detailed history. As highlighted in the introduction, people with depression vary in their age, presentation, experience and pattern of symptoms, medical and family history, psychological, relational and socioeconomic factors. To make a diagnosis of depression, NICE (2018d) recommends that symptom counting should not be used. Instead, assessment of three linked, but separate, factors: (a) severity (b) duration and (c) course should be considered, with individual symptoms assessed for their severity, impact on function and that these should be present for most of every day. A biopsychosocial assessment is, therefore, recommended. This would include assessing social support, family history, any employment or financial issues in addition to symptom experience (severity, duration and course). More on this topic can be found in Haith (2018) *Understanding Mental Health Practice*. Depression questionnaires may also contribute to the diagnosis of depression aiding the assessment of severity and/or monitoring the response to treatment (NICE, 2018d). An example is the Patient Health Questionnaire 9 (PHQ9).

The patient's symptoms and symptom experience are compared with diagnostic criteria. There are two main diagnostic systems: the *Diagnostic Statistical Manual, 5th revision* (commonly known as DSM-5) (APA, 2013), which is a system developed by the American Psychiatric Association (Table 13.1) and *The International Statistical Classification of Diseases and Related Health Problems, 10th revision,* commonly known as ICD-10. This is a World Health Organization (WHO) system. The symptoms have to be present for at least two weeks for a diagnosis to be made.

Depression is diagnosed using the *Diagnostic and Statistical Manual of Mental Disorders,* 5th edition (DSM-5) criteria

Assess for the two 'core' symptoms of depression by asking:

- During the last month have you often been bothered by feeling down, depressed or hopeless?
- Do you have little interest or pleasure in doing things?

If either of the two 'core' symptoms have been present most days, most of the time, for at least 2 weeks, ask about:

- **Other typical symptoms of depression:**
  - Fatigue/loss of energy.
  - Worthlessness/excessive or inappropriate guilt.
  - Recurrent thoughts of death, suicidal thoughts, or actual suicide attempts.
  - Diminished ability to think/concentrate or indecisiveness.
  - Psychomotor agitation or retardation.
  - Insomnia/hypersomnia.
  - Significant appetite and/or weight loss.

Table 13.1 Diagnostic criteria DSM-5: depression

More about this topic can be read at the 'Clinical knowledge summary for depression' website referred to at the end of the chapter.

Activity 13.1   Critical thinking

Re-read the case study about George and see whether you can match the signs/symptoms of depression to the DSM-5 diagnostic criteria.

An outline answer is given at the end of the chapter.

Causes of depression

We can read the case study about George and we might assume that his diagnosis of cancer caused his depression. This may be an important factor which has precipitated the depression but it would be a very simple view. As highlighted above, there are various theoretical explanations describing the risk factors for, or the causes of, depression including genetic, biochemical, endocrine, neurophysiological, psychological and social. These factors may predispose, precipitate and/or perpetuate an episode of depression. Epidemiological studies have identified some risks factors for depression. Box 13.1 lists five of the significant risk factors (NICE, 2018d; Gerhardt, 2015; Fava and Kendler, 2000). These are factors that might place a person at greater risk of developing depression.

Box 13.1   Risk factors for depression

- **Gender:** rates of depression are twice as high for women across different cultures.
- **Adverse childhood experiences:** physical and sexual abuse, poor parent–child relationship, parental discord and divorce (Gerhardt, 2015; Fava and Kendler, 2000).
- **Personality types:** 'neuroticism' – a lowered ability to deal with stressful events increase the risk of depression in the face of stressful events.
- **Major life changes:** bereavements, trauma or stress – social circumstances, such as poverty or unemployment, may increase risk of depression. Vulnerabilities to major life changes, such as lack of social network, confiding relationships, loneliness, may increase the risk of depression.
- **Certain physical illness or medication:** for example, hyper/hypothyroidism, diabetes.

Activity 13.2   Critical thinking

Consider the case of George. Suggest three possible additional risk factors he might have.

Compare your answer with the discussion below.

You might have listed a number of ideas for Activity 13.2. For example, there may be social factors involved such as isolation and loneliness. There might also be some physical causes such as increased inflammation caused by the cancer or other undiagnosed illness. George may be vulnerable to depression because of his genetic make-up or early childhood experiences. The first three risk factors identified in Box 13.1 identify some of the predisposing factors that could make a person vulnerable to an episode of depression. In a person with a vulnerability to depression, a stressful event (major life change) may then precipitate an episode of depression. George may face a number of stressors including his fears about the diagnosis, treatment and the dying process.

There is extensive research on the aetiology of depression describing the risk factors and possible psychological and biological mechanisms that produce a depressive episode. Below, we focus on some of the biological theories about what causes depression. Biological theories of depression look for changes in brain chemistry or functioning that correlate with depression. These approaches rely on the idea that symptoms of depression are caused by underlying alterations in brain function. Initially, these brain changes may be triggered by adverse life circumstances in those with an underlying vulnerability or, in some cases, by a separate disease affecting the central nervous system. An awareness of the biological changes in depression is essential for our holistic understanding of depression and to help patients understand their condition. It is particularly important for understanding pharmacological interventions.

The main theories of the biological basis of depression are (1) neurochemical dysregulation; (2) neuroendocrine dysregulation; and (3) neuroanatomical and functional abnormalities.

1. Neurochemical dysregulation: mono-amine theory of depression

The 100 billion neurones in the brain and body communicate with each other through synapses (Chapter 1, 6 and 12). These are microscopic gaps between neurones across which a neurotransmitter passes as a signalling molecule. There are many different neurotransmitters in the brain. The neurotransmitters believed to be important in depression are serotonin (also called 5 hydroxytryptamine or 5-HT), noradrenaline and dopamine. These neurotransmitters all have a similar chemical structure based upon an amine ring so are also known as monoamines.

The 'monoamine theory of depression' states that, in depression, the levels of the monoamine neurotransmitters (noradrenaline, dopamine and/or serotonin) in the brain are reduced and is the underlying cause of depression. There is evidence to support this theory. In the 1960s, a drug called reserpine was used to reduce high blood pressure. It worked by reducing the levels of monoamines in the periphery. In the brain, reserpine also reduced the levels of monoamines at the synapse. One of the side-effects caused by higher doses of reserpine was depression. Other observations identified that a class of drugs used to treat tuberculosis caused an elevation in mood. The drugs inhibit monoamine oxidase (MAO), an enzyme that breaks down the catecholamines and serotonin. Finally, the antidepressant drug imipramine was found to inhibit the reuptake of serotonin and noradrenaline, increasing the levels at the synapse. From these observations, the monoamine hypothesis was developed – that mood is linked to the levels of monoamine neurotransmitters in the brain and depression is a consequence of a deficit in one or more of these monoamines (Bear et al., 2015). We also know that the three major classes of antidepressant drugs (monoamine oxidase inhibitors, tricyclic antidepressants and selective serotonin reuptake inhibitors) share the common property, although through different mechanisms, to increase the level of monoamine neurotransmitters in the brain.

There are, however, limitations with the monoamine theory. Studies which aim to measure serotonin or noradrenaline levels in people with depression have had mixed results – some finding a reduction in levels but others not (Ferrari and Villa, 2016). In addition, antidepressants do not improve symptoms for everyone as we will discuss later in the chapter. We also know that cocaine increases monoamine neurotransmitters very quickly and causes people to feel elated. It is, however, not a useful antidepressant in the long term. Given these limitations, a new hypothesis developed that antidepressant drugs promote long-term adaptive changes in the brain.

2. Neuroendocrine dysregulation

There is significant evidence showing that chronic stress can lead to the onset or worsening of depression (Hammen, 2005) and other mental health conditions. In other words, stress can be a precipitating factor or a predisposing factor for depression. The hypothalamic–pituitary–adrenal (HPA) axis is the neuroendocrine pathway responsible for the secretion of cortisol. As we discussed in Chapter 2, the HPA axis leads to the secretion of the stress hormone cortisol. Figure 2.4 in Chapter 2 shows the HPA axis and its negative feedback regulation. Normally, physical or emotional stressors result in activation in the amygdala, an area of the brain that is part of the limbic system. The amygdala assigns 'emotional significance' to stimuli including fear and releases corticotrophin-releasing factor (CRF). This activates the hypothalamus to release CRF. The CRF activates the pituitary gland to release adrenocorticotrophic hormone (ACTH). ACTH travels in the blood to the adrenal cortex which releases cortisol. Cortisol, in the short term, enables a person to deal effectively with a stressful event. Normally, via a negative feedback system, increased cortisol levels act on glucocorticoid (cortisol) receptors in the hypothalamus. Binding of glucocorticoid receptors by cortisol inhibits the release of CRF and ACTH from the hypothalamus and pituitary respectively, to reduce the release of cortisol (Chapter 2).

Chronic stress-induced activation of the HPA axis and elevated cortisol secretion have been found in people with depression. Hyperactivity of the HPA axis, observed in a significant subgroup of patients with major depression, is one of the most consistent and important findings in the biology of depression with a link proposed between early traumatic experiences and the risk of developing depression in adulthood. People who have experienced adverse childhood experiences (Box 13.1) may have fewer cortisol and CRF receptors in their brain than those who have not developed a vulnerability to depression (Bear et al., 2015). It is possible that excessive and prolonged exposure to cortisol during childhood is responsible for this effect.

Excess cortisol may down-regulate the genes for cortisol and CRF receptors thereby reducing the number of these receptors. As a consequence, throughout their lifespan, the reduced number of receptors will reduce the effectiveness of the negative feedback mechanism during times of stress, and cortisol may continue to be produced in excessive amounts and for prolonged periods of time. The negative feedback system is 'dysregulated' and the synthesis of cortisol, instead of being reduced, continues to be secreted in large amounts (Gerhardt, 2015). It is important to remember that different people will find different situations stressful and the cause of the chronic stress might be difficult to determine. As will be discussed next, a large and sustained amount of cortisol has adverse effects on the brain which may help to explain the symptoms of depression.

Effects of increased cortisol

We saw in Chapter 2 that corticosteroid drugs can have unpleasant effects including peptic ulcers, increased body fat, muscle wasting and susceptibility to infection. These effects can all occur in chronic stress, due to excess cortisol release. Increased and sustained cortisol levels can also have adverse effects on the brain including:

- A depletion of the neurotransmitter serotonin.
- An imbalance in inflammatory cytokines in the brain which cause an increased production of CRF in the hypothalamus inducing glucocorticoid receptor tolerance and impairing the negative feedback mechanism of the HPA axis. This results in degenerative changes in the hippocampus which is involved in mood regulation with the prefrontal cortex and amygdala. The hippocampus is rich in corticosteroid receptors and normally contributes to regulation of HPA axis. Hippocampal dysfunction may be responsible for inappropriate context-dependent emotional responses. Cytokine mediated immune response may provide the link between high cortisol levels and hippocampal damage in chronic stress.
- Inhibiting neurogenesis – the brain is constantly renewing and regenerating itself, building new neural networks and repairing old ones through the development of new neurones. This process is called neurogenesis. This means that the brain is very adaptable (has plasticity) and that we can keep learning new things throughout our lives. A protein (growth factor) called brain derived neurotrophic factor (BDNF) acts to control this process. Cortisol blocks the synthesis and release of BDNF leading to reduced neurogenesis. This leads to a reduction in the volume of certain brain areas. In people with depression the hippocampus is smaller and the cerebral cortex is thinner (Gould et al., 2000). The hippocampus is involved with memory. A reduction in the size of the hippocampus might help to explain why people with depression have trouble remembering things. The cerebral cortex is involved in cognition and how we make sense of the world. As we have seen, cognitive deficits are a key feature of depression.

The findings from these studies suggest that the mechanisms responsible for dysregulation of the HPA axis and increased HPA hormone secretion contribute to the pathophysiology of depression. Box 13.2 provides further information about the stress–diathesis (vulnerability) model.

Box 13.2   Stress–vulnerability model of depression

A positive family history of depression is a risk factor for developing depression. This suggests that inheriting certain genes may predispose a person to depression. Depression does not have a clear inheritance pattern and it is clearly a multifactorial condition. Despite a possible genetic predisposition, few genes have been linked conclusively to the development of depression. Recent work by Wray et al. (2018) have carried out genome-wide association studies and found '44 risk variants' for depression. A risk variant is a site in the genome shown to have a significant link to depression. This study helps refine the basis of depression and suggests the risk for depression varies in a continuum in the population due to genetic and psychosocial factors.

The stress–diathesis or stress–vulnerability model attempts to explain a disorder as the result of an interaction between a predispositional vulnerability and a stress caused by life experiences. The medical term for predisposition is diathesis. A diathesis can take the form of genetic, biological, physiological, cognitive, personality or situational factors. The diathesis–stress model explores how these factors (*diatheses*) interact with environmental influences (*stressors*) to produce disorders such as depression. The model is considered useful for understanding the interplay of nature and nurture in a person's susceptibility to psychological disorders throughout their lifespan and explaining vulnerability to the depression.

Epigenetic factors have also been shown to modify the brain's response to stress. Parental care, including adverse childhood experiences, may affect regulation of hippocampal glucocorticoid receptor expression to cause chronically elevated cortisol levels in the brain and body to promote an individual's vulnerability to depression (Gerhardt, 2015; Goh and Agius, 2010).

The stress diathesis/vulnerability model (Box 13.2) helps us to visualise how stress and our own vulnerability to stress act together to cause depression. In the diagram (Figure 13.2) the size of the bucket represents our vulnerability; the bigger it is the more resilient we are. Our vulnerability includes our genetic make-up and external factors that can help protect us. These include issues such as early childhood experiences and current social circumstances. For example research shows people with good social networks are less likely to experience depression. The water represents the stress. There are many different kinds of stressors for example losing a job, moving house and divorce. If the stress becomes too much the 'water' overflows and we become mentally unwell, for example depressed.

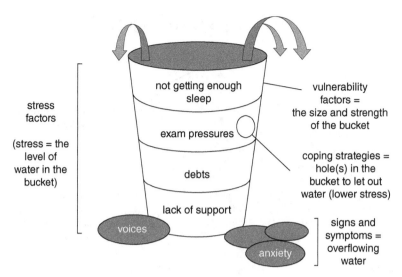

Figure 13.2   The stress bucket. Based on Brabban and Turkington (2002)

3. Neuroanatomic and functional abnormalities

In the brainstem, close to where the brain joins the spinal cord, are two regions that secrete the neurotransmitters which send signals to other areas of the brain. The raphe nuclei secrete serotonin and the locus coerulus secretes noradrenaline. Noradrenaline, serotonin and dopamine secreting neurones make up 'diffuse regulatory systems' or 'fountains' in the brain. These regulatory systems are collections of neurones which have cell bodies, originating in specific regions of the brainstem, and axons that project upwards to reach many areas of the brain. Axons are nerve fibres; a long, slender projection of a nerve cell or neurone that typically conducts electrical impulses (action potentials) away from the nerve cell body. The function of the axon is to transmit information to different neurones. When the electrical impulse along the axon reaches the synapse it causes the release of the neurotransmitter. The neurotransmitter diffuses across the synapse to an adjacent neurone where it binds with receptors to stimulate that neurone to fire or inhibit it from firing. The endings of the axon fibres release their neurotransmitters (noradrenaline, serotonin or dopamine) into areas of the brain in a diffuse manner. The neurotransmitters alter the activity of synapses – described as volume controls acting to either turn up or turn down the activity of neurones. The activity of the brain is determined by which neurones are active. The brain areas to which the 'fountains' (or projections) and their respective neurotransmitters act are diverse and include the frontal cortex for cognition and the limbic system (hypothalamus, hippocampus and amygdala) for mood and emotions (Bear et al., 2015). As these regulatory systems affect nearly every area of the brain we can see the importance for regulation of the concentration of neurotransmitters and how depletion of the monoamine neurotransmitters might lead to the range of depressive symptoms causing mood and functional changes experienced by, and observed in, people with depression.

The serotonin diffuse regulatory system (Figure 13.3)

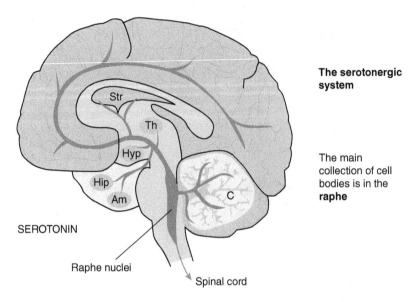

Figure 13.3 The serotonin diffuse regulatory system. Am, amygdala; C, cerebellum; Hip, hippocampus; Hyp, hypothalamus; Str, corpus striatum; Th, thalamus

Serotonin synthesising neurones are located in the brainstem raphe nuclei. These neurones project diffusely from the raphe nuclei to the cortex, limbic systems, hypothalamus, basal ganglia, cerebellum, the brainstem and spinal cord and release serotonin. Different mechanisms exist to regulate the concentration of serotonin at the synapse. These include uptake of serotonin by special transporter molecules (SERT) in the membrane of the neurones. SERT is a type of monoamine transporter protein that transports serotonin from the synaptic cleft to the presynaptic neurone. Changes in the SERT gene have been shown to influence different individual responses to stress. Serotonin release into the synapse also activates receptors that trigger BDNF gene transcription. Under stressful conditions, the BDNF gene is not activated and the lack of BDNF in the hippocampus may result in neurone atrophy or death. In addition, autoreceptors, special receptors at the synapse, act like a thermostat to monitor the concentration of serotonin. If the concentration increases, the autoreceptor inhibits the synthesis of serotonin aiming to keep a constant level. In some people, depression may reflect a dysfunctional raphe-serotonin regulatory system that normally modulates homeostasis, emotions and tolerance to aversive experiences.

The noradrenaline diffuse regulatory system (Figure 13.4)

Noradrenaline cell bodies originate in the locus coerulus of the brain. The axons project throughout the brain including the hypothalamus, the temporal lobe, the cortex,

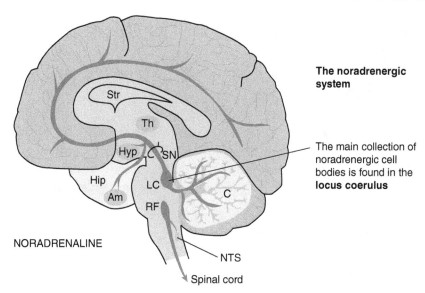

The noradrenergic system

The main collection of noradrenergic cell bodies is found in the **locus coerulus**

NORADRENALINE

Figure 13.4 The noradrenaline diffuse regulatory system. Am, amygdala; C, cerebellum; Hip, hippocampus; Hyp, hypothalamus; LC, locus coeruleus; NTS, nucleus of the tractus solitarius (vagal sensory nucleus); RF, brainstem reticular formation; SN, substantia nigra; Str, corpus striatum; Th, thalamus

cerebellum and spinal cord. The locus coerulus–noradrenaline system is implicated in the processes including attention, vigilance and orientation to aversive or threatening stimuli. Alteration in the noradrenaline system, including depletion of the neurotransmitter noradrenaline, may be linked to attention or concentration difficulties as well as sleep and arousal disturbances experienced in depression.

The dopamine diffuse regulatory system

Dopamine plays an important role in many brain functions. It affects the sleep–wake cycle, is important for goal directed behaviours and reward learning. Dopamine modulates the control of movement via the basal ganglia. Cognitive processing, such as executive function, also involves dopamine. Dopamine contributes to synaptic plasticity in brain regions such as the pre-frontal cortex. In depression, anhedonia has been associated to dysfunction (down regulation) in the dopaminergic regulatory system (Belujon and Grace, 2017). Anhedonia is defined as a loss of the ability to experience pleasure. It also includes the reward-related deficits observed in people with depression including the disruption of anticipation, motivation and decision-making processes. Imaging studies have demonstrated lower dopamine concentrations released into the synapse in people with depression.

Functional abnormalities associated with depression are also found in frontal and limbic regions. The cumulative effect of stress, with excessive cortisol, is responsible for a reduction in hippocampal and amygdala volume in MRI studies.

Inflammatory processes and depression

Activity 13.3 Reflection

Imagine you or someone you know has a viral illness such as a bad cold or flu. We know this might lead to physical symptoms such as a runny nose and a cough, but are there other symptoms you experience? For example how does it make you feel? And do you notice any changes in behaviour? Try listing some of these symptoms.

Compare your answer with the discussion.

In the exercise above you may have mentioned symptoms like feeling that you have no energy or that you might just want to sleep or lie somewhere quiet. You may have also noticed that you are less likely to want to go out and socialise with people or do things that normally give you pleasure. This is known as 'sickness behaviour' and you may have noticed that some of the symptoms are very like those that people with depression experience. Inflammation plays a major role in the pathophysiology of many conditions and diseases. A growing body of evidence suggests that psychological and social stressors increase a group of inflammatory mediators called cytokines which are thought to contribute to the pathophysiology of depression (see Box 13.2 and Chapter 2). The cytokines act on the brain to change our mood and behaviour. There is some evidence that they reduce levels of serotonin in the brain (Kopschina Feltes et al., 2017). We have already seen under the monoamine theory that a reduction in serotonin is thought to be important in depression. Elevated levels of cortisol can also lead to an imbalance in inflammatory cytokines in the brain. Increased levels of cytokines can cause an increased production of CRF in the hypothalamus (Goh and Agius, 2010). This information suggests that inflammation may be important in depression. In many patients with depression, inflammatory markers such as C-reactive protein (CRP) are increased (Howren et al., 2009). We also know that some autoimmune conditions such as rheumatoid arthritis and multiple sclerosis are associated with a higher prevalence of depression (Raison, 2014). Another interesting observation is that people treated with interferon for hepatitis can suffer from depression as a side-effect (Lucaciu and Damitrascu, 2015). Interferon is a type of cytokine involved in our immune response. Future research will help to provide insights into the process of inflammation and how this may promote the depression.

In summary, many different factors may be involved in the development of depression and there is a complex interplay between them. We have focused on some of the neurobiological theories. Monoamine neurotransmitters, the HPA axis and stress, and inflammation may all have a role to play in the neurobiology of depression. It is also possible that the neurobiology of depression might be different in different people. Beck and Bredemeier (2016) have presented a unified model of depression. The model aims to integrate the clinical features of depression with cognitive theory, recent advances in neurobiology and evolutionary perspectives. The model integrates 'seemingly disparate work across different frameworks and levels of analysis (cognitive, genetic, neural and hormonal) into a cohesive, coherent and novel fashion', acknowledging the major advances in our understanding of the nature and aetiology of depression, whilst providing recommendations for future research (Beck and Bredemeier, 2016).

Pharmacological management of depression

In this section, we will focus on the pharmacological management of depression. We will discuss the different antidepressants and how they act on the brain. Studies have shown that they can be helpful for some, but not all people with this condition and approximately 50% of people respond (Cleare et al., 2015). Antidepressants are also more effective in the treatment of moderate to severe rather than mild depression. In the UK a stepped care model for treatment of depression is suggested by NICE (2018d). Treatments are offered considering the severity of depression (Table 13.2).

Step	Intervention
Step 1 – All suspected presentations of depression	Assessment, support, psychoeducation, active monitoring and referral for further assessment and interventions
Step 2 – Persistent sub-threshold symptoms; mild to moderate depression	Low-intensity psychosocial interventions, psychological interventions, medication and referral for further assessment and interventions
Step 3 – Persistent sub-threshold symptoms or mild to moderate depression with inadequate response to initial interventions; moderate to severe depression	Medication, high-intensity psychological interventions, combined treatments, collaborative care and referral for further assessment and interventions
Step 4 – Severe and complex depression	Medication, high-intensity psychological interventions, electroconvulsive therapy, crisis service, combined treatments, multiprofessional and inpatient care

Table 13.2 Stepped care for depression (NICE, 2018d)

As Activity 13.4 shows there are some important points about antidepressants that need to be explained to patients. Patients should be informed about the side-effects they are likely to experience. This will depend on the type of antidepressant prescribed and will be discussed later in the chapter. Antidepressant use can cause an increased risk of

---

Activity 13.4   Reflection

Health professionals have a role in educating people about their antidepressant treatment. Before you read on make a list of information that a patient might find useful.

A suggested answer is given at the end of the chapter.

---

suicidal thoughts, self-harm and suicide. These risks are greatest in the 28 days before an antidepressant is started and the 28 days after it is stopped (Coupland et al., 2015). The risk is low but patients and carers need to be informed. It is important to note, however, that overall, in the long term, antidepressants reduce the risk of suicide. Patients also need to understand that they may not feel any immediate improvement in their symptoms. The common explanation is that antidepressants take 4 weeks to 'work'. However, we know that symptoms may begin to improve after as little as a week, but these might not be noticed until a longer period of time has elapsed. The length of treatment is also important. If patients discontinue their treatment too early they are more likely to become unwell again. For an initial episode of depression, a patient should continue for at least 6 months after their symptoms improve. Patients who relapse should continue antidepressants for 2 years. Some people may have multiple episodes of depression for which long-term maintenance with antidepressants can be helpful (NICE, 2018d).

Patients who wish to stop antidepressants should reduce their dose slowly over at least 4 weeks (NICE, 2018d). Many patients need to reduce the dose even more slowly than this. If antidepressants are stopped suddenly, discontinuation symptoms can occur. These include anxiety, insomnia, flu-like symptoms, electric shock like sensations and headaches. The patient may think that their depression is recurring so it is important to warn them. Because of these discontinuation symptoms, some patients might also believe that antidepressants are addictive. However in general, addictive drugs lead to additional complications such as tolerance (getting used to the dose and needing to increase it to get an effect), feelings of reward and a craving for more as the dose wears off. Tolerance and craving do not happen with antidepressants and they are not generally considered to be addictive.

In the next part of the chapter we will consider the action of antidepressants.

Mechanism of antidepressant action (pharmacodynamics)

Earlier in the chapter we discussed the monoamine theory of depression and identified that the neurotransmitters thought to be important in depression include serotonin (also known as 5HT or 5-hydroxytryptamine), noradrenaline and dopamine. In general, antidepressants increase the amount of neurotransmitters at the synapse (Figure 13.5). Different antidepressants increase different neurotransmitters by different mechanisms and we will explore this later. Despite the different pharmacological effects, all antidepressants may share 'downstream' effects on inflammatory markers and brain-derived neurotropic factor (NICE, 2018d).

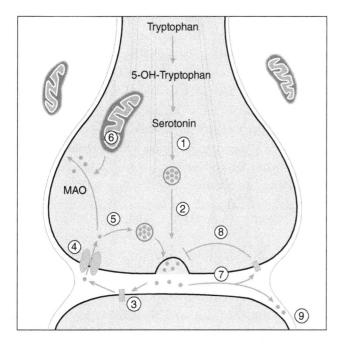

Serotonin transmitter molecules in CNS. **(1)** Serotonin is transported into synaptic vesicles. **(2)** Transmitter molecules undergo exocytosis into the synaptic cleft. **(3)** A postsynaptic serotonin receptor is being targeted. **(4)** Serotonin reuptake transporter returns transmitter to the terminal cytosol. **(5)** Some transmitter is repackaged into synaptic vesicles. **(6)** Some is degraded instead by monoamine oxidase (MAO). **(7)** Some activates presynaptic autoreceptors. **(8)** A 5-HT$_{10}$ presynaptic autoreceptor is retarding further transmitter release. **(9)** Some diffuses through the extracellular space, using 'volume transmission' to activate receptors on other neurons.

Figure 13.5   How do antidepressants work at the synapse? NB: A similar diagram is provided in Figure 1.8.

As we saw in the earlier section there are limitations with the monoamine theory. Studies examining neurotransmitter levels in depression have failed to consistently find low levels. As the science continues to make discoveries about the brain we continue to understand more about how antidepressants work. Alongside increasing levels of the monoamine neurotransmitters available at the synapse, it has been found that the monoamines (in particular serotonin), can also influence activation of the BDNF gene to increase levels of BDNF to promote neurogenesis and the number of connections between neurones. Neurogenesis leads to an improvement in memory and an increase in the size of the hippocampus. Antidepressants might also re-sensitise glucocorticoid receptors. In this way the HPA negative feedback loop is restored and cortisol levels fall (Chapter 2). As we saw previously high levels of cortisol can result in reduced neurogenesis. The role of monoamines in inflammation is yet to be determined.

Types of antidepressant

There are different types of antidepressant. These include selective serotonin reuptake inhibitors (SSRIs), tricyclics, monoamine oxidase inhibitors (MAOIs) and others such as venlafaxine and mirtazapine. We will consider the SSRIs first.

SSRIs

The SSRIs include citalopram, sertraline, escitalopram, paroxetine, fluoxetine and fluvoxamine.

Case study

Joan is a 33-year-old woman who visits the GP surgery. She has been finding work stressful due to continual reorganisations and financial cuts. Her mother is also terminally ill and she is the main carer. She is finding it difficult to socialise and go out. Her sleep is poor and as she has no appetite; she is skipping meals. Some days she finds she can barely get out of bed. She seeks the help of the GP who diagnoses moderate depression. She is on no other medication and has no other health problems. In accordance with NICE guidelines she is prescribed citalopram 20 mg each morning.

As the case study illustrates SSRIs are the first line antidepressant treatment (NICE, 2018d). They are chosen because they work as well as other antidepressants and tend to be better tolerated by patients. This means that, although they do cause side-effects, patients are less likely to discontinue them early and are more likely to continue with the treatment. They are also less toxic on overdose than some other antidepressants, especially the tricyclic drugs.

SSRIs all act in the same way. As their name suggests they selectively inhibit the reuptake of serotonin at the synapse (Figure 13.5). They have little effect on other neurotransmitters. After serotonin is released into the synapse, it is removed from the synapse by reuptake sites on the presynaptic neurone (the serotonin transporter). The SSRI blocks these sites and prevents re-uptake of serotonin (see Figure 1.8 in Chapter 1). This means that serotonin remains in the synapse for longer to exert its effect.

Side-effects and implications for practice

Common side-effects include diarrhoea, headache and agitation. These side-effects are all caused by an increase in serotonin. The brain and CNS have more than one type of serotonin receptor, for example 5HT1, 5HT2 and 5HT3 receptors. Increased activity at the 5HT1 is useful and can improve symptoms of anxiety and depression. However increased activity at other serotonin receptors (5HT2 and 5HT3 receptors) can cause side-effects. Table 13.3 shows how these side-effects are linked to activity at different receptors.

In some people SSRIs can cause extreme agitation which, alongside feeling depressed may be a factor leading to increased suicide risk when SSRIs are started. SSRIs

Side-effect	Receptor
Anxiety	5HT2
Agitation	5HT2
Akathisia	5HT2
Insomnia	5HT2
Sexual problems (e.g. delayed orgasm, erectile dysfunction)	5HT2
Nausea and vomiting	5HT3 (Chapter 7)
Diarrhoea	5HT3 (Chapter 10)

Table 13.3   Side-effects of antidepressants

can also cause hyponatraemia (low sodium). This is especially a problem for older patients on diuretics.

There are also important drug interactions to be aware of. Serotonin receptors are present on the surface of platelets. Blocking (antagonising) these receptors can make platelets less likely to clump together and form clots. This leads to an increased bleeding risk when SSRIs are used with aspirin and non-steroidal anti-inflammatory drugs (see Chapter 6). SSRIs can have an additive pharmacodynamic effect when used with other drugs that also increase serotonin. If, for example, SSRIs are used together with tramadol, the increase in serotonin can lead to serotonin syndrome. Symptoms of serotonin syndrome are shown in Table 13.4. If this occurs it can be fatal and medical intervention is needed. Serotonin syndrome can also occur if two antidepressants are used together or in cases of overdose. In some people it might occur with usual antidepressant doses; this is much rarer.

Mental state changes (e.g. confusion)	Agitation/restlessness
Sweating	Diarrhoea
Fever	Hyperreflexia
Tachycardia	Myoclonus
Hypertension	Convulsions

Table 13.4   Serotonin syndrome symptoms

Tricyclic antidepressants

Examples of tricyclic antidepressants include amitriptyline, lofepramine and nortriptyline.

These drugs were developed before SSRIs. They are called tricyclics because they all have a similar chemical structure which involves three carbon rings. Unlike the SSRIs, this group of drugs have wide ranging effects on many different receptors in the body and brain. For example, histamine, alpha and muscarinic receptors. Some of these effects are useful but some are less so and lead to side-effects. The drugs act to increase both noradrenaline and serotonin neurotransmitters by inhibiting the re-uptake of these neurotransmitters from the synapse.

Side-effects and implication for practice

Common side-effects include a pattern of side-effects known as anticholinergic side-effects. These include dry mouth, blurred vision and constipation. This happens because tricyclic antidepressants block some acetylcholine receptors (see Chapter 9 for a revision of the parasympathetic nervous system). Tricyclics also cause more weight gain than SSRIs. This side-effect may have many different causes. One explanation is that tricyclics block histamine receptors and histamine usually reduces appetite. Tricyclics can also cause a decrease in blood pressure. This is because they block alpha adrenergic receptors (see Chapter 9 for a revision of the sympathetic nervous system). Tricyclics also cause drowsiness which may be due to a combination of anticholinergic, antihistamine and alpha blocking effects. Tricyclics are more dangerous in overdose than SSRIs and newer antidepressants. This is because they affect conduction of electrical impulses in the heart. This problem also makes them unsuitable for patients with cardiac arrhythmias.

Activity 13.5   Critical thinking

Consider the side-effects of tricyclic antidepressants; can you list those that make them especially unsuitable for use in older adults, and explain the reasons why.

Which patients might benefit from tricyclics?

A suggested answer is given at the end of the chapter.

Serotonin and noradrenaline re-uptake inhibitors (SNRI)

Examples of SNRIs are venlafaxine and duloxetine.

These antidepressants are a newer group of drugs than the tricyclic and SSRI antidepressants. They inhibit the re-uptake of both noradrenaline and serotonin at the synapse. Unlike tricyclic antidepressants, the SNRIs are selective and do not block all the other receptors. As we have seen, antagonising histamine, acetylcholine and alpha receptors can cause many of the unacceptable side-effects of tricyclic antidepressants. The SNRIs cause fewer side-effects than the tricyclic antidepressants and provide an alternative to SSRIs.

Side-effects and implications for practice

In low doses venlafaxine acts to increase serotonin only. The side-effects are therefore similar to those of SSRIs. For example, agitation, nausea, vomiting, insomnia and headache. At higher doses, these side-effects can be more severe and hypertension can also occur. In addition, at higher doses, noradrenaline and dopamine neurotransmitters are increased making venlafaxine a useful antidepressant where other antidepressants have not improved patients' symptoms.

Common side-effects of duloxetine include nausea and vomiting, insomnia, dry mouth, sexual dysfunction, dizziness and constipation.

Mirtazapine

Mirtazepine increases both serotonin and noradrenaline neurotransmitters at the synapse but by a different mechanism to the other antidepressants discussed. Mirtazepine antagonises presynaptic alpha-2 receptors. These receptors usually act like a brake and inhibit the release of neurotransmitters when they are stimulated. When they are blocked by mirtazapine, the release of serotonin and noradrenaline neurotransmitters is increased. Pre-synaptic alpha-2 receptors are inhibitory and decrease the release of serotonin and noradrenaline. Mirtazepine, therefore, acts to increase the release of serotonin and noradrenaline (by antagonising the inhibitory effects of the alpha-2 receptors).

Common side-effects and implications for practice

Mirtazapine also blocks histamine receptors to cause drowsiness and weight gain. The drowsiness can be a useful side-effect in patients with insomnia, a common symptom of depression. It can also cause dry mouth and dizziness. It causes less sexual dysfunction and agitation than SSRI antidepressants. This is because mirtazapine blocks 5HT2 and 5HT3 receptors that are responsible for these effects (as we saw previously, the SSRIs lead to stimulation of these receptors).

Other antidepressants

There are other types of antidepressants. For example, monoamine oxidase inhibitors (MAOIs), reboxetine and aglomelatine. These are used much less often than other types of antidepressants and a discussion of these is outside the scope of the chapter.

Choosing an antidepressant

The first line choice of antidepressant is usually an SSRI. If a patient does not respond to this antidepressant after 3–4 weeks have elapsed, a review of antidepressant treatment is needed. This might result in a second antidepressant being tried. Normally, this is another SSRI or one of the newer antidepressants – for example mirtazapine. Some patients will have tried many different antidepressants over their life time. Choice is guided by what has worked before, as well as the different side-effect profiles the drugs have. For example, for a patient who is having difficulty sleeping, mirtazapine – which causes drowsiness – might be a better choice than an SSRI or SNRI, which can cause insomnia (NICE, 2018d). For patients who have tried at least two antidepressants without improvement, the choice of what drug to prescribe next can be difficult (Rush et al., 2006). This is why some patients might be prescribed more than one antidepressant. It is always important to discuss drug choices with a pharmacist or mental health team. Some combinations have been found to be useful such as mirtazapine and an SSRI. Other combinations might lead to serotonin syndrome. For example, MAOIs plus any other antidepressant, or tricyclic antidepressants with an SSRI.

Activity 13.6   Research

Many mental health trusts in the UK subscribe to the 'choice and medication' website which is a resource for patients and staff. If this is available from your local mental health trust, visit the website. Enter the condition depression. Under the question 'is there an easy way to compare the main medicines for depression' download the pdf summary chart. Look at the chart and consider whether, if you had depression, you would prefer to take an SSRI or mirtazapine for your depression. You can find similar charts in Bazire's *Psychotropic Drug Directory* (2018).

A suggested answer is given at the end of the chapter.

Non-pharmacological treatments for depression

This chapter has focused on pharmacological therapies. It is, however, important to remember that psychological therapies are also therapeutic interventions for depression. If you have a look again at the stepped care model (Table 13.2) you can see that for mild depression, assessment and support is offered and antidepressants are not routinely prescribed. For mild to moderate depression, psychological therapies are offered either alongside or as an alternative to antidepressants. Cognitive behavioural therapy (CBT) and interpersonal psychotherapy are some examples of therapies that might be offered. There is some evidence that antidepressant treatment plus a psychological therapy is more effective than either treatment alone (Cleare et al., 2015).

It is now time to review what you have learned within this chapter by undertaking some multiple choice questions.

Activity 13.7   Multiple choice questions

1. In addition to low mood, symptoms of depression may also include:
   a) Reduced appetite
   b) Poor concentration

   c) Loss of interest in activities

   d) All of the above

2. The role of cortisol is important in depression. It has been found that:

   a) Hyperactivity of the HPA axis leads to reduced cortisol levels.

   b) Emotional stress can reduce levels of cortisol.

   c) Increased cortisol can inhibit neurogenesis in the hippocampus.

   d) Prolonged exposure to cortisol in children can lead to reduced amygdala activity.

3. The monoamine theory of depression states that in depression:

   a) Levels of monoamines, for example serotonin, are reduced.

   b) Levels of monoamines, for example noradrenalin, are increased.

   c) Levels of monoamines, for example glutamate, are reduced.

   d) Levels of monoamines, for example acetylcholine, are increased.

4. How might inflammation be involved in depression?

   a) Histamine causes brain swelling.

   b) Cytokines act to lower levels of serotonin.

   c) Prostaglandins act to increase painful feelings.

   d) Neutrophils cause social withdrawal.

5. Which ONE of the following statements about the stress vulnerability model of depression is TRUE?

   a) It only applies to severe depression.

   b) People with a high vulnerability are more likely to become depressed at a given level of stress.

   c) People with a vulnerability to depression will have chronically reduced cortisol levels.

   d) Your genetic make-up does not influence your stress and vulnerability.

6. Which ONE of the following statements about antidepressant drug treatment is TRUE?

   a) Antidepressants are less effective than psychological therapy in severe depression.

   b) Antidepressants should be continued for at least 6 months after remission of symptoms.

   c) Antidepressants are highly addictive and should be used with caution.

   d) Antidepressants should be taken as required only when symptoms are severe.

7. What would a suitable first line antidepressant be:

   a) A tricyclic

   b) A monoamine oxidase inhibitor

(Continued)

(Continued)

    c) A selective serotonin re-uptake inhibitor
    d) A benzodiazepine

8. Which ONE of the following statements is TRUE?

    a) Amitriptyline is an example of an SSRI.
    b) Mirtazapine is an example of a tricyclic.
    c) Venlafaxine is an example of an SNRI.
    d) Fluoxetine is an example of a benzodiazepine.

9. The combination of tramadol and an SSRI is potentially dangerous because:

    a) Tramadol can increase the concentration of the SSRI causing toxicity.
    b) The combination can cause excessive drowsiness due to additive drowsiness.
    c) Suicide risk is increased.
    d) Serotonin syndrome may result as both can increase serotonin.

10. Common side-effects of SSRIs include:

    a) Insomnia, diarrhoea and headache.
    b) Dry mouth, constipation, blurred vision and urinary retention.
    c) Weight gain and drowsiness.
    d) Hypotension and hyperkalaemia.

Chapter summary

Depression is a serious health concern that severely affects people's quality of life. Our understanding of the neurobiology of depression continues to develop with advances in neuroimaging. There are a number of theories – psychological and social – as well as the neurobiological theoretical explanations that inform our understanding of the factors that may predispose, precipitate and/or perpetuate a depressive episode. The monoamine theory suggests a reduction in neurotransmitter levels may be a contributory factor. The effects of stress, dysregulation of the HPA axis and high cortisol levels are also involved. There is increasing evidence to suggest inflammation has a role. Although anyone might suffer from depression, some people appear to be more vulnerable to depression than others. Vulnerability might be due to genetic differences and early childhood experiences which lead to a dysregulation of the HPA axis and raised cortisol levels. Psychological and pharmacological interventions are useful. NICE (2018d) advocates a stepped care approach with treatment determined by the severity of symptoms. We have discussed the different types of antidepressants – including tricyclics, SSRIs, SNRIs and mirtazapine. They all act, albeit through different mechanisms, to increase neurotransmitter levels in the synapse. SSRIs are usually the first choice as they are as effective as other types and better tolerated by patients. It is important that patients are given information about their antidepressants when they start treatment including common side-effects, possible increase in suicidal thoughts, onset of action and length of treatment.

Activities: Brief outline answers

Activity 13.1 Critical thinking (p349)

Core symptoms George is experiencing

During the last month have you often been bothered by feeling down, depressed, or hopeless? (George has experienced loss of hope and belief in himself and the future.)

Do you have little interest or pleasure in doing things? (George used to enjoy watching television but now he does not really enjoy it any more.)

Other typical symptoms

Fatigue/loss of energy. (George said he feels tired all the time.)

Worthlessness/excessive or inappropriate guilt. (He felt his family would be much better off without him as he is useless.)

Recurrent thoughts of death, suicidal thoughts, or actual suicide attempts. (George attempted suicide.)

Diminished ability to think/concentrate or indecisiveness. (George finds it difficult to concentrate on reading or watching TV, finds it difficult to respond to questions.)

Psychomotor agitation or retardation. (At interview he takes time to respond to questions.)

Insomnia/hypersomnia. (George says he hardly sleeps.)

Significant appetite and/or weight loss. (He has lost a stone in weight in a month – note this could also be due to the cancer.)

Activity 13.4 Reflection (p360)

NICE (2018d) guidance outlines some of the information patients should be told. These include side-effects, explanation that there is a gradual build up to the full effect and how long treatment should be continued for. Patients should be warned about possible increased agitation and suicidal thoughts. Discontinuation symptoms should be discussed whilst addressing patient concerns that antidepressants might be addictive. What a person can expect from antidepressants and how they should take them should also be discussed.

Activity 13.5 Critical thinking (p364)

The frail older adult is particularly at risk from the side-effects of tricyclic antidepressants. Side-effects such as drowsiness and low blood pressure can be particularly problematic and could increase the risk of falls. Anticholinergic side-effects such as constipation are also a problem as older adults may already have reduced gut motility. Blocking acetylcholine can also lead to cognitive impairment which again might be a greater problem. Older adults are more likely to have co-morbidities such as heart problems, and to be prescribed other medication that could interact.

Some patients do benefit from tricyclic antidepressants. If a patient has tried other antidepressants, such as SSRIs and mirtazapine, but these have not reduced their symptoms, tricyclic antidepressants can be a useful option. A thorough investigation into past treatments should be explored. Patients who have found them helpful in the past may find them helpful again. One advantage for some is that they help with sleep. Any advantage must be carefully weighed against the potential side-effects and increased toxicity in overdose.

Activity 13.6 Research (p366)

Answer: both have side-effects but you can see that mirtazapine has three dots for feeling sleepy and weight gain whereas SSRIs have one, showing you are less likely to get these side-effects with an SSRI. However sexual problems are less likely with mirtazapine. Which side-effects are of greatest concern to you will help to determine your choice.

Activity 13.7 Multiple choice questions (pp366–8)

1. In addition to low mood, symptoms of depression may also include:

   d) All of the above

2. The role of cortisol is important in depression. It has been found that:

   c) Increased cortisol can inhibit neurogenesis in the hippocampus.

3. The monoamine theory of depression states that in depression:

   a) Levels of monoamines, for example serotonin, are reduced.

4. How might inflammation be involved in depression?

   b) Cytokines act to lower levels of serotonin.

5. Which ONE of the following statements about the stress vulnerability model of depression is TRUE?

   b) People with a high vulnerability are more likely to become depressed at a given level of stress.

6. Which ONE of the following statements about antidepressant drug treatment is TRUE?

   b) Antidepressants should be continued for at least 6 months after remission of symptoms.

7. What would a suitable first line antidepressant be:

   c) A selective serotonin re-uptake inhibitor.

8. Which ONE of the following statements is TRUE?

   c) Venlafaxine is an example of an SNRI.

9. The combination of tramadol and an SSRI is potentially dangerous because:

   d) Serotonin syndrome may result as both can increase serotonin.

10. Common side-effects of SSRIs include:

    a) Insomnia, diarrhoea and headache.

Further reading

Bazire, S (2016) *Psychotropic Drug Directory.* Warwickshire: Lloyd-Renhold.

This reference guide contains useful information about treatment options in mental health. Includes drug interactions, management of side-effects and drug-induced psychiatric disorders.

Cleare, A, et al. (2015) Evidence-based guidelines for treating depressive disorders with antidepressants: a revision of the 2008 British Association for Psychopharmacology guidelines. *Journal of Psychopharmacology, 29* (5): 459–525.

An alternative to NICE explores treatments choices in depression.

Mental Health Foundation (2016) *Fundamental Facts about Mental Health.* Available at: **www. mentalhealth.org.uk/publications/fundamental-facts-about-mental-health-2016/**

A useful webpage from the Mental Health Foundation giving facts and figures from a summary of mental health research.

NICE (2018d) CG90. *Depression in Adults: Recognition and Management.* Available at: **www.nice.org. uk/guidance/cg91/**

Renal conditions

Chapter aims

After reading this chapter, you will be able to:

- explain the role of the kidney in homeostasis;
- recognise the risk factors for acute kidney injury and chronic renal disease;
- identify the main mechanisms of acute kidney injury and identify the main causes of chronic renal failure;
- explain the main complications of acute kidney injury and chronic renal failure and their clinical manifestations;
- explain the rationale for drug treatments for acute kidney injury and chronic kidney disease.

Introduction

Case study

Penny, aged 52 years, is involved in a skiing accident and receives fractures to her left tibia, fibula and femur. She has lacerations on her body and has lost two units of blood. On admission to the emergency department Penny is conscious but in severe pain.

Her vital signs are: blood pressure: 90/60 mmHg; pulse: 120 bpm; temperature: 36.5°C. Following examination Penny has no other fractures, no evidence of intra-abdominal bleeding and on palpation her abdominal organs are soft with no tenderness or rigidity.

Prior to the skiing accident, Penny was taking the following medication: ibuprofen – an NSAID, which she takes for chronic shoulder pain, and Lisinopril, an ACE inhibitor, which she takes for hypertension. Normally, Penny's blood pressure is well controlled at 130/90 mmHg.

In the emergency department Penny is given fluid resuscitation. Over the next four hours Penny's blood pressure responds well but her urine output remains very low (5–10 mL/h).

In the case study above, Penny has experienced physiological trauma in a skiing accident. She has gone on to develop acute kidney injury (AKI). AKI is a common, serious problem which is often poorly managed. Early recognition and action are essential.

In this chapter we examine acute kidney injury and chronic renal disease. Acute kidney injury (AKI) and chronic kidney disease (CKD) can arise through various types of trauma and/or disease-processes occurring to the kidney or from systemic disease. Both AKI and CKD manifest through a reduction in kidney function that can lead to a range of complications including those of fluid and electrolyte balance, and those from the build-up of metabolic wastes, such as creatinine and urea in the body.

We begin this chapter by reviewing aspects of kidney function needed to understand AKI and CKD. We then move on to examining acute kidney injury and chronic kidney disease and their pharmacological management.

Overview of kidney function

The main function of the kidney is to regulate the extracellular fluid environment. The regulation of the extracellular fluid environment is an important aspect of homeostasis. The importance of homeostasis for maintaining the function of the body cells – and therefore the health of the individual – was introduced in Chapter 1.

The extracellular fluid (ECF) is the fluid outside the cells. The ECF supplies the cell with nutrients – such as glucose and amino acids – and oxygen. The ECF also removes the waste products of cellular metabolism – such as carbon dioxide, lactate and urea. The ECF must have the right balance of electrolytes and water to ensure cell functioning. In addition, the ECF must be at the optimum pH to maintain the function of the body cells. The pH of the ECF is maintained between 7.35–7.45. The composition and normal ranges of the ECF electrolytes, as well as the pH and concentrations of key waste metabolites is discussed further below.

Plasma is an important part of the extracellular fluid. Specifically, plasma is the fluid part of the blood – that part of the extracellular fluid component that circulates around the body in the vascular system. The plasma is in constant exchange with the interstitial fluid at capillary beds. The interstitial fluid is the other main component of the extracellular fluid. 'Interstitial' means 'between the cells'. Interstitial fluid is the part of the extracellular fluid that is outside the vascular system. It is present in the spaces between the cells and therefore sometimes termed 'tissue fluid'.

At the arteriole end of capillary beds, water, electrolytes and nutrients are squeezed out of the plasma to become interstitial fluid. At the venous end, water, electrolytes and waste metabolites return to the plasma. The constant exchange of fluid between the plasma and interstitial fluid, and the circulation of plasma around the body, ensures that the composition of the extracellular fluid remains relatively constant throughout the body, (Hall, 2015; Chapter 1). By filtering the plasma and excreting waste metabolites, excess water and electrolytes, the kidney regulates the composition of the plasma and through its exchange with the interstitial fluid, regulates the extracellular fluid as a whole.

Table 14.1 shows the normal ranges of the main components of the plasma. The most important electrolyte in plasma is sodium, but other key electrolytes are: potassium, magnesium, phosphate and chloride.

Component	Reference range
Sodium (Na^+)	133–146 mmol/L
Potassium (K^+)	3.5–5.3 mmol/L
Chloride (Cl^-)	95–108 mmol/L
Magnesium (Mg^{2+})	0.7–1.0 mmol/L
Bicarbonate (HCO_3^-)	22–29 mmol/L
Phosphate (PO_4^{2-})	0.8–1.5 mmol/L
pH	7.35–7.45
Urea	2.5–7.8 mmol/L
Creatinine	60–120 µmol/L
Serum osmolality	275–295 mmol/kg

Table 14.1 Normal ranges of the main electrolytes, creatinine and urea in the plasma

Serum 'osmolality' (Table 14.1) refers to the concentration of osmotically active particles in the plasma. Sodium (and its associated anions – chloride and phosphate) are the main osmotically active particles in extracellular fluid. This is because sodium is the most abundant electrolyte in the extracellular fluid and tends to be kept out of the cells through the action of the sodium–potassium pump (Lote, 2012). Any changes in the osmolality of the plasma will cause water to enter, or leave, the cells by osmosis. This is potentially harmful to the cells as it may cause cell-swelling or cell-shrinkage. The osmolality of the plasma must be maintained within a fairly narrow range (275–295 mmol/kg) to prevent excess fluid movement into or out of the cells. The kidney regulates serum osmolality by excreting more, or less, water. This is described further below (under 'Regulation of plasma osmolality').

We have noted above that the pH of the extracellular fluid is kept within a very narrow range (pH 7.35–7.45). The regulation of plasma pH falls under the physiological concept of acid–base balance. Acid–base balance is complex, involving buffers in the blood such as haemoglobin, and compensatory changes made by the renal and respiratory system (Tortora and Derrickson, 2017).

Another very important function of the kidney is to maintain the blood volume. Blood volume is around 3 L in adults and proportionally less in children. Blood volume must be maintained to ensure an adequate blood pressure for the circulation of blood around the body. Blood volume is determined by the amount of water and sodium ingested (from the diet) – and the amount lost by the body (largely in urine by the kidneys). To maintain a normal blood volume, the kidneys regulate the amount of sodium and water lost in urine. This is described further below, under 'Blood volume regulation'.

In addition to its role in homeostasis of the extracellular fluid, the kidney produces several hormones. These include erythropoietin, renin and active vitamin D (calcitriol). These regulate, respectively, red blood cell production, blood pressure and calcium absorption from the GI tract.

Table 14.2 summarises the main functions of the kidney.

Function	Mechanism
Regulation of electrolyte concentrations of the plasma	Through the processes of filtration, selective reabsorption and secretion in the kidney tubules excess electrolytes will be excreted from the plasma.
	Fine-tuning of Na^+, K^+, Ca^{2+}, PO_4^{2-} excretion is under hormone regulation (aldosterone, parathyroid hormone, and vitamin D).
Regulation of acid–base balance of the plasma	Through secretion of hydrogen ions (H^+) and the conservation and/or generation of additional HCO_3^- ions.
Excretion of waste products of metabolism, including urea, creatinine, drugs	Filtration into the tubules without active reabsorption. Some wastes and drugs are actively secreted into the tubules.
Regulation of the osmolality of the plasma	Through excretion of more, or less, water from kidney: antidiuretic hormone (ADH) regulates the amount of water reabsorbed from the distal tubules and collecting duct.
Regulation of blood volume	Through the reabsorption of more, or less, sodium (Na^+) from the tubules. Various mechanisms regulate sodium excretion, including the renin angiotensin aldosterone system (RAAS) – described under 'Production of the hormone renin', in this table, below.
Production of the hormone erythropoietin	Erythropoietin stimulates the production of erythrocytes (red blood cells) in the bone marrow. Erythropoietin is produced in response to low oxygen levels (PO_2) in arterial blood.
Production of the hormone renin	Renin is involved in regulating blood volume and therefore blood pressure. Renin is part of a larger cascade of hormone signalling called the renin angiotensin aldosterone system (RAAS). RAAS functions to prevent sodium and fluid loss from the kidneys and to cause widespread vasoconstriction.
Production of active vitamin D (calcitriol)	Active vitamin D functions in calcium homeostasis and bone growth and maintenance.

Table 14.2   An overview of the main functions of the kidney

Many of these functions of the kidney become compromised in acute kidney injury and chronic kidney disease. It is important, therefore, to look more closely at the components of the renal system and nephron function. The nephron is the functional unit of the kidney.

The components of the renal system

Figure 14.1A shows the main components of the renal system. The main organs are the two kidneys. The two ureters collect urine from their respective kidney and convey it to the bladder where it is stored temporarily; the urethra takes urine from the bladder to the outside world. The blood supply to each kidney comes from the right and left renal arteries. The right and left renal veins return blood from the kidneys to the heart via the inferior vena cava.

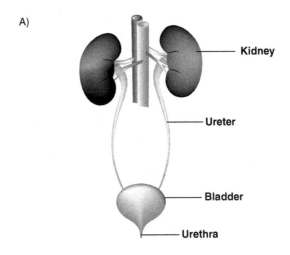

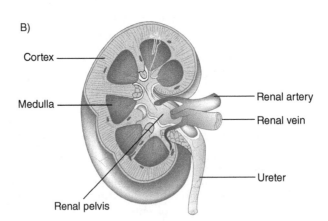

Figure 14.1 The renal system. (A) Shows the right and left kidney; the ureters which take urine from the kidneys to the bladder where urine is stored temporarily; and the urethra – the tube carrying urine to the outside world. (B) Shows a section through the right kidney

The renal artery is a direct branch of the abdominal aorta. The kidney has a high blood supply in relation to its size. It receives around 20% of the cardiac output even though it is much less than 25% mass of the body. This disproportionately high blood supply arises from the kidney's function which is to filter the blood; effective filtration requires this high blood supply. As you shall see shortly, compromises to the blood supply to the kidney may cause acute kidney injury.

Figure 14.1B shows a section through the right kidney. The outer part of the kidney is called the cortex and the inner part is called the medulla. Urine collects in the renal pelvis where it enters the ureter to be taken to the bladder.

As noted above, the kidney carries out its function by filtering the plasma. Filtration is carried out by microscopic tubules called nephrons. The filtered fluid (the filtrate) is modified as it travels downs the nephron by two processes: tubular reabsorption and tubular secretion. Tubular reabsorption is the process that returns substances to the plasma. Reabsorbed substances include: nutrients, water, most of the electrolytes. By contrast, wastes and toxins remain in the tubules and are passed to the bladder as urine where they will be removed to the outside world via the urethra. Additional wastes and drugs can be added to the filtrate from the surrounding blood capillaries. This is called tubular secretion.

Figure 14.2 illustrates the processes of filtration, reabsorption and secretion.

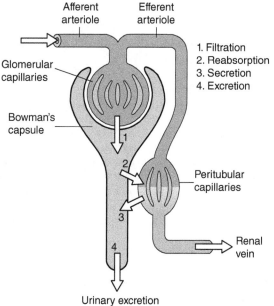

Figure 14.2 Filtration, reabsorption and secretion in a single nephron. The figure shows a single nephron and its blood supply. Arrows show the processes of (1) filtration; (2) reabsorption; and (3) secretion. For a given substance, the amount (4) excreted in urine is determined by the amount filtered minus the amount reabsorbed plus the amount secreted. Some substances, for example glucose, are completely reabsorbed (with no secretion); some substances, such as potassium, are both reabsorbed and secreted. See text for details.

The kidney can regulate the individual excretion of water and electrolytes (such as sodium and potassium) through changes in tubular reabsorption or tubular secretion. For example, if too much sodium is consumed in the diet, the kidney can excrete the excess without altering the excretion of water or other electrolytes. We will look more closely at these functions in the next section.

The nephron

Figure 14.3 shows a single kidney tubule or nephron and its blood supply. Each kidney contains around 1 million nephrons.

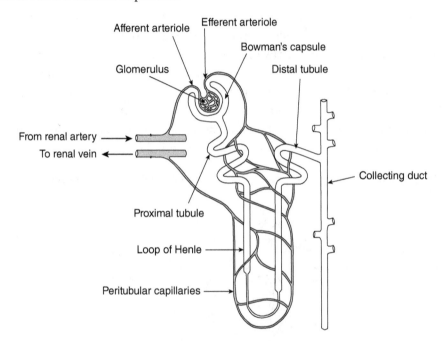

Figure 14.3 A single kidney tubule or nephron and its blood supply. The figure shows a single nephron and its blood supply. There are about 1 million nephrons in each kidney. The nephron is a filtering unit. Blood entering the glomerulus is filtered under high pressure into the Bowman's capsule. The filtrate is successively modified as it passes down the tubule. Several nephrons join with a collecting duct. From the collecting ducts, urine is delivered to the renal pelvis to enter the ureter.

The nephron is divided into four sections:

- **Bowman's capsule** – the site of filtration of the plasma.
- **Proximal tubule** – the first winding tubule and site of most tubular reabsorption.
- **Loop of Henle** – a hairpin loop – the site of further water and sodium reabsorption and the formation of a 'salt' gradient in the medulla. This gradient is essential for water conservation (reabsorption) from the collecting ducts.
- **Distal tubule and collecting ducts** – the second winding tubule and collecting duct. This is where 'fine-tuning' of the filtrate occurs. Fine-tuning is particularly important for sodium, potassium balance and water conservation. Several distal tubules connect to a collecting duct. The connecting duct drains into the renal pelvis.

Each of the 1 million or so nephrons is fed by a knot of capillaries called a glomerulus. Blood enters the glomerulus from the afferent arteriole and blood leaves the glomerulus via the efferent arteriole. The efferent arteriole then branches forming the peritubular capillaries. Re-absorbed nutrients, water and electrolytes enter the peritubular capillaries in their return to the systemic circulation.

Glomerular filtration

Glomerular filtration is the filtration of plasma in the glomerulus. The pressure of blood in the glomerulus (the hydrostatic pressure) must be high to filter the plasma. (The hydrostatic pressure in the glomerulus is around 50–55 mmHg compared to around 32 mmHg in other capillaries.) Under this high pressure, water and solutes from the plasma are forced through the wall of the glomerulus into the Bowman's capsule. This process is an 'ultrafiltration' because small molecules (such as water, glucose, electrolytes) pass through the filtration barrier but larger molecules (such as the plasma proteins) do not. These larger molecules and blood cells remain in the plasma.

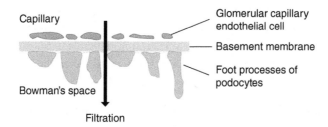

Figure 14.4   The filtration membrane. This is made from the wall of the glomerulus and the wall of the Bowman's capsule. The basement membrane joining the two layers of cells makes up the main barrier to filtration. Only water and small solutes (such as glucose, electrolytes, urea and creatinine) can pass through the filtration barrier

Figure 14.4 shows the structure of the filtration barrier. The barrier is very delicate and can be easily damaged. Damage can arise from high blood pressure (hypertension) or from diabetic nephropathy (Chapter 12). A damaged filtration barrier may result in protein appearing in the urine. Glomerular damage may also be caused by immune complexes lodging in the glomerulus. This can lead to various forms of glomerular disease and eventually to chronic kidney disease. Detection of even microscopic amounts of protein (microproteinuria) in the urine can indicate damage to the glomerular filtration barrier. The albumin:creatinine ratio (ACR) is one such test (see section on 'Chronic kidney disease', below).

The high pressure within the glomerulus is dependent upon an effective blood supply to the kidney. Blood flow to the glomerulus is maintained by altering the diameter of the afferent and efferent arterioles. This is called autoregulation and will be discussed further when we look at the causes of acute kidney injury (Table 14.3).

The glomerular filtration rate, or GFR, is the rate at which fluid is filtered from the blood into the Bowman's capsule. The normal ranges for GFR are from 130 L to 145 L/day in women and 165 L to 180 L/day in men. On a daily basis, virtually all the filtered solutes and water (around 99%) are returned to the circulation through tubular reabsorption.

An estimated glomerular filtration rate (eGFR) is used to determine kidney function from plasma creatinine concentration. eGFR is discussed in the box below.

Estimated GFR (eGFR) is used to measure kidney function

The glomerular filtration rate (GFR) is used routinely to assess kidney function and monitor the course of renal disease. GFR refers to the sum of the filtration rates in all the functioning nephrons. GFR is therefore an index of the *functioning renal mass* – a measure of how much of the kidney is functional (Rennke and Denker, 2013).

Plasma creatinine concentration is used to enable an estimate of GFR (eGFR). Creatinine is a waste metabolite produced by skeletal muscle. The level of creatinine in the plasma depends upon the rate of production of creatinine and its rate of excretion by the kidneys. The rate of production of creatinine is approximately constant (in an individual at a given time). The rate of excretion depends upon the rate of filtration, or GFR. Very little creatinine is reabsorbed or secreted from the tubules. As such, the plasma creatinine level can be used to estimate GFR.

Plasma creatinine levels in men are higher than in women because men (generally) have a greater muscle mass and a higher rate of creatinine production. Similarly, people of African origin have a higher muscle mass and a higher rate of creatinine production. By contrast, muscle mass is reduced in the older adult. Algorithms have been devised to take account of the variables age, sex and ethnicity. A standardised eGFR is reported in $mL/min/1.73\ m^2$.

The eGFR forms part of the diagnosis and staging of acute kidney injury and chronic kidney disease, as will be described below under the sections on acute kidney injury and chronic kidney disease.

Having reviewed eGRF, we turn to look at how the filtrate is processed in the renal tubules (or nephrons).

Tubular processing

Tubular processing refers to the modification of the filtrate within the tubules and includes the processes of reabsorption and secretion (Figure 14.2). Figure 14.5 shows in more detail the main sites of reabsorption of sodium, potassium and water and the main sites of hormone regulation.

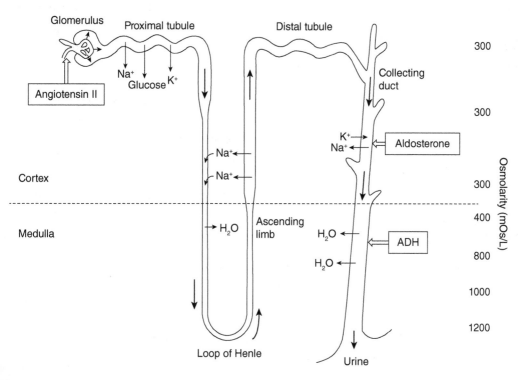

Figure 14.5 Tubular processing of the filtrate. The figure shows a single nephron. The main sites of reabsorption of sodium, glucose potassium and water are shown. Secretion of potassium in the distal tubule is also shown. The main sites of action of the hormones angiotensin II, ADH and aldosterone are shown. For details see text

The mechanisms by which tubular processing occur are complex, involving ion pumps and carrier molecules in the membrane of the cell lining the tubules. In the sections below, we highlight the main processes. For further details of membrane transport mechanisms, we recommend that you consult one of the texts in the Further reading section at the end of this chapter.

Following filtration in the Bowman's capsule, most of the electrolytes, nutrients and water are re-absorbed in the proximal tubule. Figure 14.5 shows the reabsorption of sodium, glucose and potassium as key examples of substances reabsorbed in the proximal tubule. Active transport by the sodium-potassium pump is used to 'drive' much of the reabsorption of electrolytes and nutrients, such as glucose and amino acids. Water follows passively by osmosis.

The loop of Henle produces a 'salt' (or osmotic) gradient in the medulla of the kidney. Figure 14.5 shows that the osmolality in the cortex of the kidney is 300 mOsm/kg but in the medulla, at the tip of the loop, the osmolality reaches as high as 1200 mOsm/L. The high osmolality in the medulla enables a concentrated urine to be produced.

This is how the kidney is able to conserve water (as will be described under 'Regulation of plasma osmolality', below).

The salt gradient is produced by a 'counter-current' mechanism which is dependent on the hairpin shape of the loop of Henle. The mechanism of the counter-current system is complex and it is beyond the scope of this book to give a detailed description. Details of the mechanism can be found by consulting one of the physiology textbooks given in the Further reading section at the end of this chapter. In essence, there is active transport of sodium from the filtrate as it ascends the thick ascending loop (Figure 14.5). This part of the loop and the subsequent distal tubule and collecting ducts are (normally) impermeable to water. As such, water will not leave these parts of the tubule. The active removal of sodium from the ascending loop without the loss of water ensures a dilute filtrate reaches the distal tubule and collecting ducts. Without further water reabsorption in the distal tubule or collecting duct, *a dilute urine is produced*. However, under the influence of the hormone ADH, the distal tubule and collecting duct become permeable to water.

The active transport of sodium from the ascending loop creates the osmotic gradient within the medulla, which as noted above, can reach as high as 1200 mOsm/L at the tip of the loop and the collecting duct. In the presence of ADH, the collecting ducts become permeable to water. The high osmolality in the medulla promotes water reabsorption by osmosis from the collecting ducts. As a result, in the presence of ADH, a concentrated urine is produced.

In the next section, we will look at how 'fine-tuning' of the filtrate in the distal tubule and collecting duct is regulated by hormones. We look first at how ADH helps regulate plasma osmolality, and then at the role of the renin angiotensin adrenal system in regulating blood pressure.

Regulation of plasma osmolality

We have seen that ADH determines the volume of water lost from the kidney, through increasing the permeability of the collecting ducts. The release of ADH is dependent on the osmolality of the plasma. In effect, ADH works to regulate the osmolality of the plasma, by regulating the volume of water lost from the kidney.

ADH is synthesised in the hypothalamus and released from the posterior pituitary gland. In the kidney, ADH binds to receptors on the cell membrane of cells lining the collecting ducts. This causes specialised water channels called 'aquaporins' to be inserted into the cell membrane which make the collecting duct permeable. Water now moves out of the collecting ducts and into the interstitial space and plasma.

The main stimulus for ADH release is a rise in plasma osmolality (above 285 mOsm/kg). Raised osmolarity is detected by osmoreceptors located in the hypothalamus. Thirst is also triggered by a raised osmolality and should lead to a greater fluid intake from drinking. Dehydration, or an increased sodium intake, can raise plasma osmolality and trigger the release of ADH and the feeling of thirst. The release of ADH works through a negative feedback loop. Once the osmolality returns to the normal (285 mOsm/kg) the stimulus for release is removed and ADH release will reduce/cease.

Activity 14.1 asks you to consider the diuretic effects of alcohol.

Activity 14.1   Critical thinking

You may be aware that alcohol is a diuretic. A diuretic is a substance that increases urine production. Alcohol exerts a diuretic effect through affecting antidiuretic hormone (ADH). From your understanding of ADH suggest two ways alcohol might cause diuresis.

A suggested answer is given at the end of the chapter.

Completing Activity 14.1 should help you to develop your understanding of ADH and therefore of fluid balance. We now look at blood pressure regulation and the role of the renin angiotensin aldosterone system.

Blood pressure regulation

The maintenance of blood pressure is essential for life, relying on an effective volume of circulating blood. The kidney has a very important role in preserving blood volume and therefore blood pressure. Blood volume is regulated by adjusting the body's sodium content. The body's sodium content is a balance between the sodium intake through the diet and the amount of sodium excreted. The kidneys regulate the latter, by excreting more, or less, sodium.

Sodium is the main cation in the plasma and the main contributor to plasma osmolality (Table 14.1). Plasma osmolality, as noted above, is regulated through the reabsorption of more, or less, water from the kidney under the influence of ADH. Therefore, the reabsorption of more sodium by the kidney will increase the osmolality of the plasma. Through the ADH system, a decrease in water loss will return plasma osmolality to normal and increase blood volume. Similarly, if less sodium is reabsorbed by the kidney, plasma osmolality will decrease. Less ADH will be secreted and more water will be excreted from the kidney. The result will be a decrease in blood volume.

The renin–angiotensin–aldosterone system (RAAS) is one of the most important regulators of blood pressure over the long term. We have previously introduced the RAAS in Chapter 8 under 'Drugs used to treat hypertension'. The RAAS is also important as a compensatory mechanism in heart failure, which was also introduced in Chapter 8. RAAS is a regulatory hormone cascade, which starts with the release of renin from the kidney. Several stimuli cause the release of renin. These include a low perfusion pressure in the glomerulus, and a low delivery of sodium to the tubules. Renin is an enzyme which converts the plasma protein angiotensinogen to angiotensin I. Angiotensin I is converted to angiotensin II by angiotensin converting enzyme (ACE). Angiotensin II has a range of effects that help restore circulating volume and blood pressure. These include:

- Increased ADH secretion – increases water reabsorption by the distal tubule and collecting ducts.
- Increased sodium reabsorption in the proximal tubule.
- Aldosterone secretion from the cortex of the adrenal glands.
- Widespread vasoconstriction.

These effects all increase blood pressure and/or blood volume. Aldosterone acts on the distal tubule and medullary collecting ducts to stimulate the reabsorption of sodium and to promote the secretion of potassium. This raises the plasma sodium levels and decreases the plasma potassium level. The increase in sodium increases the volume of the plasma and therefore the blood pressure.

You have now completed this review of the normal functions of the kidney. You will be able to use this knowledge to understand the effects of kidney injury and to understand what the priorities for management are. In the next sections, we therefore move on to examine acute kidney injury.

Acute kidney injury (AKI)

Penny in the case study at the start of this chapter developed AKI following a skiing accident. Acute kidney injury is defined as a sudden decrease in kidney function over hours or days. Tests will show a drop in glomerular filtration rate (GFR) with rapid increases in blood urea and creatinine levels. There is often, but not always, a decrease in urine output. AKI can present in a mild form but in its severest form, renal replacement therapy may be needed.

Acute kidney injury is most often seen in patients who are in hospital for a separate serious condition. It is usually reversible or partially reversible, but some patients may experience long-term consequences including chronic kidney disease (Woodward and Oliveira, 2017). Acute kidney injury occurs in around 13–18% of all those admitted to hospital. It can affect any age group, although older adults are more likely to be affected. The focus for AKI is on early intervention with a focus on risk assessment, early recognition and treatment.

Acute kidney injury is classified into three stages based upon GFR, serum creatinine concentration and urine output. The current consensus classification is the Kidney Disease: Improving Global Outcomes (KDIGO) (Woodward and Oliveira, 2017).

The following criteria are used to define stage 1 acute kidney injury:

- A rise in serum creatinine of 26 μmol/L or greater within 48 hours.
- A 50% or greater rise in serum creatinine known or presumed to have occurred within the past 7 days.
- A fall in urine output to less than 0.5 ml/kg/hour for more than 6 hours in adults and more than 8 hours in children and young people.
- A 25% or greater fall in eGFR in children and young people within the past 7 days.

Stages 2 and 3 are detailed in NICE (2013c).

The rapid rise in serum creatinine is the direct consequence of a drop in glomerular filtration rate. The relationship between serum creatinine and GFR was described in the box above on glomerular filtration rate. The fall in urine output will also reflect a drop in GFR.

The causes (or aetiology) of acute kidney injury are classified by mechanism into three groups:

1. **Prerenal:** ('before the kidney') any cause of a decreased blood supply to the kidneys – these account for around 35% of AKI cases.
2. **Intrarenal (renal or intrinsic):** ('within the kidney') any injury that lies within the kidney itself – these account for around 45% of cases.
3. **Postrenal:** ('after the kidney') any cause of obstruction to the passage of urine from the kidney to the outflow through the urethra to outside world (20%) (Figure 14.1, above).

The categorisation by cause of acute renal injury helps the professional care team choose the most appropriate treatment. Most cases of AKI in the hospital setting involve a combination of prerenal and renal factors. This produces a pattern of injury known as acute tubular necrosis.

We will look at the three types of causes in turn.

1. Prerenal

Table 14. 3 shows some of the main prerenal causes of AKI.

Prerenal causes of AKI are those that affect renal blood flow (perfusion). As described above, the blood supply to the kidney is high (around 20% cardiac output). This is necessary to maintain the glomerular filtration rates needed for kidney function. Any reduction in blood flow to the kidney will produce a reduced GFR and a decreased urine output. The blood flow to the kidneys is carefully regulated under normal physiological conditions. This is called renal autoregulation. Some drugs which can interfere with this mechanism of autoregulation are mentioned in Table 14.3.

Causes	Examples
Volume depletion	Haemorrhage (trauma, surgery, postpartum)
	Diarrhoea or vomiting (leading to dehydration)
	Burns
Reduced effective circulating volume (actual volume is not lost but circulation is reduced or inappropriately distributed)	Heart failure
	Cardiogenic shock
	Sepsis
	Liver cirrhosis
Renal hypoperfusion	Renal artery stenosis
	Embolism or thrombosis of renal artery or vein
Drugs (alter renal autoregulation – see text)	NSAIDS
	ACE inhibitors; angiotensin II receptor blockers (ARBs)

Table 14.3　Main causes of prerenal acute kidney injury

Data from Woodward and Oliveira, 2017; Rennke and Denker, 2014.

Drugs that affect renal autoregulation

The blood flow to each glomerulus is maintained in normal circumstances within a narrow range despite changes to renal artery blood pressure. This maintenance of a relatively constant blood flow despite changes to blood pressure is called autoregulation. Autoregulation ensures that glomerular filtration rate is constant over a range of renal artery pressures.

The blood flow to the glomerulus is from the afferent arteriole (Figures 14.2 and 14.3, above). Blood leaves the glomerulus via the efferent arteriole. Constriction of the afferent arteriole decreases the pressure in the glomerulus and decreases the filtration pressure and the GFR. Conversely, constriction of the efferent arteriole increases the pressure in the glomerulus and increases filtration pressure and GFR.

NSAIDS can interfere with the autoregulation of the kidney. Prostaglandins whose production is inhibited by NSAIDS (Chapter 6) cause vasodilation of the afferent arteriole. In healthy individuals the effect of prostaglandins on maintaining renal blood flow is minimal. However, in those with volume depletion, such as heart failure or dehydration, the vasodilatory effect from prostaglandins is essential for maintaining GFR by increasing blood flow to the glomerulus. NSAIDS should be avoided in anyone with renal impairment or reduced circulating volume.

Angiotensin II normally causes vasoconstriction of the efferent arteriole. This, as described, increases the filtration pressure and promotes glomerular filtration. ACE inhibitors and angiotensin II receptor blockers prevent efferent arteriole vasoconstriction. This reduces blood flow to the glomerulus which can induce prerenal acute kidney injury in certain settings.

In most circumstances a reduced blood flow to the kidney can be reversed without causing permanent damage to the cells of the kidney. Prerenal causes are often 'volume responsive' and kidney function can be improved or resolved with appropriate fluid resuscitation. However, a significantly decreased blood flow to the kidneys (20–25%) will result in ischaemic injury. The cells become hypoxic because of the ischaemia (low blood supply) and may die or be permanently damaged. Ischaemic injury from a low blood supply is one of the causes of renal (intrinsic) AKI – which is discussed next.

2. Renal (intrinsic)

Table 14.4 shows the main causes of renal AKI.

Cause	Example
Ischaemic injury	Any cause reducing renal perfusion (see prerenal causes above)
Nephrotoxic injury	Endogenous toxins (produced by body cells) – massive haemolysis (breakdown of red blood cells); massive tumour lysis; rhabdomyolysis (breakdown of muscle)
	Exogenous toxins – antibiotics (especially aminoglycosides), chemotherapy agents, e.g. cisplatinum, radiocontrast agents, bacterial endotoxins
Immune-mediated injury	Antibodies and immune complexes can damage the glomerulus of the nephrons
	Systemic lupus erythematosus
Vascular disease	Vasculitis
	Atheroemboli to the kidney

Table 14.4   Main causes of renal (intrinsic) acute kidney injury

Data from Woodward and Oliveira, 2017; Rennke and Denker, 2014.

Renal causes of acute kidney injury involve actual damage to the kidney tissue. As can be seen from Table 14.4 injury is often divided according to the location of injury: glomerular, tubular, blood vessel or interstitium. Acute tubular necrosis is one of the major causes of intrinsic injury and results from ischaemia and/or nephrotoxicity.

3. Postrenal

A number of abnormalities can cause obstruction to the lower urinary tract and cause postrenal injury. These include:

- The presence of a tumour, for example compressing the ureter, urethra or bladder outflow.
- Renal stones (renal calculus).

- Blood clot.
- Enlarged prostate (men).

Obstruction can be full or partial. Complete obstruction is likely to cause *anuria* – a cessation of urine output. Partial obstruction may present with symptoms of difficulty voiding urine (needing to strain, or hesitancy and poor stream). Obstruction of urine outflow will in turn increase pressure in the Bowman's capsule and oppose glomerular filtration. As a result, GFR will reduce with consequent adverse effects on kidney function.

Clinical features of acute kidney injury

A patient with AKI may present with non-specific symptoms such as nausea and lethargy. They may have a history of decreased urine output. Depending upon the severity, the patient may develop fluid overload (oedema and hypertension), electrolyte imbalances, acid–base disturbances and a build-up of toxic (uraemic) wastes. Raised potassium (hyperkalaemia), fluid overload and metabolic acidosis can be life-threatening. Severe hyperkalaemia can cause arrhythmia and can lead to cardiac arrest.

These presentations represent the loss of significant kidney function and will be discussed further, in the context of chronic kidney disease, below.

Activity 14.2   Critical thinking

You have seen that hypovolaemia is a potential cause of acute kidney injury. Nurses have a pivotal role in recognising a patient with hypovolaemia. How would you recognise potential hypovolaemia during your assessment of a patient's vital signs?

A suggested answer is given at the end of the chapter.

We now move onto examining the pharmacological management of AKI.

Pharmacological management of acute kidney injury

There are few pharmacological therapies used in acute kidney injury. Supportive treatment is given in an attempt to maintain fluid balance, treat electrolyte disturbances and maintain acid–base balance. The treatment given will depend on the cause and stage of AKI.

Fluid management

In some cases, fluid replacement therapy might be needed, especially if the cause is hypovolaemia – for example, the case study of Penny. A blood transfusion might be necessary. Intravenous fluids – for example normal saline, might also be used.

In other cases, the body might become overloaded with fluid leading to oedema as the kidneys fail to excrete fluids. In these cases the loop diuretic furosemide might be useful. It is called a loop diuretic because it acts on the loop of Henle in the kidney. Specifically, furosemide inhibits the active transport of sodium, chloride and potassium from the ascending limb of the loop. The reduction in sodium (and chloride) removal from the ascending loop decreases the osmotic 'salt' gradient in the medulla (Figure 14.4). This, in turn, reduces the volume of water that is reabsorbed from the collecting ducts. As a result, more water is excreted in urine. Important side effects include hypokalaemia which occurs if too much potassium is lost in the urine. Also if the volume loss is too great, dehydration leading to hypotension and shock may occur.

Renal replacement therapy

In some cases, supportive therapies fail to control the consequences of AKI. For example, the potassium level may continue to rise, or the patient has life-threatening fluid overload despite diuretics. In such cases renal replacement therapy may be needed to take over the role of the failing kidneys (NICE, 2013c). There are different types of renal replacement therapy. For example, in continuous veno-venous haemodialysis an extracorporeal circuit is formed which means the patient's blood is passed through a dialysis machine and then back into the patient (Gemmell et al., 2017). The machine removes excess water and solutes from the blood, correcting electrolyte abnormalities and restoring acid–base balance. The hope is that the patient will recover some kidney function and will not need renal replacement in the long term but some patients will need long-term dialysis or a renal transplant after AKI.

Medicines review and kidney injury

Some medication can make AKI worse. Examples are NSAIDs, diuretics and antihypertensive medication. All these drugs can potentially reduce blood flow to the kidney and consideration should be given to stopping these in patients with suspected AKI. Drugs that are excreted by the kidney will also accumulate in AKI, for example opioids where accumulation can lead to respiratory depression. These drugs may need to be stopped or the dosage reduced. It is also important to consider whether the patient has started any new nephrotoxic drugs which could be causing the AKI. These should be reviewed or stopped. More information about problematic medication and many aspects of AKI can be found at the 'Think kidney' website given at the end of the chapter.

Chronic kidney disease (CKD)

Scenario

Kate is a 33-year-old woman who has just registered at the GP practice where you are a student on clinical placement. You attend Kate's appointment with the advanced clinical practitioner. Kate has no specific symptoms.

On examination, Kate is pale, has hypertension (BP 180/105 mmHg) with blood and protein in her urine. Retinopathy is present bilaterally. A subsequent renal ultrasound shows small, non-obstructive kidneys.

Blood investigations show:

- Haemoglobin: 85 g/L
- Urea: 18.0 mmol/L
- Creatinine: 310 μmol/L; eGFR = 20 mL/min/1.73 m²

Chronic kidney disease is a gradual and often progressive loss of renal function. NICE (2014c) describes chronic kidney disease as 'common and frequently unrecognised, and often exists together with other conditions (such as cardiovascular disease and diabetes)'.

Kate in the case study above has stage 4 chronic kidney disease. Stage 4 CKD represents a severe decrease in kidney function. Despite this, Kate had no specific symptoms and her kidney disease was picked up through a routine appointment. Kate's kidney disease is likely to be due to hypertension. Without further intervention it is likely that Kate will progress to end-stage renal disease (ESRD) and require renal replacement therapy.

CKD can result from any disease affecting the kidney including systemic conditions like hypertension and diabetes. Currently in the UK, the three main causes of CKD are:

- diabetes
- hypertension
- glomerulonephritis.

Other causes include:

- chronic pyelonephritis
- polycystic kidney disease
- renovascular disease.

For a more extensive list please see Woodward and Oliveira (2017).

Despite the high prevalence of CKD only a minority of those with CKD will progress to end-stage renal disease (ESRD). The majority of patients with CKD will be identified and managed within the primary care setting. Early identification and management of CKD are important to prevent or delay progression to ESRD, and to minimise complications.

As described, CKD is often asymptomatic in its early stages. NICE (2014c) recommends testing eGFR and ACR (albumin:creatinine ratio) in those in the following risk factors:

- Diabetes.
- Hypertension.
- Cardiovascular disease.
- Structural renal tract abnormalities, renal calculi and prostatic hypertrophy.
- Multisystem disease with potential kidney involvement, e.g. systemic lupus erythematosus.
- Family history of stage 5 CKD or hereditary kidney disease.
- Opportunistic detection of haematuria.
- Regular use of nephrotoxic drugs (e.g. lithium, NSAIDS).

Albumin:creatinine ratio (ACR) is a sensitive test of proteinuria (protein in the urine) and is suggestive of certain types of renal damage such as diabetic nephropathy.

A diagnosis of chronic kidney disease is made by establishing a chronic reduction in kidney function and/or structural damage to the kidney. The nature of the kidney damage is often ascertained following biopsy. A definition of CKD is glomerular filtration rate less than 60 mL/min/1.73 m² or markers of kidney damage, or both, of at least three months duration.

CKD is classified into five stages (Table 14.5).

Stage	Description	eGFR (ml/min)
1	Normal or increased GRF with other evidence of kidney damage	> 90
2	Slight decrease in GRF with other evidence of kidney damage	60–89
3a	Moderate decrease in GRF, with or without other evidence of kidney damage	45–59
3b		30–44
4	Severe decrease in GRF, with or without other evidence of kidney damage	15–29
5	End-stage renal disease	< 15

Table 14.5 Stages of chronic kidney disease

See NICE (2014c)

Clinical presentation of chronic kidney disease

The early stages (1–3b) of kidney disease are usually asymptomatic. It is likely that CKD will only be picked up if eGFR is measured in patients known to be at risk, for example, those with diabetes, or hypertension. The list above, from NICE (2014c), gives the risk factors for which renal testing is recommended.

The kidney has considerable renal reserve and maintains GFR in the early stages of renal disease, despite injury and nephron loss. GFR is maintained through increased filtration and enlargement of the remaining nephrons. However, these adaptations lead to further nephron loss and disease progression (Woodward and Oliveira, 2017).

As the disease progresses patients can develop non-specific symptoms such as tiredness, lethargy, weight-loss and nausea. These are due in part to the build-up of toxic metabolic wastes in the body which have not been excreted. The build-up of metabolic wastes is called uraemia and the resultant symptoms called uraemic symptoms.

Further reduction in GRF can lead to salt and water retention, acid retention, raised serum potassium (hyperkalaemia) and raised serum phosphate (hyperphosphataemia). Other major complications include anaemia, mineral bone disease and cardiovascular disease. The major complications are given in Table 14.6 and discussed below.

Abnormality	Pathophysiological effect	Clinical presentation
Abnormal excretory function	Fluid retention	Hypertension
		Peripheral oedema
		Pulmonary oedema
	Potassium retention	Hyperkalaemia
		Arrhythmia
	Acid retention	Metabolic acidosis
	Phosphate retention	Hyperphosphataemia
Decreased synthesis erythropoietic	Impaired erythropoiesis	Tiredness
		Left ventricular hypertrophy
Decreased production active vitamin D (calcitriol)	Hypocalcaemia	Bone pain
	Increased parathyroid hormone	Osteomalacia
		Osteitis fibrosa
		Fractures
Cardiovascular disease	Increased risk of atherosclerosis (see text) leading to stroke, myocardial infarction	Symptoms may include: chest pain, breathlessness, dizziness, nausea

Table 14.6 Major complications of chronic kidney disease

Modified from Woodward and Oliveira (2017).

Fluid and electrolyte retention

Sodium levels are normally maintained within normal levels until late-stage disease (stage 5). Compensatory mechanisms – which include increased excretion of sodium – can help prevent excessive sodium levels. However, activation of the RAAS, along with a decline in kidney function, may lead to water and sodium retention in late-stage disease.

Sodium and water retention can lead to oedema, hypertension and heart failure. Salt restriction can help with fluid overload, but a diuretic may be needed.

Potassium retention in late-stage disease is a potentially life-threatening complication. Dietary restriction of potassium can help prevent hyperkalaemia along with the avoidance of potassium-sparing drugs.

Calcium and phosphate are described under bone and mineral disease, below.

Anaemia

Anaemia is a common complication of CKD and is largely due to impaired red blood cell production (erythropoiesis) due to reduction in synthesis of erythropoietin from a damaged kidney. Other factors may be present such as malnutrition, iron deficiency and hyperparathyroidism.

The activity below asks you to identify whether Kate – in the earlier case study – has anaemia.

Activity 14.3   Critical thinking

Kate, in the case study at the start of the section on chronic kidney disease, has a haemoglobin level of 85 g/L.

Does she have anaemia?

What symptoms does anaemia produce? What treatment might be offered?

A suggested answer is given at the end of the chapter. The treatment of anaemia is discussed below under 'Pharmacological management of chronic kidney disease'.

Following Activity 14.3 on anaemia, we look at two further complications of CKD: bone and mineral disease and cardiovascular disease.

Bone and mineral disease

These are a common complication of CKD even in the early stages. Changes to bone are initially asymptomatic but bone pain and fractures can occur in late-stage disease (Table 14.6). The main mineral in bone is calcium phosphate ($CaPO_4$). Free ionised calcium (Ca^{2+}) and phosphate (PO_4^{2-}) are present in the plasma and come originally from the diet. Calcium ions are the most abundant ions in the body and have roles in muscle contraction, nerve impulses and cell signalling. The bone provides a store of both calcium and phosphate ions. The level of calcium in the plasma must be carefully regulated. Excess calcium, not absorbed in bone, is normally excreted by the kidneys.

The levels of plasma calcium and phosphate are regulated by parathyroid hormone (PTH) and active vitamin D. In response to low plasma calcium levels, the parathyroid glands release PTH. PTH increases the level of plasma calcium in the following ways:

- Release of calcium and phosphate from bone. (This is called bone resorption.) This occurs in the presence of active vitamin D.
- Promoting the synthesis of active vitamin D (calcitriol) by the kidney. Calcitriol stimulates the absorption of calcium and phosphate from the gut.
- Promoting reabsorption of calcium in the proximal tubule of the kidney.

PTH also promotes phosphate excretion by the kidney by decreasing the reabsorption from the distal tubule. However, this effect is balanced by release of phosphate from bone and increased reabsorption from the gut (Rennke and Denker, 2013).

Active vitamin D (calcitriol) has the following effects on calcium and phosphate metabolism:

- It stimulates the absorption of calcium and phosphate from the gut.
- It promotes the release of calcium and phosphate from bone (bone resorption) in the presence of PTH.
- It may decrease urinary calcium and phosphate excretion.

In chronic kidney disease, mineral bone disease can present as abnormalities in calcium, phosphate, parathyroid hormone, or vitamin D metabolism (Webster et al., 2017). Phosphate retention is common and reflects the reduction in GFR (a reduced ability to filter and therefore excrete phosphate). CKD is associated with raised PTH levels. The reasons for this raised level are unclear but may be in response to reductions in calcitriol. Enhanced PTH causes increased bone resorption. This in turn causes the characteristic bone and mineral disease of CKD and contributes to the raised plasma phosphate levels (Table 14.6). Hypocalcaemia results from diminished production of vitamin D by the damaged kidney which reduces calcium absorption from the gut and from increased phosphate levels which sequester the calcium.

Cardiovascular complications

Cardiovascular complications are a serious and common complication of all stages of CKD. Patients with chronic kidney disease are more likely to have one or more traditional risk factors, such as diabetes and hypertension. In addition, patients have non-traditional risk factors of anaemia, disorders of calcium and phosphorous metabolism, and increased chronic low-grade inflammation. These factors increase the rate of atherosclerosis which can lead to various cardiovascular diseases, such as myocardial infarction and stroke (Chapter 8).

In late-stage kidney disease (stages 4–5) symptoms of uraemia worsen, and the patient is likely to experience anorexia, nausea and vomiting, itching, and neuromuscular symptoms such as restless legs. At this stage renal replacement therapy may be needed. For further information on late-stage disease and renal replacement therapy, please see the Further reading section.

Pharmacological management of chronic kidney disease

As we have seen from the pathophysiology, impaired kidney function can cause widespread complications. Treatments are aimed at rectifying these abnormalities, for example treating anaemia and normalising phosphate, calcium and vitamin D levels. Once damage is done it cannot be reversed. It is however important that steps are taken to prevent the CKD getting worse and treatment of cardiovascular risk is important. We will look at all these in this part of the chapter.

Management of risk factors

Complete Activity 14.4 which concerns Rasool who has CKD.

Activity 14.4   Critical thinking

Rasool has chronic kidney disease. He was seen in clinic for an annual review of his renal function. His glomerular filtration rate is 51 ml/min/1.73 m² which is considered a mild to moderate reduction and his albumin creatinine ratio is 5 which is considered moderately increased (NICE, 2014c). Before his diagnosis he had hypertension but his blood pressure is now controlled by Losartan at 131/82 mm/Hg. He has diabetes but this is also well-controlled. He used to smoke but gave that up after his diagnosis. He also uses ibuprofen gel for knee pain.

Before diagnosis Rasool had a number of risk factors for progression of CKD. What are they?

Is there any advice you would give Rasool about his current medication?

A suggested answer is given at the end of the chapter.

As we can see from the Activity 14.4, hypertension, diabetes and smoking are all risk factors which can increase the likelihood that the CKD will get worse; it is therefore important that hypertension and diabetes are managed, and smoking cessation supported. These factors all increase the risk of progression of CKD and/or the risk of cardiovascular disease. Chronic use of NSAIDs (See Chapter 6) can also lead to progression of CKD and these drugs should be avoided.

Secondary prevention of cardiovascular disease

As we saw in Chapter 8 statins and antiplatelet drugs are used to help prevent cardiovascular disease in those at risk. Patients with CKD are often prescribed a statin such as atorvastatin and an antiplatelet such as aspirin. As CKD progresses, bleeding time is prolonged and patients are more likely to bleed with an antiplatelet, so this needs to be monitored. It is also important to treat hypertension. In general ACE inhibitors or angiotensin receptor blockers (Chapter 8) are the drugs of choice, especially in diabetes or where proteinuria is present, as they reduce progression of CKD and reduce proteinuria.

Treatment of complications

Anaemia

A patient is at risk of anaemia if their eGFR falls below 45 ml/min/1.73 m². Anaemia is monitored by measuring the haemoglobin and a low haemoglobin concentration indicates anaemia. As we have seen, the kidneys produce a hormone called erythropoietin that stimulates red blood cell production in the bone marrow. As kidney disease progresses, the production of this hormone decreases leading to anaemia. Erythropoietin stimulating agents (ESA), also called epoetins, are used in place of the body's natural erythropoietin to stimulate red blood cell formation. Examples of epoetins are Darbepoetin alfa, Epoetin alfa and Epoetin beta. No epoetin has been proved to be more effective than any other and the choice of agent depends on cost, dialysis status and local availability.

Increased bleeding and reduced absorption of iron may also occur in CKD. Iron is needed for haemoglobin synthesis and red blood cell formation. If iron levels are low this is treated with ferrous sulphate until they return to normal. Patients on dialysis often receive IV iron as this replenishes stores more rapidly.

Treatment of anaemia improves patient symptoms such as fatigue, weakness, depression and dizziness. It also reduces cardiovascular mortality.

Side-effects and implications for practice

In some patients epoetins increase blood pressure causing hypertension or make existing hypertension worse. Epoetins can also suddenly increase blood pressure to a very high level even in patients with a normal blood pressure. This is called a hypertensive emergency and can be life-threatening. It is important that haemoglobin levels are monitored during treatment and that anaemia is not over treated. If haemoglobin levels are too high the patient is more at risk from cardiovascular diseases such as stroke and myocardial infarction. Some people are resistant to epoetins and they may need blood transfusions to treat anaemia instead.

Epoetins are usually administered subcutaneously and patients may self-administer. If a patient is on dialysis they can be given intravenously at the same time as the dialysis. The dosage interval varies. Darbepoetin, for example, is given once every one or two weeks. Epoetin alfa is given three times a week.

Bone and mineral disease

CKD leads to imbalances in calcium, phosphate, parathyroid hormone and vitamin D levels. If these are left untreated the strength and growth of bones can be adversely affected. Calcification of soft tissues can also occur. Bone and mineral disease are a frequent complication of late-stage disease.

Vitamin D

The kidneys play an important part in transforming inactive vitamin D to active vitamin D (calcitriol). As CKD progresses the amount of active vitamin D falls and supplements are needed. If vitamin D deficiency was left untreated hypocalcaemia would result. Vitamin D deficiency in severe renal impairment is treated with alfacalcidol or calcitriol (BNF, 2018). These are active forms of vitamin D which do not need metabolism by the kidneys to be activated. Treatment can help correct calcium levels (reverse hypocalcaemia) and prevent secondary hyperparathyroidism.

Side-effects and implications for practice

Vitamin D can cause hypercalcaemia, increase cardiovascular risk and cause vascular calcification (NICE, 2014c).

Phosphate binders

As CKD progresses, phosphate levels rise. It is important that patients reduce their dietary intake of phosphate. Foods rich in phosphate include oily fish and dairy products. Patients also need phosphate binders to reduce the amount of phosphate absorbed from the GI tract. Examples of phosphate binders include calcium acetate, sevelamer and lanthanum.

Side-effects and Implications for practice

Calcium acetate can increase calcium levels. This can be useful if a patient's calcium levels are low. However, it can also cause hypercalcaemia. Sevelamer and lanthanum do not increase calcium levels; lanthanum can in fact cause hypocalcaemia. Side-effects of lanthanum and sevelamer include abdominal pain, constipation or diarrhoea, nausea and vomiting, dyspepsia and flatulence.

Renal replacement therapies

As CKD progresses the use of drugs and dietary restriction alone is not enough to control the accumulation of metabolic wastes and fluid in the body. A patient will need renal replacement therapy. These include dialysis (renal dialysis or peritoneal dialysis) or a kidney transplant. For more information on these topics visit the suggested reading at the end of the chapter.

Other medicines issues to consider in patients with CKD

There are important considerations in prescribing drugs for patients with renal impairment. The doses of some drugs need to be reduced. This is the case if a drug or an active metabolite is excreted by the kidney (Chapter 1). The BNF often gives information about the doses of drugs used in renal impairment.

Some people with renal impairment may also become more sensitive to the side-effects of drugs such as codeine, antihistamines and benzodiazepines.

As described above, hyperkalaemia can occur in CKD. Drugs which cause hyperkalaemia as a side-effect can further increase hyperkalaemia. Such drugs include potassium sparing diuretics, ACE inhibitors, angiotensin receptor blockers, NSAIDs and trimethoprim.

It is now time to review what you have learned within this chapter by undertaking some multiple choice questions.

Activity 14.5　Multiple choice questions

1. The kidney tubules carry out which three processes?
   a) Filtration, reabsorption, excretion
   b) Filtration, reabsorption, secretion
   c) Filtration, secretion, excretion
   d) Filtration, autoregulation, reabsorption

2. Which of the following electrolytes is responsible for plasma osmolality?
   a) Sodium
   b) Potassium
   c) Calcium
   d) Phosphate

3. Which of the following hormones regulates plasma osmolarity?
   a) Renin
   b) Aldosterone
   c) ADH
   d) Angiotensin II

4. An enlarged prostate may cause which of the following kidney disorders?

    a) Prerenal acute kidney injury
    b) Intrinsic acute kidney injury
    c) Postrenal acute kidney injury
    d) Chronic kidney disease

5. Which of the following complications of chronic kidney disease is due to a reduction in hormone secretion from the kidney?

    a) Anaemia
    b) Fluid overload
    c) Hyperkalaemia
    d) Itching

6. Which of the following statements is true for the treatment of chronic kidney disease?

    a) Treatments help to reverse the damage to the kidneys
    b) Treatments can help to maintain homeostasis and improve symptoms
    c) Treatments completely stop further deterioration of the kidneys
    d) Treatments are placebos only

7. Erythropoetin stimulating agents help to correct anaemia by:

    a) Stimulation of red blood cell production
    b) Replenishing stores of iron in the body
    c) Increasing absorption of iron in the gastrointestinal tract
    d) Increasing the effectiveness of haemoglobin

8. Which vitamin supplement may be needed in patients with CKD?

    a) Vitamin A
    b) Vitamin C
    c) Vitamin D
    d) Vitamin E

9. Other medication that might be useful to help prevent chronic kidney disease includes:

    a) Phosphates
    b) NSAIDs
    c) Antibiotics
    d) Antihypertensives

10. Patients with kidney disease may need to reduce the dose of some medication because:

    a) Absorption of drugs will be increased
    b) Distribution of drugs will be increased
    c) Metabolism of drugs will be increased
    d Excretion of drugs will be increased

Chapter summary

The kidney is responsible for maintaining the homeostasis of the extracellular fluid (ECF). This includes fluid and electrolyte balance, and acid–base balance. The kidney maintains the ECF homeostasis through filtering the plasma. The filtering units of the kidney are called nephrons. Each nephron is a microscopic tubule. The filtrate is modified as it passes along the nephron through the processes of tubular reabsorption and tubular secretion. Ninety-nine per cent of the filtrate is returned to the plasma through tubular reabsorption. Fine-tuning of the filtrate which occurs mostly in the proximal tubule enables the pH, fluid and electrolyte balance of the plasma to be maintained in homeostasis. Much of the fine-tuning of the filtrate is under hormonal control and ensures the excretion of excess water and electrolytes through tubular secretion and/or reabsorption.

Acute kidney injury is a sudden drop in glomerular filtration rate. There are three mechanisms producing AKI: pre-renal, renal and postrenal. Prerenal kidney injury is the most common and arises through any mechanism affecting renal perfusion. AKI causes disturbances to homeostasis of the ECF. This may present as non-specific symptoms such as nausea and lethargy. There is often a history of decreased urine output. Depending upon the severity, fluid overload (oedema and hypertension), electrolyte imbalances, acid–base disturbances and a build-up of toxic (uraemic) wastes may develop. Raised potassium (hyperkalaemia), fluid overload and metabolic acidosis can be life-threatening. Severe hyperkalaemia can cause arrhythmia and can lead to cardiac arrest.

Chronic kidney disease can result from any condition affecting kidney function. Currently, in the UK, diabetes, hypertension and glomerulonephritis are the most common causes of CKD. All kidney disease can progress to end-stage renal failure when renal replacement therapy is needed.

Activities: Brief outline answers

Activity 14.1 Critical thinking (p383)

Alcohol could in theory reduce ADH secretion from the posterior pituitary gland – that is, it could be centrally acting. Alternatively, it could block the binding of ADH to its receptors on the collecting duct – that is, it could act peripherally. Alcohol is known to act centrally to reduce the circulating levels of ADH.

Activity 14.2 Critical thinking (p388)

A patient with hypovolaemia may have the following signs:

- Low blood pressure
- Postural hypotension
- Tachycardia

- Loss of skin turgor
- Dry mucus membranes

The patient may report thirst, dizziness and weakness. There may have been a recent history of vomiting, diarrhoea or poor fluid intake, or major bleeding (Woodward and Oliveira, 2017).

Activity 14.3 Critical thinking (p393)

Kate has a haemoglobin level of 85 g/L which indicates anaemia. The normal range is 115–155 g/L in women. Anaemia in chronic kidney disease is diagnosed if haemoglobin is below 110 gL (NICE, 2015). The symptoms of anaemia may include: tiredness, shortness of breath, lethargy, palpitations. Depending upon the cause, anaemia in CKD may be treated with erythropoietic stimulating agents. See 'Treatments for complications', above.

Activity 14.4 Critical thinking (p395)

Smoking, diabetes and hypertension are all risk factors for chronic renal disease and cardiovascular disease.

You might want to advise Rasool to stop the ibuprofen gel and use an alternative such as paracetamol or physiotherapy depending on the cause of the knee pain. NSAIDs can worsen CKD. Even though this drug is being given topically some of the drug will still be absorbed systemically.

Activity 14.5 Multiple choice questions (pp398–9)

1. The kidney tubules carry out which three processes?

    b) Filtration, reabsorption, secretion

2. Which of the following electrolytes is responsible for plasma osmolality?

    a) Sodium

3. Which of the following hormones regulates plasma osmolarity?

    c) ADH

4. An enlarged prostate may cause which of the following kidney disorders?

    c) Postrenal acute kidney injury

5. Which of the following complications of chronic kidney disease is due to a reduction in hormone secretion from the kidney?

    a) Anaemia

6. Which of the following statements is true for the treatment of chronic kidney disease?

    b) Treatments can help to maintain homeostasis and improve symptoms

7. Erythropoetin stimulating agents help to correct anaemia by:

    a) Stimulation of red blood cell production

8. Which vitamin supplement may be needed in patients with CKD?

    c) Vitamin D

9. Other medication that might be useful to help prevent chronic kidney disease includes:

    d) Antihypertensives

10. Patients with kidney disease may need to reduce the dose of some medication because:

    d) Excretion of drugs will be increased

Further reading

Lote, C (2012) *Principles of Renal Physiology* (5th edition). Berlin: Springer.

A clearly written textbook covering the principles of normal renal physiology.

Woodward, S and Oliveira, D (2017) *Renal Medicine.* London: JP Medical.

This is a very useful and clearly written introduction to both biomedical principles and clinical applications. Primarily designed for medical students but useful to nursing students wanting further information of both the science and clinical applications.

Useful websites

The following NICE websites provide guidance on the assessment and management of CKD.

www.nice.org.uk/guidance/ng8/

NICE (2015) *Chronic Kidney Disease. Managing Anaemia.*

https://cks.nice.org.uk/chronic-kidney-disease-not-diabetic#!scenariorecommendation:5/

NICE (2016) *Clinical Knowledge Summary. Chronic Kidney Disease – Not Diabetic.*

www.nhs.uk/conditions/dialysis/

For more information on dialysis.

www.thinkkidneys.nhs.uk/aki/wp-content/uploads/sites/2/2016/07/Primary-Care-Advice-for-medication-review-in-AKI-.pdf/

For information on acute kidney injury including problematic drugs.

Glossary

acid–base balance: the balance between acidic and basic (alkaline) compounds in the blood. The acid–base balance of blood is maintained between pH 7.35 and 7.45. This is essential for health.

acidosis: low pH of blood.

action potential: a momentary change in electrical charge across a cell membrane. It results in an electric current which creates the nerve impulse which flows along the **neurone**.

adaptive immune response: part of the immune response mediated by B- and T-lymphocytes.

adrenergic receptor: membrane protein that binds and responds to neurotransmitters noradrenaline and adrenaline.

agonist: substance that binds to a receptor and stimulates a response.

allergen: a substance that causes an allergic reaction.

analgesia: relief from pain.

analgesics: any group of drugs used to achieve **analgesia**, relief from pain.

aneurysm: a localised widening or 'bulge' of a blood vessel wall.

antagonist: substance that binds to a receptor without causing a response.

antigen: a substance that stimulates the production of antibodies.

atheroma: a fatty deposit in the wall of an artery. It is also referred to as a fatty plaque.

atherosclerosis: a disease of the arteries in which fatty plaques build up inside the artery walls.

autoimmune: a disease which is caused by the immune response targeting its own body tissues.

autonomic nervous system: part of the nervous system responsible for controlling the internal organs and is involved in many aspects of homeostasis.

bactericidal: an antibacterial which acts to kill bacteria.

bacteriostatic: an antibacterial which acts to inhibit growth.

beta adrenergic receptor: cell membrane receptor that can bind with drugs/chemicals that activate or block the action of cells which increase heart rate and force of contraction of the heart as well as relaxing bronchi and vascular smooth muscle.

blood–brain barrier: a highly selective barrier that separates the circulating blood from the brain and spinal cord. It acts to protect the central nervous system from potentially harmful chemicals.

broad spectrum: a term applied to antibacterials indicating they act against a wide range of bacteria.

bronchoconstriction: reduction in the diameter of the bronchial tubes in the lungs.

bronchodilation: increase in the diameter of the bronchial tubes in the lungs.

cardiac output: the volume of blood pumped out of the ventricles each minute.

cell body: part of a neurone containing the cell nucleus.

cellular respiration: a set of chemical reactions taking place inside the cells, in which energy from nutrients is used to make adenosine triphosphate (ATP) molecules.

ciliated epithelium: a tissue which lines the airways containing tiny hair-like structure called cilia. The cilia move in one direction to remove mucus and trapped dust particles from the lungs.

clone: a group of genetically identical cells which originate by cell division of one parent cell.

complement: asset of plasma proteins which help fight infection as part of the innate immune response.

corticosteroid: a group of chemicals including the steroid hormones produced by the adrenal cortex, and synthetic analogues used as medicines.

cytokine: a small protein that affects the behavior of other cells.

descending modulation: the **modulation** of pain at the dorsal horn in the **spinal cord** from nerve fibres coming from the brain.

dorsal horn: an area of the spinal cord that receives the nerve endings of sensory neurones, present at all levels of the spinal cord.

dorsal root ganglion: swelling in a spinal nerve containing the cell bodies of sensory neurones that bring information from the periphery into the spinal cord.

endogenous: substances or processes that originate from within the body.

endorphin: endogenous opioids produced by the central nervous system.

enzyme: a chemical, usually a protein, which speeds up a chemical reaction.

eukaryotic: any organism whose cells contain a nucleus and other organelles enclosed within membranes.

exhalation: breathing out (removing air from the lungs).

exudate: fluid with a high protein content leaking out of a capillary because of injury or inflammation.

fatty streak: the first visible lesion in atherosclerosis.

fight or flight response: a physiological response which occurs in response to a perceived harmful event, attack or threat to survival. It physiologically prepares us to 'fight' or 'take flight'. It involves activation of the sympathetic nervous system.

first pass metabolism: the metabolism by the intestine and liver of a drug taken orally which affects the amount that enters the general circulation.

formulate: put together according to a **formulation**.

formulation: the way different ingredients, including a drug, are combined to make a medicine which can be taken by a patient. Different formulations include tablets, liquids and injections for example.

gas exchange: the exchange of oxygen and carbon dioxide between the blood and the lungs, or the blood and the internal tissues.

glucocorticoid: any corticosteroid that is involved in glucose metabolism and has anti-inflammatory effects.

growth factor: a chemical, usually a protein, which signals to a cell to cause a response, usually cell division.

hematopoietic stem cell: the stem cells in the bone marrow which give rise to all the blood cells.

hormone: chemical messenger which travels in the blood from an endocrine cell to its target receptor.

hyperlipidaemia: raised levels of lipids (fats) in the blood.

hypersensitivity: a set of immune responses which cause damage to the body. Damage can be mild, severe or even fatal.

hypertension: raised blood pressure.

hypertrophy: an enlargement of an organ or tissue in response to an increase in the size of its cells.

immunity: the ability to resist a particular infection or toxin through the immune system.

immunocompromised: weakened immune response as a result of administration of drugs, irradiation, malnutrition or certain disease processes.

immunodeficiency: impairment of the immune system which results in a reduced ability to fight infections.

immunoglobulin: proteins produced by plasma cells which function as antibodies.

inflammatory mediator: a chemical, e.g. histamine, which contributes to an inflammatory response by acting on blood vessels, immune cells, or other cells involved in inflammation.

inhalation: breathing in (taking air into the lungs).

innate immune response: non-specific immune defence mechanisms that appear immediately or within hours of an infection.

integration: bringing different components together to form a whole.

interstitial fluid: the fluid in the spaces between the cells of a tissue. Also referred to as tissue fluid.

intima: the inner lining of a blood vessel (artery or vein).

ion channel: a membrane protein containing a central pore through which charged particles (ions) pass into or out of the cell.

ischaemia: insufficient blood supply to an organ or tissue.

ischaemic heart disease: heart disease caused by insufficient blood supply to the heart muscle. It is most commonly caused by atherosclerosis of the coronary arteries.

lipoprotein particle: a microscopic particle made from lipids and protein.

media: the middle layer of an artery or vein.

metabolism: chemical processes in an organism which maintain life. Drug metabolism refers to the conversion, by enzymes, of a drug into more water-soluble compounds. This occurs mainly in the liver.

metabolites: chemicals formed during metabolism, created by the chemical reactions occurring in every cell (metabolism).

modulation: regulate or adjust to a certain degree – such as **pain modulation**.

monoclonal antibody: an antibody produced by a single clone of cells and consisting of identical antibody molecules.

muscarinic receptor: membrane receptor that contains a recognition site for neurotransmitter acetycholine.

myocardial infarction: 'death of heart tissue' due to an absence of blood flow to the tissue. Often referred to as a 'heart attack'.

narrow spectrum: a term applied to anti-microbial drugs indicating only a narrow range of different organisms are affected.

nerve fibre: another name for a single nerve cell or neurone.

neurone: a single nerve cell. Often called a nerve fibre.

neuropathic pain: pain arising from nerve damage or damage to the central nervous system.

neurotransmitter: a chemical substance released from a nerve fibre which acts to transmit the signal to another nerve fibre.

neutrophil: a type of white blood cell and major component of the white blood cell count in humans. Neutrophils are phagocytic and have an important role in entering the tissues and engulfing and killing extracellular pathogens.

nociception: conversion of pain stimuli into nerve impulses by nociceptors.

nociceptive pain: pain arising from the stimulation of nociceptors.

nociceptor: a type of sensory neurone activated by pain-causing stimuli such as intense pressure or extremes of temperature.

noradrenaline: a chemical that functions as a hormone and neurotransmitter.

nucleus: organelle that contains the genetic material.

obstructive pulmonary disorder: a respiratory disease caused by airway obstruction. This includes asthma and chronic obstructive pulmonary disease.

oedema: an abnormal build-up of interstitial fluid.

opioid: a chemical that resembles morphine in its pharmacological effects.

organelle: structure in the cell that carries out a particular function, e.g. nucleus.

pain fibre: another name for a nociceptor.

pain modulation: an increase or decrease in the sensation of pain.

parasympathetic nervous system: one of two divisions of the autonomic nervous system responsible for slow heart rate and increased intestinal and glandular activity. Complementary to sympathetic nervous system which is responsible for stimulating activities associated with fight or flight response.

partial agonist: a drug that binds to and activates a receptor but has only partial effect.

pathogen: disease-causing microorganism.

pathogenic: disease-causing.

phagocyte: a cell, e.g. macrophage capable of phagocytosis.

phagocytosis: the process in which a cell ingests a solid particle to form an internal vesicle.

pharmacodynamics: the study of what drugs do to the body, including their mechanism of action.

pharmacokinetics: the study of what the body does to drugs, including absorption, distribution, metabolism and excretion.

pharmacology: the study of drugs in living organisms.

prokaryotic: any organism that has no nuclear membrane, no organelles and no nucleus, e.g. bacteria.

pseudomembranous colitis: a serious inflammation of the large intestine caused by toxins produced by *Clostridium difficile.*

pulmonary ventilation: movement of air into and out of the lungs. It includes inhalation and exhalation.

receptor: a molecule, usually on the surface of the cell, that selectively receives and binds to another molecule. A receptor can also be used to refer to an organ or cell in the nervous system (e.g. the eye) that can detect a stimulus such as light.

relay neurone: a neurone which conveys an impulse from one part of the central nervous system to another.

respiratory membrane: the thin layer of tissue separating the air in the lungs from the blood in the capillaries.

restrictive: a respiratory disease that reduces lung volume or expansion.

ribosomes: macromolecular structure in the cell cytoplasm responsible for protein synthesis.

signal transduction: a process which occurs when a receptor on the cell membrane is activated to trigger a chain of events inside the cell creating a response.

spinal cord: bundles of nerve fibres enclose by the vertebral column (or spine), part of central nervous system.

spinal nerve: a mixed nerve carrying sensory, motor and autonomic signals from the spinal cord to the body. There are 31 pairs of spinal nerves in humans.

stenosis: an abnormal narrowing of a passage in the body or blood vessel.

stimulus: something that causes a reaction in an organ or cell.

subclinical: without symptoms.

sympathetic nervous system (SNS): one of two divisions of the autonomic nervous system. The SNS is constantly active to maintain homeostasis and stimulate the body's fight or flight response.

synapse: the microscopic gap between two neurones across which a neurotransmitter acts.

systemic: refers to a substance that is spread throughout the body through the systemic circulation.

systemic vascular resistance: sometimes referred to as 'total peripheral resistance' and is the resistance to blood flow by the systemic blood vessels.

thrombosis: the formation of a blood clot inside a blood vessel and obstructs blood flow through the circulatory system.

thrombus: a blood clot that forms in a vessel resulting from blood coagulation (or platelet aggregation).

tissue fluid: another name for interstitial fluid: the solution which bathes and surrounds cells.

tracheobronchial tree: refers to the trachea, bronchi and bronchioles as a system of airways that allow passage of air into the lungs.

vascular permeability: the degree to which small blood vessels, e.g. capillaries, allow movement of substances (e.g. water, nutrients, proteins) across their wall.

vasoconstriction: narrowing of the blood vessels that results from contraction of the muscular wall of the blood vessels and leads to slowing of blood flow.

vasodilation: widening or dilatation of the blood vessels that results from relaxation of the muscular walls of the blood vessels.

visceral: internal organ of the body.

white matter tracts: bundle of nerve fibres following a path through the brain or spinal cord.

zoonotic: infection that has come from an animal.

References

Ahmad, AS, Ormiston-Smith, N and Sasieni, PD (2015) Trends in the lifetime risk of developing cancer in Great Britain: comparison of risk for those born in 1930 to 1960. *British Journal of Cancer, 112* (5): 943–7.

Alaeddini, J and Shirani, J (2015) *Medscape: Angina Pectoris.* Available at: http://emedicine.medscape.com/article/150215-overview#showall/

Alzheimer's Society (2014) Dementia UK Update. Available at: https://www.alzheimers.org.uk/sites/default/files/migrate/downloads/dementia_uk_update.pdf

American Psychiatric Association (2013) *Diagnostic and Statistical Manual of Mental Disorders: DSM-5.* Arlington, TX: American Psychiatric Publishing.

Baker, G, Brooks, J, Buck, D and Jacoby, A (2000) The stigma of epilepsy: a European perspective. *Epilepsia, 41* (1): 98–104.

Balk, R (2014) Systemic inflammatory response syndrome (SIRS): where did it come from and is it still relevant today? *Virulence, 5*(1): 20–6.

Bannister, M (2011) Time to prepare for Passport Control. *Journal of Diabetes Nursing.* Available at: www.thejournalofdiabetesnursing.co.uk/media/content/_master/1515/files/pdf/jdn15-10-369-70.pdf/

Barnes, PJ (2005) Theophylline in chronic obstructive pulmonary disease: new horizons. *Proceedings of the American Thoracic Society, 2* (4): 334–9.

Bazire, S (2016) *Psychotropic Drug Directory 2016: The Professionals' Pocket Handbook and Aide Memoire 2016.* Warwickshire: Lloyd-Renhold.

Bear, MF, Connors, BW and Paradiso, MA (2015) *Neuroscience: Exploring the Brain* (4th edition). Philadelphia, PA: Lippincott Williams and Wilkins.

Beck, AT and Bredemeier, K (2016) A unified model of depression: integrating clinical, cognitive, biological, and evolutionary perspectives. *Clinical Psychological Science, 4* (4): 596–619.

Belujon, P and Grace, AA (2017) Dopamine system dysregulation in major depressive disorders. *International Journal of Neuropsychopharmacology, 20* (12): 1036–46. Available at: www.ncbi.nlm.nih.gov/pmc/articles/PMC5716179/#/

Bladder and Bowel Foundation (2016) Bristol Stool Chart. Available at: www.bladderandbowel.org/wp-content/uploads/2017/05/BBC002_Bristol-Stool-Chart-Jan-2016.pdf/

BLF (2018) *British Lung Foundation Asthma Statistics*. Available at: https://statistics.blf.org.uk/asthma/

British Heart Foundation (2016) *Heart Statistics*. Available at: www.bhf.org.uk/research/heart-statistics/

British Medical Journal Best Practice (2018) *Sepsis in Adults*. Available at: https://bestpractice.bmj.com/topics/en-us/245/

British National Formulary (BNF) 76 (2018) London: Pharm Press. Available at: www.bnf.org/

British Pain Society (BPS) (2010) *Opioids for Persistent Pain: Good Practice*. Available at: www.britishpainsociety.org/static/uploads/resources/files/book_opioid_main.pdf/

British Pain Society (2014) *FAQs*. Available at: www.britishpainsociety.org/people-with-pain/frequently-asked-questions/

BTS/SIGN (2016) *British Guideline on the Management of Asthma*. Available at: www.brit-thoracic.org.uk/document-library/clinical-information/asthma/btssign-asthma-guideline-2016/

Burn, D (2000) Parkinson's disease: treatment. *Pharmaceutical Journal*, 264 (7089): 476–9.

Carton, J (2012) *Oxford Handbook of Clinical Pathology*. Oxford: Oxford University Press.

Charman, CR, Morris, AD and Williams, HC (2000) Topical corticosteroid phobia in patients with atopic eczema. *British Journal of Dermatology*, *142*: 931–6.

Cleare, A and Pariante, CM, et al. (2015) Evidence-based guidelines for treating depressive disorders with antidepressants: a revision of the 2008 British Association for Psychopharmacology Guidelines. *Journal of Psychopharmacology*, *29* (5): 459–525.

Cortelli, P, Giannini, G, Favoni, V, Cevoli, S and Pierangeli, G (2013) Nociception and the autonomic nervous system. *Neurological Sciences*, *34* (supplement 1): 44–6.

Coupland, C, Hill, T, Morris, R, et al. (2015) Antidepressant use and risk of suicide and attempted suicide or self harm in people aged 20 to 64: cohort study using a primary care database. *BMJ*, *350*: h517.

CRUK (2018a) *Children's Cancer Types*. Available at: www.cancerresearchuk.org/about-cancer/childrens-cancer/types/

CRUK (2018b) *Lifetime Risk of Cancer*. www.cancerresearchuk.org/cancer-info/cancerstats/incidence/risk/statistics-on-the-risk-of-developing-cancer#source4/

Daniels, R, Nutbeam, I, McNamara, G, et al. (2011) The sepsis six and the severe sepsis resuscitation bundle: a prospective observational cohort study. *Emergency Medicine Journal*, *28* (6): 507–12.

Dawes, JM, Calvo, M, Perkins, JR, et al. (2011) CXCL5 Mediates UVB irradiation-induced pain. *Science Translational Medicine*, *3* (90): 90ra60. Available at: www.ncbi.nlm.nih.gov/pmc/articles/PMC3232447/

Department of Health (2000) *Coronary Heart Disease: National Service Framework 2000*. Available at: www.gov.uk/government/uploads/system/uploads/attachment_data/file/198931/National_Service_Framework_for_Coronary_Heart_Disease.pdf/

Dhalla, I, Persaud, N and Juurlink, D (2011) Facing up to the prescription opioid crisis. *British Medical Journal, 343*: d5142. Available at: www.bmj.com/content/343/bmj.d5142/

Diabetes Control and Complications Trial Research Group (1993) The effect of intensive treatment of diabetes on the development and progression of long-term complications in insulin-dependent diabetes mellitus. *New England Journal of Medicine* Sep 30; 329 (14): 977–86.

Diabetes UK (2014) *Diabetes Complications.* Available at: www.diabetes.org.uk/Guide-to-diabetes/Complications/

Diabetes UK (2015) *Diabetes Risk Factors.* Available at: www.diabetes.org.uk/Guide-to-diabetes/What-is-diabetes/Know-your-risk-of-Type-2-diabetes/Diabetes-risk-factors/

Diabetes UK (2017) *Diabetes Prevalence 2017.* Available at: www.diabetes.org.uk/professionals/position-statements-reports/statistics/

Diabetes UK (2018) *Emotional and Psychological Support for People with Diabetes.* Available at: www.diabetes.org.uk/resources-s3/2018-08/Our%20position%20on%20emotional%20and%20psychological%20support%20for%20people%20with%20diabetes.pdf/

Diabetes UK (2019) Diagnostic criteria for diabetes. Available at: https://www.diabetes.org.uk/professionals/position-statements-reports/diagnosis-ongoing-management-monitoring/new_diagnostic_criteria_for_diabetes

Dillorio, C, Shafer, PO, Letz, R, et al. (2004) Project EASE: a study to test psychological model of epilepsy medication management. *Epilepsy and Behaviour, 5*: 926–36.

Eller, M, Vergani, K, Saraiva-Romanholo, B, Antonangelo, L, Leone, C and Rodrigues, J (2018) Can inflammatory markers in induced sputum be used to detect phenotypes and endotypes of pediatric severe therapy-resistant asthma? *Pediatric Pulmonology, 53*: 1208–17.

Epidemiology of Diabetes Interventions and Complications (EDIC) (1999) Design, implementation, and preliminary results of a long-term follow-up of the Diabetes Control and Complications Trial cohort. *Diabetes Care* Jan; *22* (1): 99–111.

Epilepsy Society (2018) What is epilepsy? Available at: https://www.epilepsysociety.org.uk/what-epilepsy#.XK-XwS-ZM6g

Fava, M and Kendler, KS (2000) Major depressive disorder. *Neuron, 28* (2): 335–41.

Ferrari, F and Villa, RF (2016) The neurobiology of depression: an integrated overview from biological theories to clinical evidence. *Molecular Neurobiology, 54* (7): 4847–65.

Fisher, R, Acevedo, C, Arzimanoglou, A, et al. (2014) ILAE official report: a practical clinical definition of epilepsy. *Epilepsia, 55* (4): 475–82.

Flather, MD, Yusuf, S, Kober, L, et al. (2000) Long-term ACE-inhibitor therapy in patients with heart failure or left-ventricular dysfunction: a systematic overview of data from individual patients. *Lancet, 355* (9215): 1575–81.

Freynhagen, R, Geisslinger, G and Schug, SA (2013) Opioids for chronic non-cancer pain. *British Medical Journal, 346.* Available at: www.bmj.com/content/346/bmj.f2937/

Gedzelman, E and Meador, KJ (2012) Antiepileptic drugs in women with epilepsy during pregnancy. *Therapeutic Advances in Drug Safety, 3*: 71–87.

Gemmell, L, Docking, R and Black, E (2017) Renal replacement therapy in critical care. *BJA Education, 17* (3): 88–93.

Gerhardt, S (2015) *Why Love Matters: How Affection Shapes a Baby's Brain* (2nd edition). Hove, East Sussex: Routledge.

Goering, R, Dockrell, H, Zuckerman, M, Roitt, I and Chiodini, P (2013) *Mims' Medical Microbiology* (5th edition). London: Elsevier.

Goh, C and Agius, M (2010) The stress–vulnerability model: how does stress impact on mental illness at the level of the brain and what are the consequences? *Psychiatrica Danubina, 22* (2): 198–202.

Gould, E, Tanapat, P, Rydell, T and Hastings, N (2000) Regulation of hippocampal neurogenesis in adulthood. *Biological Psychiatry, 48*: 715–20.

Haith, M (2018) *Understanding Mental Health Practice.* Exeter: Learning Matters (Sage).

Halban, PA, Polonsky, KS, Bowden, DW, et al. (2014) Cell failure in type 2 diabetes: postulated mechanisms and prospects for prevention and treatment. *Diabetes Care 37* (6): 1751–8. Available at: http://care.diabetesjournals.org/content/37/6/1751.full/

Hall, J (2015) *Guyton and Hall Textbook of Medical Physiology* (13th edition). Oxford: Elsevier.

Hammen, C (2005) Stress and Depression Annual. *Review of Clinical Psychology, 1*: 293–319.

Hanahan, D and Weinburg, RA (2000) The hallmarks of cancer. *Cell, 100* (1): 57–70. Available at: www.cell.com/cell/fulltext/S0092-8674(00)81683-9?_returnURL=https%3 A%2F%2Flinkinghub.elsevier.com%2Fretrieve%2Fpii%2FS0092867400816839%3Fsho wall%3Dtrue/

Hanahan, D and Weinburg, RA (2011) Hallmarks of cancer: the next generation. *Cell,* 4 March, DOI 10.1016/j.cell.2011.02.013. Available at: www.cell.com/abstract/S0092-8674%2811%2900127-9/

Hawthorne, AB, Rubin, G and Ghosh, S (2008) Review article: Medication nonadherence in ulcerative colitis – strategies to improve adherence with mesalazine and other maintenance therapies. *Alimentary Pharmacology and Therapeutics, 27*: 1157–66.

Holst, JJ (2007) The physiology of glucagon-like peptide 1. *Physiological Reviews, 87*: 1409–39.

Horn, C (2008) Why is the neurobiology of nausea and vomiting so important? *Appetite, 50* (2–3): 430–4.

Horne, R, Parham, R, Driscoll, R and Robinson, A (2009) Attitudes to medicines and adherence to maintenance treatment in inflammatory bowel disease. *Inflammatory Bowel Diseases, 15* (6): 837–44.

House of Commons (2012) Committee of Public Accounts Department of Health: The Management of Adult Diabetes Services in the NHS; Seventeenth Report of Session 2012–13. Available at: www.publications.parliament.uk/pa/cm201213/cmselect/cmpubacc/289/289. pdf/

Howren, MB, Lamkin, DM and Suls, J (2009) Associations of depression with C-reactive protein, IL-1, and IL-6: a meta-analysis. *Psychosomatic Medicine, 71*: 171–86.

Hughes, AJ, Daniel, SE, Ben-Shlomo, Y and Lees, AJ (2002) The accuracy of diagnosis of Parkinson's syndromes in a specialist movement disorder service. *Brain*, 125: 861–70.

IASP (2012) *IASP Taxonomy.* Available at: www.iasp-pain.org/AM/Template.cfm? Section=Pain_Definitions/

IASP (2014) *IASP Curriculum Outline on Pain for Nursing.* Available at: www.iasp-pain.org/ Education/CurriculumDetail.aspx?ItemNumber=2052/

Iliopoulou, A, Abbas, A and Murray, R (2013) How to manage withdrawal from glucocorticoid therapy. *Prescriber, 24* (10): 23–9.

Independent Mental Health Task Force to the NHS in England (2016) *The Five Year Forward View for Mental Health.* Available at: www.england.nhs.uk/wp-content/ uploads/2016/02/Mental-Health-Taskforce-FYFV-final.pdf/

ISIS-2 (1988) Second International Study of Infarct Survival. Collaborative Group. Randomised trial of intravenous streptokinase, oral aspirin, both or neither among 17187 cases of suspected acute myocardial infarction. *The Lancet, 332* (8607): 349–60.

Janeway, C and Murphy, K (2012) *Janeway's Immunobiology* (8th edition). London: Taylor and Francis.

Joint British Diabetes Societies Inpatient Care Group (2012) The management of the hyperosmolar hyperglycaemic state (HHS) in adults with diabetes. Available at: https://diabetes-resources-production.s3-eu-west-1.amazonaws.com/diabetes-storage/ migration/pdf/JBDS-IP-HHS-Adults.pdf

Joint British Diabetes Societies Inpatient Care Group (2013) The management of diabetic ketoacidosis in adults. Available at: https://www.diabetes.org.uk/resources-s3/2017-09/ Management-of-DKA-241013.pdf

Joint British Diabetes Societies Inpatient Care Group (2018) The Hospital Management of Hypoglycaemia in Adults with Diabetes Mellitus, 3rd edition Revised April 2018. Available at: https://diabetes-resources-production.s3.eu-west-1.amazonaws.com/ resources-s3/2018-05/JBDS_HypoGuidelineRevised2.pdf%2008.05.18.pdf

Joint British Thoracic Society/Scottish Intercollegiate Guidelines Network (SIGN) (2016) *British Guideline on the Management of Asthma.* Available at: www.sign.ac.uk/sign-153-british-guideline-on-the-management-of-asthma.html/

Kopschina, Feltes P, Doorduin, J, Klein, H, et al. (2017) Anti-inflammatory treatment for major depressive disorder: implications for patients with an elevated immune profile and non-responders to standard antidepressant therapy. *Journal of Psychopharmacology, 31* (9): 1149–65.

Kumar, V, Abbas, A, Fausto, N and Mitchell, R (2014) *Robbins Basic Pathology* (9th edition). Philadelphia, PA: Saunders Elsevier.

Kuruvilla, M, Lee, F and Lee, G (2018) Asthma phenotypes, endotypes and mechanisms of disease. *Clinical Reviews in Allergy and Immunology.* Available at: https://doi.org/10.1007/ s12016-018-8712-1/

Lote, C (2012) *Principles of Renal Physiology* (5th edition). Berlin: Springer.

Lucaciu, LA and Dumitrascu, DL (2015) Depression and suicide ideation in chronic hepatitis C patients untreated and treated with interferon: prevalence, prevention, and treatment. *Annals of Gastroenterology, 28* (4): 440–7.

MacLean, P (1990) *The Triune Brain in Evolution: Role in Paleocerebral Functions.* New York: Plenum Publishing.

Mannix, KA (2010) Palliation of nausea and vomiting. In: Hanks, G, Cherny, NI, Christakis, NA, et al. (eds) *Oxford Textbook of Palliative Medicine* (4th edition). Oxford: Oxford University Press, pp. 801–12.

Marson, A, Appleton, R, Baker, GA, et al. (2007) A randomised controlled trial examining the longer-term outcomes of standard versus new antiepileptic drugs. The SANAD trial. *Health Technology Assessment, 11* (37): 1–134.

Mayberg, HS (2003) Modulating dysfunctional limbic-cortical circuits in depression: towards development of brain-based algorithms for diagnosis and optimized treatment. *British Medical Bulletin, 65* (1): 193–207.

Melzack, R and Wall, PD (1965) Pain mechanisms: a new theory. *Science 150* (3699): 971–9.

Mental Health Foundation (2016) *Fundamental Facts About Mental Health.* Available at: www.mentalhealth.org.uk/publications/fundamental-facts-about-mental-health-2016/

MHRA (2004) *Atypical Antipsychotics and Stroke.* Available at: http://webarchive. nationalarchives.gov.uk/20141205212951/http://www.mhra.gov.uk/Safetyinformation/ Safetywarningsalertsandrecalls/Safetywarningsandmessagesformedicines/CON1004298/

MHRA (2009) *Antiepileptics: Adverse Effects on Bone. Drug Safety Update.* Available at: www. gov.uk/drug-safety-update/antiepileptics-adverse-effects-on-bone/

MHRA (2017) *Anti-Epileptic Drugs: Changing Products.* Available at: www.gov.uk/drug-safety-update/antiepileptic-drugs-updated-advice-on-switching-between-different-manufacturers-products/

Mind (2018) *Understanding Mental Health Problems.* Available at: www.mind.org.uk/ media/23634461/understanding-mental-health-problems-2018.pdf/

Mitchell, R, Kumar, V, Abbas, A and Aster, J (2016) *Pocket Companion to Robbins & Cotran Pathologic Basis of Disease* (9th edition) (*Robbins Pathology*). Oxford: Elsevier.

Naish, J and Syndercombe, D (2018) *Medical Sciences* (3rd edition). London: Elsevier.

National Cancer Institute (2015) *Definition of Solid Tumor.* Available at: www.cancer.gov/ publications/dictionaries/cancer-terms?cdrid=45301/

National Cancer Institute (2018) *Targeted Cancer Therapies.* Available at: www.cancer.gov/ about-cancer/treatment/types/targeted-therapies/targeted-therapies-fact-sheet/

National Clinical Guideline Centre (2013) *Epilepsies: Diagnosis and Management.* Available at: www.nice.org.uk/Guidance/CG137/

National Diabetes Inpatient Audit (NaDIA) (2018) Available at: https://digital.nhs.uk/ data-and-information/clinical-audits-and-registries/national-diabetes-inpatient-audit

NHS Scotland (2014) *Scottish Palliative Care Guidelines: Nausea and Vomiting.* Available at: www.palliativecareguidelines.scot.nhs.uk/media/1183/nausea-and-vomiting.pdf/

NICE (2008) *Familial Hypercholesterolaemia: Identification and Management. CG71.* Available at: www.nice.org.uk/guidance/CG71/

NICE (2011a) *Hypertension in Adults: Diagnosis and Management. CG127.* Available at: www.nice.org.uk/guidance/cg127/

NICE (2011 updated 2018) *Donepezil, Galantamine, Rivastigmine and Memantine for the Treatment of Alzheimer's Disease.* Available at: www.nice.org.uk/guidance/TA217/chapter/1-Guidance/

NICE (2011b) *Common Mental Health Problems: Identification and Pathways to Care. CG123.* Available at: www.nice.org.uk/guidance/cg123/resources/common-mental-health-problems-identification-and-pathways-to-care-pdf-35109448223173/

NICE (2012 updated 2018) *Epilepsies: Diagnosis and Management. CG137.* Available at: www.nice.org.uk/guidance/cg137/

NICE (2013a) *National Institute for Care Excellence: Asthma: Quality Standard QS25.* Available at: www.nice.org.uk/guidance/qs25/

NICE (2013b) *Ulcerative Colitis: Management. CG166.* Available at: www.nice.org.uk/guidance/cg166/

NICE (2013c) *Acute Kidney Injury: Prevention, Detection and Management. Clinical Guideline [CG169].* Available at: https://www.nice.org.uk/guidance/cg169

NICE (2014a) *Cardiovascular Disease: Risk Assessment and Reduction, Including Lipid Modification. CG181.* Available at: www.nice.org.uk/guidance/CG181/

NICE (2014b) *Gastro-oesophageal Reflux Disease and Dyspepsia in Adults: Investigation and Management. CG184.* Available at: www.nice.org.uk/guidance/CG184/

NICE (2014c) *Chronic Kidney Disease in Adults. Assessment and Management. CG 182.* Available at: https://nice.org.uk/guidance/cg182/

NICE (2014d) *Management of Vomiting in Children and Young People with Gastroenteritis: Ondansetron.* Available at: www.nice.org.uk/advice/esuom34/chapter/Key-points-from-the-evidence/

NICE (2016a) *Palliative Care: Nausea and Vomiting.* Available at: https://cks.nice.org.uk/palliative-care-nausea-and-vomiting#!topicsummary/

NICE (2016b) *Crohn's Disease: Management. CG152.* Available at: www.nice.org.uk/guidance/cg152/

NICE (2016c) *Type 1 Diabetes in Adults: Diagnosis and Management. NG17.* Available at: www.nice.org.uk/guidance/ng17/

NICE (2016d) *Sepsis: Recognition, Diagnosis and Early Management.* Available at: www.nice.org.uk/guidance/ng51/resources/sepsis-recognition-diagnosis-and-early-management-pdf-1837508256709/

NICE (2017a) *Corticosteroids.* Available at: https://cks.nice.org.uk/corticosteroids-oral/

NICE (2017b) *Clinical Knowledge Summary: Constipation.* Available at: https://cks.nice.org.uk/constipation#!scenario/

NICE (2017c) *Type 2 Diabetes in Adults: Management. NG 28.* Available at: www.nice.org.uk/guidance/ng28/

NICE (2017d) *Parkinson's Disease in Adults. NG71.* Available at: www.nice.org.uk/guidance/ng71/

NICE (2018a) *Nausea/Vomiting in Pregnancy.* Available at: https://cks.nice.org.uk/nauseavomiting-in-pregnancy#!topicsummary/

NICE (2018b) *Chronic Obstructive Pulmonary Disease in Over 16's: Diagnosis and Management.* Available at: www.nice.org.uk/guidance/ng115/

NICE (2018c) *Dementia: Assessment, Management and Support for People Living With Dementia and Their Carers.* Available at: www.nice.org.uk/guidance/ng97/

NICE (2018d) *Depression in Adults: Recognition and Management. CG 90.* Available at: www.nice.org.uk/guidance/cg91/

NMC (2018) *Nursing and Midwifery Council: Future Nurse: Standards of Proficiency for Registered Nurses.* Nursing and Midwifery Council. Available at: www.nmc.org.uk/standards/standards-for-nurses/

Packham, B (2009) How to improve compliance with antiepileptic drugs. *Prescriber, 20* (3): 12–20.

Pecorino, L (2012) *Molecular Biology of Cancer: Mechanisms, Targets and Therapeutics* (3rd edition). Oxford: Oxford University Press.

Public Health England (2018a) *Gastrointestinal Infections: Guidance, Data and Analysis.* Available at: www.gov.uk/government/collections/gastrointestinal-infections-guidance-data-and-analysis/

Public Health England (2018b) *Guidelines for the Management of Norovirus Outbreaks in Acute and Community Health and Social Care Settings.* Available at: www.gov.uk/government/uploads/system/uploads/attachment_data/file/322943/Guidance_for_managing_norovirus_outbreaks_in_healthcare_settings.pdf/

Raison, CL (2014) Inflammatory depression: a trifecta of trouble. *Journal of Clinical Psychiatry, 75*: 663–4.

Ramrakha, P and Hill, J (eds) (2012) *Oxford Handbook of Cardiology* (2nd edition). Oxford: Oxford University Press.

Rang, H, Ritter, JM, Flower, RJ and Henderson, G (2015) *Rang and Dale's Pharmacology* (8th edition). London: Elsevier.

Rennker, H and Denker, BM (2013) *Renal Pathophysiology* (4th edition). New York: Lippincott Williams & Wilkins.

Rhodes, VA and McDaniel, RW (2001) Nausea, vomiting, and retching: complex problems in palliative care. *CA Cancer Journal Clinicians, 51* (4): 232–48.

Rodrigo, GJ and Castro-Rodriguez, JA (2005) Anticholinergics in the treatment of children and adults with acute asthma: a systematic review with meta-analysis. *Thorax, 60* (9): 740–6.

Rush, AJ, Trivedi, MH, Wisniewski, S, et al. (2006) Acute and longer-term outcomes in depressed outpatients requiring one or several treatment steps: a STAR*D report. *American Journal of Psychiatry, 163*: 1905–17.

Singer, M, Deutschman, C, Seymour, C, et al. (2016) The Third International Consensus Definitions for Sepsis and Septic Shock (Sepsis-3). *JAMA, 315* (8): 801–10.

Spiers, N, Qassem, T, Bebbington, P, et al. (2016) Prevalence and treatment of common mental disorders in the English national population, 1993–2007. *British Journal of Psychiatry, 209*: 150–6.

Taibjee, S and Charman, C (2009) *Steroid Phobia, A Major Obstacle in Caring for Eczema Sufferers.* Available at: http://pdfsr.com/pdf/steroid-phobia-a-major-obstacle-in-caring-for-eczema-sufferers/

The Health Foundation (2016) *Person-Centred Care Made Simple: What Everyone Should Know About Person-Centred Care.* Available at: www.health.org.uk/sites/health/files/PersonCentredCareMadeSimple.pdf/

The Immune System. In: *Defence of our Lives.* Nobelprize.org. Nobel Media AB 2014. Web. 6 Mar 2019. Available at: http://educationalgames.nobelprize.org/educational/medicine/immuneresponses/overview/index.html/

Tortora, G and Derrickson, B (2017) *Principles of Anatomy and Physiology* (17th edition). Oxford: Wiley.

Turner, H and Wass, J (2007) *Oxford Handbook of Diabetes.* Oxford: Oxford University Press.

UK Prospective Diabetes Study (UKPDS) Group (1998) Tight blood pressure control and risk of macrovascular and microvascular complications in type 2 diabetes: UKPDS 38. *BMJ, 317*: 703–13.

Vleeming, W, van Amsterdam, JG, Stricker, BH and de Wildt, DJ (1998) ACE inhibitor-induced angioedema: incidence, prevention and management. *Drug Safety: An International Journal of Medical Toxicology and Drug Experience, 18*: 171–88.

Vogt, B (2005) Pain and emotion interactions in subregions of the cingulate gyrus. *Nature Reviews Neuroscience, 6* (7): 533–44.

Waller, DG and Sampson, AP (2018) *Medical Pharmacology and Therapeutics* (5th edition). London: Elsevier.

Warner, B, Johnston, E, Arenas-Hernandez, M, et al. (2016) *Frontline Gastroenterology.* Available at: https://fg.bmj.com/content/flgastro/early/2016/08/29/flgastro-2016-100738.full.pdf/

Webster, A, Nagler, E, Morton, R and Masson, P (2017) Chronic kidney disease. *Lancet,* *389*: 1238–52.

Woodward, S and Oliveira, D (2017) *Renal Medicine.* London: JP Medical.

World Anti-Doping Agency (2015) *List of Prohibited Substances and Methods.* Available at: http://list.wada-ama.org/

World Health Organization (2010) *Pain Relief Ladder for Cancer Pain Relief.* Available at: www.who.int/cancer/palliative/painladder/en/

World Health Organization (2011) *Definition and Diagnosis of Diabetes Mellitus and Intermediate Hyperglycemia.* Available at: www.who.int/diabetes/publications/ Definition%20and%20diagnosis%20of%20diabetes_new.pdf/

World Health Organization (2014) *Diabetes Fact Sheet N° 312.* Available at: www.who.int/ mediacentre/factsheets/fs312/en/

World Health Organization (2015) *World Health Organization Fact Sheet: Antibiotic Resistance.* October. Available at: www.who.int/mediacentre/factsheets/antibiotic-resistance/en/

World Health Organization (2018a) *Top 10 Causes of Death in the World.* Available at: www. who.int/news-room/fact-sheets/detail/the-top-10-causes-of-death/

World Health Organization (2018b) Diarrhoea. Available at: www.who.int/topics/ diarrhoea/en/

World Health Organization (n.d.) ICD-10 classification of mental and behavioural disorders. Available at: https://www.who.int/substance_abuse/terminology/icd_10/en/

Wray, NR, Ripke, S, Mattheisen, M, Trzaskowski, M, et al. (2018) Genome-wide association analyses identify 44 risk variants and refine the genetic architecture of major depression. *Nature Genetics, 50*: 668–81.

Yusuf, S, Hawken, S, Ôunpuu, T, et al. (2004) Effect of potentially modifiable risk factors associated with myocardial infarction in 52 countries (the INTERHEART study): case-control study. *The Lancet, 364*: 937–52.

Index

Locators in *italics* refer to figures and those in **bold** to tables though these are not distinguished where they are interspersed with relevant text.

CPSIA information can be obtained
at www.ICGtesting.com
Printed in the USA
LVHW052344280322
714614LV00011B/489

9 781526 432117